EARLY INTERVENTION FOR TRAUMA AND TRAUMATIC LOSS

Early Intervention for Trauma and Traumatic Loss

edited by

Brett T. Litz

THE GUILFORD PRESS
New York   London

© 2004 The Guilford Press
A Division of Guilford Publications, Inc.
72 Spring Street, New York, NY 10012
www.guilford.com

Printed in the United States of America

This book is printed on acid-free paper.

Last digit is print number: 9 8 7 6 5 4 3 2

Library of Congress Cataloging-in-Publication Data
Early intervention for trauma and traumatic loss / edited by Brett T. Litz.
    p. cm.
Includes bibliographical references and index.
   ISBN-10: 1-57230-953-9   ISBN-13: 978-1-57230-953-1 (alk. paper)
   1. Psychic trauma—Treatment.   2. Post-traumatic stress disorder—
Treatment.   I. Litz, Brett T.
   RC552.P67E256 2004
   616.85′2106—dc22
                      2003017547

About the Editor

Brett T. Litz, PhD, is an Associate Professor in the Department of Psychiatry at Boston University School of Medicine and the Department of Psychology at Boston University, as well as the Associate Director of the Behavioral Sciences Division of the National Center for Posttraumatic Stress Disorder at the Boston Department of Veterans Affairs Medical Center. Dr. Litz is also Principal Investigator on several research studies funded by the National Institutes of Health and the Department of Defense to explore the efficacy of early intervention strategies in trauma, and he is currently studying adaptation to traumatic loss as a result of 9-11. In addition to conducting research on early intervention for trauma, Dr. Litz studies the mental health adaptation of U.S. military personnel across the lifespan, the assessment and treatment of posttraumatic stress disorder, and emotional numbing in trauma.

Contributors

Amy B. Adler, PhD, U.S. Army Medical Research Unit–Europe, Walter Reed Army Institute of Research, Heidelberg, Germany

Edward B. Blanchard, PhD, Center for Stress and Anxiety Disorders, Department of Psychology, University at Albany, State University of New York, Albany, New York

John Broderick, MD, Department of Emergency Medicine, Albany Medical College, Albany, New York

Richard A. Bryant, PhD, School of Psychology, University of New South Wales, Sydney, Australia

Carl Andrew Castro, PhD, Department of Psychiatry and Behavioral Science, Division of Neuropsychiatry, Walter Reed Army Institute of Research, Silver Spring, Maryland

Judith A. Cohen, MD, Drexel University School of Medicine, Allegheny General Hospital, Pittsburgh, Pennsylvania

Charles C. Engel, Jr., MD, MPH, Department of Psychiatry, Uniformed Services University, Bethesda, Maryland; Deployment Health Clinical Center, Walter Reed Army Medical Center, Washington, DC

Cynthia B. Eriksson, PhD, The Headington Program, Graduate School of Psychology, Fuller Theological Seminary, Pasadena, California

Edna B. Foa, PhD, Department of Psychiatry, Center for the Treatment and Study of Anxiety, University of Pennsylvania, Philadelphia, Pennsylvania

David W. Foy, PhD, Graduate School of Education and Psychology, Pepperdine University, Encino, California; The Headington Program, Graduate School of Psychology, Fuller Theological Seminary, Pasadena, California

Matt J. Gray, PhD, Department of Psychology, University of Wyoming, Laramie, Wyoming

Edward J. Hickling, PsyD, Center for Stress and Anxiety Disorders, Department of Psychology, University at Albany, State University of New York, Albany, New York

Daniel W. King, PhD, National Center for Posttraumatic Stress Disorder, Boston Department of Veterans Affairs Medical Center, and Departments of Psychiatry and Psychology, Boston University, Boston, Massachusetts

Lynda A. King, PhD, National Center for Posttraumatic Stress Disorder, Boston Department of Veterans Affairs Medical Center, and Departments of Psychiatry and Psychology, Boston University, Boston, Massachusetts

Eric Kuhn, MA, Center for Stress and Anxiety Disorders, Department of Psychology, University at Albany, State University of New York, Albany, New York

Linnea C. Larson, MA, MPH, The Headington Program, Graduate School of Psychology, Fuller Theological Seminary, Pasadena, California

Alicia F. Lieberman, PhD, Department of Psychiatry, University of California–San Francisco, San Francisco, California

Brett T. Litz, PhD, National Center for Posttraumatic Stress Disorder, Boston Department of Veterans Affairs Medical Center; Department of Psychiatry, Boston University School of Medicine; and Department of Psychology, Boston University, Boston, Massachusetts

Randall D. Marshall, MD, Department of Psychiatry, Columbia University, and New York State Psychiatric Institute, New York, New York

Yuval Neria, PhD, Departments of Psychiatry and Epidemiology, Columbia University, and New York State Psychiatric Institute, New York, New York

Amy R. Olson, BS, BSOSEH, Department of Psychology, University of Wyoming, Laramie, Wyoming

Holly G. Prigerson, PhD, Departments of Psychiatry, Epidemiology, and Public Health, Yale University School of Medicine, New Haven, Connecticut

Beverley Raphael, MD, Centre for Mental Health, NSW Health Department, Sydney, Australia

Sheila A. M. Rauch, PhD, Department of Psychiatry, Center for the Treatment and Study of Anxiety, University of Pennsylvania, Philadelphia, Pennsylvania

Eun Jung Suh, PhD, Department of Psychiatry, Columbia University, and New York State Psychiatric Institute, New York, New York

Patricia Van Horn, PhD, Department of Psychiatry, University of California–San Francisco, San Francisco, California

Dawne S. Vogt, PhD, National Center for Posttraumatic Stress Disorder, Boston Department of Veterans Affairs Medical Center, and Department of Psychiatry, Boston University School of Medicine, Boston, Massachusetts

Amy Wagner, PhD, Department of Psychiatry and Behavioral Science, University of Washington School of Medicine, Seattle, Washington

Sally Wooding, PhD, Centre for Mental Health, NSW Health Department, Sydney, Australia

Douglas Zatzick, MD, Department of Psychiatry and Behavioral Science and Harborview Injury Prevention and Research Center, University of Washington School of Medicine, Seattle, Washington

Acknowledgments

This book is dedicated to survivors of any form of trauma and traumatic loss and to clinicians at every level motivated to learn how best to help them. If research ideas are generated and new research is initiated in early intervention for trauma and traumatic loss, we will have done our job. I wish to thank Julie Wang and Lawrence Williams for their essential help vetting and editing and Jamie Suvak for providing feedback. Finally, I would like to thank Jayne and Emily for being so patient, understanding, and supportive.

BRETT T. LITZ

Contents

III

Special Topics

1

Introduction

BRETT T. LITZ

Traumatic life events are unpredictable, uncontrollable, and devastating. Suddenly, persons or groups are exposed to unimaginable suffering and threats to themselves or others, resulting in terror, panic, frailty, and vulnerability. Traumatic events violate core tacit beliefs and assumptions that otherwise promote safety, stability, well-being, purposefulness, and personal and collective agency. Unfortunately, trauma is not rare and as a result represents a major public health problem. Population estimates in the United States vary, as do methods and definitions of trauma across epidemiological studies, but approximately 5 of every 10 individuals will be exposed to a major, severe life stressor or trauma at some point in their lives (Breslau et al., 1998; Kessler, Sonnega, Bromet, Hughes, & Nelson, 1995). At the time of the event, and for a varying period of time afterward, trauma eviscerates normal functioning and consumes consciousness, physiology, and coping resources.

While the prevalence of trauma across the lifespan suggests that it is part of the human condition, on average, people are remarkably resilient and adept at recovering over time. The risk of long-term, untoward mental health problems implicated by exposure to trauma is surprisingly low. Although time does not heal all wounds, most individuals will heal psychologically, socially, and morally with the passage of time. Though the majority of people exposed to trauma are initially overwrought, epidemiological studies show that between

8% and 9% are at risk for chronic mental health problems stemming from all forms of trauma (Breslau et al., 1998; Kessler et al., 1995). Those who experience chronic posttraumatic symptoms and problems pose a major international mental health challenge. The chronic psychological and social difficulties that stem from trauma are pernicious, disabling, and resistant to change (e.g., Kessler et al., 1995; Kulka et al., 1990).

For many, psychological recovery and adjustment from trauma are not linear, static processes but, rather, unfolding lifelong challenges. In the aftermath of trauma and traumatic bereavement, clinicians and public health officials need to be concerned with how long a person suffers acutely and how much time passes before a relatively normal routine is reestablished (the rate of recovery) and the risk for enduring functional impairment and specific chronic mental health problems that may require professional intervention (e.g., posttraumatic stress disorder [PTSD]; American Psychological Association, 1994), as well as symptom flare-ups after periods of effective functioning (e.g., Bryant & Harvey, 2002; Harvey & Bryant, 2002). Yet, for some, after an initial period of disruption, trauma can lead to personal growth, more effective coping with minor life hassles, as well as a greater sense of connection with loved ones (Frazier, Conlon, & Glaser, 2001; Tedeschi, 1999; Williams & Yule, 1993). A variety of complex, interrelated (and yet to be researched) factors moderate the rate and form of recovery from trauma across the lifespan. The psychological and psychiatric effects of a given trauma depend on temperament, psychological and physiological individual differences, developmental period, culture, gender, and social context (e.g., Breslau et al.; 1998; Kessler et al., 1995; Shalev, 1999; True et al., 1993). Characteristics of the traumatic event are also important predictors of outcome—severe, malicious, and grotesque traumas as well as traumatic bereavement are associated with much greater risk for posttraumatic adjustment problems than for other forms of trauma (e.g., Breslau et al., 1998; Kessler et al., 1995; Kulka et al., 1990).

In the mix of causal factors that create or attenuate risk for lasting problems from exposure to trauma is the quality of the recovery environment (e.g., how friends, family members, coworkers, and the community at large respond; e.g., Bolton et al., 2003; Campbell, Ahrens, Sefl, Wasco, & Barnes, 2001; Ullman, 1997) and the professional care provided to people immediately and soon after trauma, otherwise referred to as *early intervention*. This book is devoted to the public health, clinical, and research issues relevant to early intervention for trauma and traumatic loss.

Unfortunately, people suffer through most traumatic experiences in anonymous isolation because of the nature of the event (e.g., incest), the stigma attached (e.g., sexual assault), the social context (e.g., punitive significant others), or some combination of these factors. In all too many cases, no one is around to assist in recovery, and care is never provided. For example, most sexual assaults are unreported; victims receive neither medical attention nor mental health intervention (Rennison, 2002). When trauma and traumatic loss are associated with a public emergency or become public for any number of reasons, a wide variety of professionals may intervene with people immediately or soon following the experience. Most early responders on the scene of an incident are emergency services personnel or medical care professionals (police officers, emergency medical technicians, emergency room staff, assistant district attorneys, firefighters, Red Cross personnel, etc.) whose priority is ensuring physical safety, securing basic needs (shelter, water, food, etc.), or gathering evidence to process a crime, not attending to victims' emotional needs or current mental health. Some *first* or *early responders* may be called on to assist in a time of disaster and tragedy simply because they happened to be there or because of professional training of some kind. Other individuals who assist people soon after tragedy have a formal mental health role providing immediate emotional support, screening, and triage for severity of psychological response and risk for chronic difficulties and assisting individuals in planning for the days, weeks, and months of recovery and reemergence into daily routines. Some of these specialists have advanced training in acute trauma and its care, some have advanced degrees in the allied health professions (e.g., social work, psychology, psychiatry, and nursing), and others do not have specialized training per se.

As would be expected, there is great variability in training background, role, philosophy, approach to emergency services, and mental health background in personnel who work with trauma survivors at various points in the response chain. However, in the aftermath of trauma, all professionals, regardless of the services they provide or the context in which they provide it, are part of a collective invested, in one way or another, in facilitating recovery. Arguably, from a mental health perspective, one of the guiding assumptions shared by all professionals stems from implicit theories of crisis intervention and grief counseling: If a trauma or loss is not resolved in a healthy manner, the experience can create lasting psychological and social problems (e.g., Roberts, 1991). This may be true. Initially, victims of trauma and traumatic loss experience tremendous emotional shock and upheaval. Unexpectedly, their routines, their sense of fairness and goodness, and their expectations about how things work and how they should be treated or how human beings should be treated have been shattered and disrupted tragically, which could taint their life course in completely unanticipated and disorienting ways. There is no doubt that trauma and traumatic loss are implicated as causes of chronic and severe mental health problems, such as PTSD (e.g., Kessler et al., 1995). Furthermore, early mental health interventions could prove to be an important tool to prevent problems implicated by exposure to trauma (see Litz, Gray, Bryant, & Adler, 2002). In addition, because individuals' decisions about seeking care in the weeks and months after trauma may be influenced by the way they were treated and the things they learned immediately after the trauma occurred, it is important for all professionals in the response chain to appreciate how they might be constructive and not inadvertently destructive. In the early intervention for trauma and traumatic loss arena, there is consensus about why early intervention is important, but more questions remain with respect to how, when, and with whom interventions should take place.

This disturbing state of affairs is due to a variety of factors. First, there is a dearth of naturalistic, prospective studies of the course of posttraumatic recovery, especially the course of adjustment to mass violence and traumatic loss. Although research has illustrated convincingly that, following trauma, after a period of intense distress, approximately 90% of individuals recover effectively without professional intervention, many questions remain (e.g., Rothbaum, Foa, Riggs, Murdock, & Walsh, 1992). For example, it is unclear how resilient people naturally cope with severe trauma and whether resilience is lifelong or phasic (e.g., a period of adjustment could be followed by a period of severe impairment).

Second, there is much conjecture about what puts people at risk for chronic PTSD, but there are few well-designed, empirical studies. Furthermore, there are no cogent conceptual frameworks to draw from when considering practical screening programs for early trauma intervention. At present, studies have examined correlates of chronic PTSD (e.g., Harvey & Bryant, 1999), but there are very few focused investigations of specific risk mechanisms. If risk mechanisms could be identified, secondary prevention programs could be designed to address the factors that place people at risk for chronic PTSD.

Third, although there is good evidence to support the use of multisession, therapist-intensive, cognitive-behavioral interventions in the secondary prevention of PTSD (e.g., Bryant, Sackville, Dang, Moulds, & Guthrie, 1999), the necessary and sufficient elements for successful prevention remain unstudied. In the context of traumas that affect large numbers of individuals (e.g., mass violence) and in medical care contexts where well-trained professionals may be scarce, evaluating efficient methods of delivering the key elements of early interventions is crucial.

Fourth, there is scant descriptive, epidemiological, or clinical research on the unique psychosocial needs and outcomes of individuals who suffer traumatic loss or those who suffer the dual burden of losing a loved one through trauma while experiencing their own acute trauma (e.g., Raphael, Dobson, & Minkov, 2001). Although there are some promising uncontrolled trials (e.g.,

Shear et al. 2001; Sireling, Cohen, & Marks, 1988), there are no randomized controlled trials of early interventions for traumatic bereavement.

However, when disaster, trauma, and traumatic loss strike individuals and communities, professionals of goodwill with various background and so-called trauma specialists are on the scene to assist victims as early as possible. For example, the tragic mass violence on 9-11-01 and the loss incurred created an assumed huge demand for brief early intervention and other mental health services, and a strong desire for professionals, many of whom also suffered pain and sorrow on that terrible day, to help in some way during a time of great tragedy and suffering. Large sums of money were devoted to meeting the acute mental health aftermath of 9-11. For example, the Federal Emergency Management Agency awarded $132 million for "crisis counseling" in New York City, which was the largest grant in the agency's history, nearly the total amount awarded for emergency mental health in disasters since 1974. Yet, there was uncertainty in many circles about how to use the vast resources—the question that arose was, "What best practices are recommended based on scientific evidence?" The disquieting answer to this question is that there is little valid research from which to draw practical recommendations.

The field of early mental health intervention for trauma was at a cross-roads and approaching a paradigm shift well before 9-11. The early intervention field is dominated by non-evidence-based practices, poorly defined and anachronistic notions about recovery from trauma and risk for trauma-linked disorders, and an apparent unresponsiveness to scientific inquiry. It is perfectly understandable for professionals to attempt to help people cope with the immediate and enduring aftermath of personal and collective tragedy. It is also understandable that special disaster and victims' assistance organizations such as the Red Cross routinely provide early counseling and grief intervention services to affected individuals. Communities and governmental agencies are intensely motivated to take care of those affected by trauma and traumatic loss, often funding and mandating early intervention for people in their charge. For example, personnel in all five boroughs in the New York City Police Department were provided formal psychological debriefing after the 9-11 terrorist attack. Added to this mix are entrepreneurs and organizations that routinely offer early interventions such as *critical incident stress debriefing* (Mitchell & Everly, 1996), even though there is insufficient evidence to support its efficacy (e.g., Litz et al., 2002; Rose, Brewin, Andrews, & Kirk, 1999). Because of this lack of sufficient scientific evidence, the community of mental health professionals and consumers of services (e.g., government officials, private agencies, school boards, and hospitals) need to be considerably more cautious about the type of acute care recommended on the scene of a trauma or in various contexts soon afterward (e.g., the workplace). Offering or requiring services with-

out evidence for their efficacy could, in the best case, waste much time and resources, and in the worst case thwart natural recovery. It is not acceptable that
early interventions for trauma be based exclusively on the understandable human need to help people who appear to be suffering or out of the motivation
to promote organizational or corporate goals. A model of care needs to be ar-
ticulated such that, in the absence of evidence-based screening and intervention strategies, victims should be assisted in the least intrusive manner possible and in a way that respects their natural resourcefulness.

As it turns out, the crisis counseling doctrine that healthy recovery from
trauma and traumatic loss reduces risk for chronic problems is mostly true,
but professional intervention in most instances is not needed to make this
happen (Litz et al., 2002). In addition, there are myriad ways that individuals
process and recover from trauma and loss, and initial suffering or the lack of
overt strong emotional upheaval does not imply that anything is wrong (e.g.,
Wortman & Silver, 1989). Some people do not share their emotional experience of loss and trauma, as a personal preference, not necessarily as a result of
denial or avoidance. In fact, recovery from trauma and loss can be hampered
by poorly timed and overly intrusive demands for emotional expression and
sharing (e.g., Stroebe, Stroebe, Schut, Zech, & van den Bout, 2002).

Nevertheless, the crisis counseling approach assumes that something
needs to be "done to" *any* survivor of trauma. The approach taken is that soon
after trauma, all victims need some kind of education, guidance, support, or
emotional outlet, assuming that people cannot find these things in their natural environment. In addition, crisis counseling assumes that some kind of brief
intervention soon after trauma can have lasting impact in the course of adjustment to trauma. However, there is no evidence to support this view, and there
are several well-designed research trials that suggest that, at best, early brief interventions are inert with respect to affecting the course of coping with the
psychological aftermath of trauma (e.g., Bisson, Jenkins, Alexander, & Bannister, 1997).

Old assumptions about early interventions are being challenged from a
variety of fronts. Because it is unclear how best to serve the immediate and
acute needs of trauma sufferers and there is little agreement how best to facilitate recovery from trauma, a reckoning of where we are and where we need to
go is required. As there is little research on early interventions to prevent
chronic posttraumatic difficulties, it is critical to set forth a research agenda for
the future. It is also important to glean important lessons learned from past
practical field experience in early intervention—there have been, and continue
to be, well-meaning efforts to assist individuals following trauma and traumatic loss. Future research must examine the necessary and sufficient ingredients
(and the unique meaningful clinical and functional outcome indicators) of

effective mental health first-aid care and formal secondary prevention of chronic psychopathology.

The goal of this book is to comprehensively address the conceptual, empirical, and applied issues pertaining to early intervention for trauma and traumatic loss. The intent is to clarify the available evidence supporting various types of interventions, and when an evidentiary base does not exist, to use researchers with extensive clinical experience to generate conceptual frameworks that will guide future studies in an area that desperately needs empirical research. Another goal is to cover the issues and content areas essential to an understanding of early intervention, focus on clarifying empirical and methodological issues, and set forth a research agenda for the next phase of early intervention research. We anticipate that the information in this volume will be useful to various care providers and professionals in all disciplines and organizations that are concerned with how best to help people adapt to trauma, as well as decision makers and consumer groups. Additional intended audiences include graduate students and postdoctoral trainees in the allied health professions interested in evaluating the state of the art in empirical research on early intervention, in service of conducting further research (e.g., public health, clinical social work, psychiatry, and clinical psychology).

TYPES OF TRAUMA AND TRAUMATIC LOSS COVERED IN THIS BOOK

Although we do not address early intervention for all possible types or categories of trauma in this book (war zones, natural disasters, technological disasters, etc.), we do not systematically limit the scope and type of trauma discussed. The principals discussed in this volume are applicable to most traumatic events, large or small, experienced at any age, in isolation or shared by all of humanity. On the other hand, different types of traumatic events are distinguished by unique exigencies in the immediate environment and the acute recovery context. In addition, the degree of public awareness and civic or legal involvement, the number of victims, the extent of the devastation, the breadth of the shared experience, and the resources available are among the many factors that determine the extent to which early intervention is possible or feasible. Thus, this book will not entail recommendations for various specific logistical "how-tos" germane to all possible traumatic contexts (which would be nearly an impossible task). Our goal is to explicate the state of the empirical literature and recommend evidence-based early intervention strategies as well as to set forth an extensive agenda for future research. Clinicians and clinical researchers will need to mold these principles and empirical methods into tasks and agendas applicable to various unique traumatic contexts. We are confident that this is possible.

ORGANIZATION OF THIS BOOK

The book has three parts. The first part, "Predictors and Course of Acute Stress Disorder, Posttraumatic Stress Disorder, and Traumatic Grief," provides a depiction of the psychological demands of trauma and traumatic loss, the course of acute adaptation and recovery, and what research has shown places individuals at risk for chronic posttraumatic difficulties, including acute stress disorder, PTSD, and traumatic grief. First, in Chapter 2, Bryant describes the clinical course, epidemiology, and the assessment and treatment of acute stress disorder, which is ostensibly PTSD in the first month after exposure to trauma. The presence of acute stress disorder (ASD) is a powerful predictor of those who will go on to develop chronic psychosocial disturbance stemming from exposure to trauma. Bryant argues that early intervention should be provided exclusively to individuals with ASD soon after a traumatic event so that scarce secondary prevention resources can be devoted to those most at risk for chronic PTSD and least likely to get better on their own. In the next chapter, King and colleagues review research that has explored personal, traumatic event, and social factors that promote or impede effective recovery from trauma, so-called resilience and risk factors, respectively. One of the most important new lines of research on trauma and PTSD will be the identification of specific temperamental, personality, psychological, physiological, and social mechanisms or processes that impede recovery from trauma. Once these factors can be reliably assessed in logistically feasible ways in the acute aftermath of trauma, their mitigation will prove effective as a secondary prevention strategy. King, Vogt, and King (in Chapter 3) also provide a conceptual framework to advance empirical research on risk and resilience factors. In the last chapter in this part, Chapter 4, Gray, Prigerson, and Litz discuss conceptual and definitional issues in traumatic grief. When people lose intimates unexpectedly, and from malicious acts of violence in particular, they are at risk for complicated or chronic grief-related problems and mental health disturbances (Raphael & Martinek, 1997). In this bereavement context, recovery demands and mental health outcomes are represented by a synergy of psychological trauma and grief. The study of loss by traumatic means, and, in particular, the psychological and psychiatric sequelae implicated by loss due to malicious violence, is relatively new. At present, there is no single paradigmatic approach but, rather, several competing theories conceptualizing the causes of chronic grief implicated by bereavement by traumatic loss. Nevertheless, research has shown that loss by traumatic means can lead to chronic grief, which can be horrifically functionally impairing.

The next part, "Empirical Research on Early Interventions for Trauma and Traumatic Loss," summarizes the state of the art in research on early intervention for trauma and traumatic loss across the lifespan (in very young children, older children, and adults). In each chapter, the authors describe existing research and explicate a set of empirical questions for future research as well as propose methods of study. In Chapter 5, Litz and Gray critically review the history and current state of early intervention for trauma, distinguish psychological first aid from the methods and goals of formal secondary prevention interventions, and make a set of recommendations for research and practice. In Chapter 6, Van Horn and Lieberman describe research on early intervention for trauma and traumatic loss in the most vulnerable of individuals: infants, toddlers, and preschoolers. Early physical and sexual abuse and, in particular, a combination of brutality, neglect, and sexual abuse or incest can have a profoundly devastating impact on emotional and intellectual development, the quality of adult attachments, self-care, self-esteem, a variety of psychopathologies, and substance abuse (e.g., Cohen, Brown, & Smaile, 2001; Dube et al., 2001; MacMillan et al., 2001). Unfortunately, there is little research on secondary prevention interventions for traumatized children, which is extraordinary given the societal problem of child neglect and abuse. Van Horn and Lieberman also describe their treatment approach, which systematically incorporates parents to promote and restore trust and healing. In Chapter 7, Cohen describes the best way to target trauma in school-age children and adolescents. The reader needs only to recall the terrible tragedy of Columbine to appreciate the important work of Cohen and others. Fortunately, such mass violence episodes are statistically rare. However, assaults among school-age children as well as suicide and motor vehicle accidents are not rare. For example, in 2001, 17.4% of students in the United States carried a weapon to school and 6.6% of students reported missing at least 1 day of school in approximately 30 days because they felt unsafe at school or on their way to or from school (Centers for Disease Control and Prevention, 2001). In Chapter 8, Raphael and Wooding discuss ways of conceptualizing and treating traumatic loss in adults. Although loss by traumatic means (e.g., homicide, mass violence, and suicide) is considered in the diagnostic nosology as a psychological trauma that can result in PTSD, the PTSD construct fails to capture the unique psychological and social burden of traumatic bereavement. Raphael and Wooding also discuss the psychological, social, and psychiatric sequelae of loss by traumatic means and discuss the unique early intervention needs of individuals bereaved in such tragic circumstances. Finally, in Chapter 9, Gray, Litz, and Olson discuss various ways early intervention can be studied in scientifically sound ways. There are a host of practical barriers and ethical considerations unique to the early posttraumatic context that creates hurdles and roadblocks to research efforts. Nevertheless, empirically sound and internally valid early intervention investigations can, and have been, conducted.

The last part, "Special Topics," has a series of chapters germane to early intervention. First, in Chapter 10, Neria, Suh, and Marshall summarize the lessons learned from providing mental health care after the 9-11 attack on the World Trade Center in New York City and describe a series of steps taken to respond to this enormous tragedy. Next, in Chapter 11, Rauch and Foa discuss the unique psychological and interpersonal challenges women face in the immediate aftermath of sexual violence and describe their research on secondary prevention of PTSD using cognitive-behavioral therapy. Third, in Chapter 12, Eriksson, Foy, and Larson discuss ways of intervening with a population of individuals affected chiefly by bearing witness to the trauma of others, such as emergency services personnel and relief organization workers. Fourth, in Chapter 13, Zatzick and Wagner address an underresearched but important topic—the enduring psychological burden created from physical trauma—and address ways of assisting individuals before they leave the hospital to prevent chronic PTSD. Fifth, Blanchard, Hickling, Kuhn, and Broderick, in Chapter 14, discuss their research on early mental health intervention for motor vehicle accident survivors. In the United States, motor vehicle accidents account for over 3 million injuries a year and are among the most common traumatic events (Blanchard & Hickling, 1997). Finally, in Chapter 15, Castro, Engel, and Adler, all of whom are clinicians and researchers in the U.S. military, address empirical and practical issues in early intervention for soldiers in the field of battle and when they return from war. The demands, stressors, and conflicts of participation in war can be traumatizing, spiritually and morally devastating, and transformative in potentially damaging ways, the impact of which can be manifest across the lifespan. The U.S. military has learned many important lessons about training and intervening early so as to reduce the mental health impact of combat. The U.S. military is also the largest user of psychological debriefing as an early intervention, in part because "after-action" debriefing has a long history in the military culture. The book ends with some concluding and summarizing remarks.

REFERENCES

American Psychiatric Association. (1994). *Diagnostic and statistical manual of mental disorders* (4th ed.). Washington, DC: Author.

Bisson, J. I., Jenkins, P. L., Alexander, J., & Bannister, C. (1997). Randomized controlled trial of psychological debriefing for victims of acute burn trauma. *British Journal of Psychiatry, 171,* 78–81.

Blanchard, E. B., & Hickling, E. J. (1997). *After the crash.* Washington, DC: American Psychological Association.

Bolton, E. E., Glenn, D. M., Orsillo, S., Roemer, L., & Litz, B. T. (2003). The relationship between self-disclosure and symptoms of posttraumatic stress disorder in peace-keepers deployed to Somalia. *Journal of Traumatic Stress, 16,* 203–210.

Breslau, N., Kessler, R., Chilcoat, H., Schultz, L, Davis, G., & Andreski, P. (1998). Trauma and posttraumatic stress disorder in the community: The 1996 Detroit area survey of trauma. *Archives of General Psychiatry, 55,* 626–632.

Bryant, R. A., & Harvey, A. G. (2002). Delayed-onset posttraumatic stress disorder: A prospective evaluation. *Australian and New Zealand Journal of Psychiatry, 36,* 205–209.

Bryant, R. A., Sackville, T., Dang, S. T., Moulds, M., & Guthrie, R. (1999). Treating acute stress disorder: An evaluation of cognitive behavior therapy and supporting counseling techniques. *American Journal of Psychiatry, 156,* 1780–1786.

Campbell, R., Ahrens, C. E., Sefl, T., Wasco, S. M., & Barnes, H. E. (2001). Social reactions to rape victims: Healing and hurtful effects on psychological and physical health outcomes. *Violence and Victims, 16,* 287–302.

Centers for Disease Control and Prevention. (2002, June). Youth Risk Behavior Surveillance—United States, 2001. *Morbidity and Mortality Weekly Report Surveillance Summaries, 51,* SS-4.

Cohen, P., Brown, J., & Smaile, E. (2001). Child abuse and neglect and the development of mental disorders in the general population. *Development and Psychopathology, 13,* 981–999.

Dube, S. R., Anda, R. F., Felitti, V. J., Chapman, D. P., Williamson, D. F., & Giles, W. H. (2001). Childhood abuse, household dysfunction, and the risk of attempted suicide throughout the life span: Findings from the adverse childhood experiences study. *Journal of the American Medical Association, 286,* 3089–3096.

Frazier, P., Conlon, A., & Glaser, T. (2001). Positive and negative life changes following sexual assault. *Journal of Consulting and Clinical Psychology, 69,* 1048–1055.

Harvey, A. G., & Bryant, R. A. (1999). The relationship between acute stress disorder and posttraumatic stress disorder: A 2-year prospective evaluation. *Journal of Consulting and Clinical Psychology, 67,* 985–988.

Harvey, A. G., & Bryant, R. A. (2002). Acute stress disorder: A synthesis and critique. *Psychological Bulletin, 128,* 886–902.

Kessler, R. C., Sonnega, A., Bromet, E., Hughes, M., & Nelson, C. B. (1995). Posttraumatic stress disorder in the National Comorbidity Survey. *Archives of General Psychiatry, 52,* 1048–1060.

Kulka, R. A., Schlenger, W. E., Fairbank, J. A., Hough, R. L., Jordan, B. K., Marmar, C. R., & Weiss, D. S. (1990). *Trauma and the Vietnam war generation: Report of the findings from the National Vietnam Veterans Readjustment Study.* New York: Brunner/Mazel.

Litz, B. T., Gray, M. J., Bryant, R. A., & Adler, A. B. (2002). Early intervention for trauma: Current status and future directions. *Clinical Psychology: Science and Practice, 9,* 112–134.

MacMillan, H. L., Fleming, J. E., Streiner, D. L., Lin, E., Boyle, M. H., Jamieson, E., Duku, E. K., Walsh, C. A., Wong, M. Y., & Beardslee, W. R. (2001). Childhood abuse and lifetime psychopathology in a community sample. *American Journal of Psychiatry, 158,* 1878–1883.

Mitchell, J. T., & Everly, G. S. (1996). *Critical incident stress debriefing: An operations manual for the prevention of traumatic stress among emergency services and disaster workers* (2nd ed.). Ellicott City, MD: Chevron.

Raphael, B., Dobson, M., & Minkov, C. (2001). Psychotherapeutic and pharmacological interventions for bereaved people. In M. S. Stroebe, R. O. Hansson, W. Stroebe, & H. Schut (Eds.), *Handbook of bereavement research: Consequences, coping, and care* (pp. 587–612). Washington, DC: American Psychological Association.

Raphael, B., & Martinek, N. (1997) Assessing traumatic bereavement and posttraumatic stress disorder. In J. Wilson & T. Keane (Eds.), *Assessing psychological trauma and PTSD* (pp. 373–395). New York: Guilford Press.

Rennison, C. M. (2002, August). *Rape and sexual assault: Reporting to police and medical attention, 1992–2000* (NCJ 194530). Washington, DC: U.S. Department of Justice, Bureau of Justice Statistics Selected Findings.

Roberts, A. R. (1991). Delivery of services to crime victims: A national survey. *American Journal of Orthopsychiatry, 61,* 128–137.

Rose, S., Brewin, C. R., Andrews, B., & Kirk, M. (1999). A randomized controlled trial of individual psychological debriefing for victims of violent crime. *Psychological Medicine, 29,* 793–799.

Rothbaum, B., Foa, E., Riggs, D., Murdock, T., & Walsh, W. (1992). A prospective examination of post-traumatic stress disorder in rape victims. *Journal of Traumatic Stress, 5,* 455–475.

Shalev, A. Y. (1999). Psychophysiological expression of risk factors for PTSD. In R. Yehuda (Ed.), *Risk factors for posttraumatic stress disorder* (pp. 143–161). Washington, DC: American Psychiatric Association.

Shear, M. K., Frank, E., Foa, E., Cherry, C., Reynolds, C. F. III, Vander Bilt, J., & Masters, S. (2001). Traumatic grief treatment: A pilot study. *American Journal of Psychiatry, 158,* 1506–1508.

Sireling, L., Cohen, D., & Marks, I. (1988). Guided mourning for morbid grief: A controlled replication. *Behavior Therapy, 19,* 121–132.

Stroebe, M., Stroebe, W., Schut, H., Zech, E., & van den Bout, J. (2002). Does disclosure of emotions facilitate recovery from bereavement? Evidence from two prospective studies. *Journal of Consulting and Clinical Psychology, 70,* 169–178.

Tedeschi, R. G. (1999). Violence transformed: Posttraumatic growth in survivors and their societies. *Aggression and Violent Behavior, 4,* 319–341.

True, W. R., Rice, J., Eisen, S. A., Heath, A. C., Goldberg, J., Lyons, M. J., & Nowak, J. (1993). A twin study of genetic and environmental contributions to liability for posttraumatic stress symptoms. *Archives of General Psychiatry, 50,* 257–265.

Ullman, S. E. (1997). Attributions, world assumptions, and recovery from sexual assault. *Journal of Child Sexual Abuse, 6,* 1–19.

Williams J. S., & Yule, R. W. (1993). Changes in outlook following disaster: The preliminary development of a measure to assess positive and negative responses. *Journal of Traumatic Stress, 6,* 271–279.

Wortman, C. B., & Silver, R. C. (1989). The myths of coping with loss. *Journal of Consulting and Clinical Psychology, 57,* 349–357.

I

Predictors and Course of Acute Stress Disorder, Posttraumatic Stress Disorder, and Traumatic Grief

2

Acute Stress Disorder

Course, Epidemiology, Assessment, and Treatment

RICHARD A. BRYANT

Increasing attention has been paid in recent years to the management of acute stress reactions following trauma. One important contributor to this interest has been the introduction of the acute stress disorder (ASD) diagnosis, which has caused considerable controversy and has stimulated much research on acute responses to trauma. This chapter outlines the rationale for this diagnosis, reviews the evidence supporting its utility, describes available assessment tools for ASD, and critiques treatment options for ASD.

THE COURSE OF PSYCHOLOGICAL RESPONSES

Before addressing the issue of ASD, it is important to review our knowledge of the normal course of posttraumatic adjustment. There is strong evidence that most people who are recently exposed to a traumatic experience report a broad array of anxiety symptoms in the initial weeks after exposure. For example, there are reports of high rates of emotional numbing (Feinstein, 1989; Noyes, Hoenk, Kuperman, & Slymen, 1977), reduced awareness of one's environment (Berah, Jones, & Valent, 1984; Hillman, 1981), derealization (Cardeña & Spiegel, 1993; Freinkel, Koopman, & Spiegel, 1994; Noyes & Kletti, 1977; Sloan, 1988), depersonalization (Cardeña & Spiegel, 1993; Freinkel et al., 1994; Noyes et al., 1977; Sloan, 1988), dissociative amnesia (Cardeña & Spiegel, 1993; Feinstein, 1989; Madakasira & O'Brien, 1987), intrusive thoughts (Cardeña & Spiegel, 1993; Feinstein, 1989; Sloan, 1988), avoidance behaviors (Bryant & Harvey, 1996; Cardeña & Spiegel, 1993; North, Smith, McCool, & Lightcap, 1989), insomnia (Cardeña & Spiegel, 1993; Feinstein, 1989; Sloan, 1988), concentration deficits (Cardeña & Spiegel, 1993; North et al., 1989), irritability (Sloan, 1988), and autonomic arousal (Feinstein, 1989; Sloan, 1988). There is little doubt that psychological distress is commonplace in the weeks after a traumatic experience.

Although acute stress reactions are common, there is also strong evidence that the majority of these stress responses are transient. That is, the majority of people who initially display distress naturally adapt to their experience in the following months. For example, whereas 94% of rape victims in one study displayed symptoms of posttraumatic stress disorder (PTSD) 2 weeks posttrauma, this rate dropped to 47% 11 weeks later (Rothbaum, Foa, Riggs, Murdock, & Walsh, 1992). In another study, 70% of women and 50% of men were diagnosed with PTSD at an average of 19 days after an assault; the rate of PTSD at 4-month follow-up dropped to 21% for women and zero for men (Riggs, Rothbaum, & Foa, 1995). Similarly, half of a sample meeting criteria for PTSD shortly after a motor vehicle accident had remitted by 6 months and two-thirds had remitted by 1 year posttrauma (Blanchard et al., 1996). A similar pattern was observed in community studies of residents of New York following the terrorist attacks on the World Trade Center. Whereas 9% of residents reported PTSD within 1 month after the attacks (Galea, Resnick, et al., 2002), the rate dropped to 4% 4 months later (Galea, Ahern, Resnick, Kilpatrick, & Vlahov, 2002). These patterns suggest that the normative response to trauma is to experience a range of PTSD symptoms initially with the majority of these reactions remitting in the following months.

THE RATIONALE FOR ACUTE STRESS DISORDER

In an attempt to avoid pathologizing transient stress reactions, the fourth edition of the *Diagnostic and Statistical Manual of Mental Disorders* (DSM-IV; American Psychiatric Association, 1994) stipulated that PTSD could only be recognized at least 1 month after a trauma. This resulted in a nosological gap because people distressed by a traumatic event could not be readily described in existing diagnostic categories. In 1994, DSM-IV introduced the ASD diagnosis to describe stress reactions in the initial month after a trauma. One goal of this diagnosis was to fill the diagnostic gap that existed in the initial month following trauma. A second goal was to discriminate between recent trauma survivors who are experiencing transient stress reactions and those who are suffering reactions that will persist into long-term PTSD (Koopman, Classen, Cardeña, & Spiegel, 1995). The goal of the ASD diagnosis to predict PTSD contrasts with the conceptualisation of acute stress reactions in the tenth edition of the *International Classification of Diseases* (ICD-10; World Health Organization, 1992). ICD-10 describes acute stress reaction as a transient reaction that occurs in the initial 48 hours after a trauma and encompasses a broad range of anxiety and depressive reactions.

The ASD diagnosis was strongly influenced by the perspective that dissociative reactions are a crucial mechanism in posttraumatic adjustment. Tracing its origins to Janet (1907), this perspective argues that dissociative responses following trauma lead to psychopathological responses because they impede access to, and processing of, memories and emotions associated with the traumatic experience (van der Kolk & van der Hart, 1989). According to this view, dissociative responses shortly after trauma exposure will impede integration and resolution of traumatic memories, and this process will directly lead to PTSD (Koopman et al., 1995). The proposal that dissociation in the acute phase leads to PTSD is supported by prospective studies that indicate a relationship between peritraumatic dissociation and subsequent pathology (Koopman, Classen, & Spiegel, 1994; Marmar et al., 1994; Shalev, Peri, Canetti, & Schreiber, 1996; Solomon & Mikulincer, 1992). This evidence needs to be considered, however, in the context of other prospective work that suggests that peritraumatic dissociation is not necessarily linked to subsequent psychopathology (Dancu, Riggs, Hearst-Ikeda, Shoyer, & Foa, 1996; Marshall & Schell, 2002; for review, see Keane, Kaufman, & Kimble, 2000).

DEFINITION OF ACUTE STRESS DISORDER

DSM-IV stipulates that ASD can occur after a fearful response to experiencing or witnessing a threatening event (Cluster A). The requisite symptoms to meet criteria for ASD include three dissociative symptoms (Cluster B), one re-experiencing symptom (Cluster C), marked avoidance (Cluster D), marked anxiety or increased arousal (Cluster E), and evidence of significant distress or impairment (Cluster F). The disturbance must last for a minimum of 2 days and a maximum of 4 weeks (Cluster G), after which time a diagnosis of PTSD should be considered. The primary difference between the criteria for ASD and PTSD is the time frame and the former's emphasis on dissociative reactions to the trauma. ASD refers to symptoms manifested during the period from 2 days to 4 weeks posttrauma, whereas PTSD can only be diagnosed from 4 weeks. The diagnosis of ASD requires that the individual has experienced at least three of the following: (1) a subjective sense of numbing or detachment, (2) reduced awareness of one's surroundings, (3) derealization, (4) depersonalization, or (5) dissociative amnesia.

Criticisms of the Acute Stress Disorder Diagnosis

The introduction of the ASD diagnosis has resulted in a strong debate about its utility (Bryant & Harvey, 2000; Butler, 2000; Koopman, 2000; Marshall, Spitzer, & Liebowitz, 2000; Simeon & Guralnik, 2000; Spiegel, Classen, & Cardeña, 2000). Critics of the diagnosis have focused on the following potential flaws with the new diagnosis. First, it was introduced with little evidence to support its inclusion (Keane et al., 2000). At the time of its introduction, even the proponents of the diagnosis admitted that the alleged relationship between ASD and PTSD was "based more on logical arguments than on empirical research" (Koopman et al., 1995, p. 38). Second, the ASD diagnosis was one of the few diagnoses that were included without being subjected to the empirical or peer-review scrutiny given to other potential diagnoses (Bryant, 2000). Third, the emphasis on dissociation as a necessary response to trauma was criticized on the grounds that there was insufficient evidence to support the idea that this construct plays such a pivotal role in acute trauma response (Bryant & Harvey, 1997; Keane et al., 2000; Marshall et al., 2000). Fourth, some objected to the notion that the primary role of the ASD diagnosis was to predict another diagnosis (Bryant, 2000). Fifth, there was concern that the diagnosis may pathologize transient stress reactions (Marshall, Spitzer, & Liebowitz, 1999). Sixth, it was argued that distinguishing between two diagnoses (ASD and PTSD) that have comparable symptoms on the basis of the duration of these symptoms is not justified (Marshall, Spitzer, & Liebowitz, 1999). Seventh, it was suggested that the broader conceptualisation adopted by ICD-10 was more useful for clinicians than the more focused DSM-IV criteria (Marshall et al., 1999; Solomon, Laor, & McFarlane, 1996).

Incidence of Acute Stress Disorder

A number of studies have now reported the incidence of ASD following a range of traumatic events. ASD has been reported in 13%–21% of victims following motor vehicle accidents (MVAs; Harvey & Bryant, 1998a; Holeva, Tarrier, & Wells, 2001), in 14% following mild brain injury (Harvey & Bryant, 1998b), in 16%–19% of people following assault (Brewin, Andrews, Rose, & Kirk, 1999; Harvey & Bryant, 1999a), in 16% following traumatic loss (Green,

Krupnick, Stockton, & Goodman, 2001), and in 10% of those suffering burns (Harvey & Bryant, 1999a), in between 6 and 12% following industrial accidents (Creamer & Manning, 1998; Harvey & Bryant, 1999a), in 33% following a mass shooting (Classen, Koopman, Hales, & Spiegel, 1998), and in 7% following a typhoon (Staab, Grieger, Fullerton, & Ursano, 1996) Overall, the reported incidence of ASD is generally lower than the rate of acute PTSD (e.g., Feinstein, 1989; Rothbaum et al., 1992), which probably reflects the more stringent criteria for the ASD diagnosis.

Does Acute Stress Disorder Predict Posttraumatic Stress Disorder?

There are now 10 prospective studies (Brewin et al., 1999; Bryant & Harvey, 1998; Harvey & Bryant, 1998a, 1999b, 2000; Holeva, Tarrier, & Wells, 2001; Kangas & Bryant, 2002; O'Donnell, Creamer, Pattison, & Atkin, 2001; Schnyder, Moergeli, Klaghofer, & Buddeberg, 2001; Staab et al., 1996) that have prospectively assessed the relationship between ASD in the initial month after trauma and subsequently assessed PTSD. Table 2.1 presents a summary of the 10 studies in terms of (1) the proportion of people who initially had ASD and who subsequently developed PTSD, and (2) the proportion of people who eventually developed PTSD who initially met criteria for ASD. In terms of people who initially display ASD, a significant number of studies have found that approximately three-quarters of trauma survivors who display ASD subsequently develop PTSD (see Table 2.1). These studies suggest that the ASD di-

TABLE 2.1. Summary of Prospective Studies of Acute Stress Disorder

Trauma type	Study	Proportion of ASD who develop PTSD	Proportion of PTSD who had ASD
MVA	Harvey & Bryant (1998a)	78%	39%
Brain injury	Bryant & Harvey (1998)	83%	40%
Assault	Brewin et al. (1999)	83%	57%
MVA	Holeva et al. (2001)	72%	59%
MVA	O'Donnell et al. (2001)	30%	34%
MVA	Schnyder et al. (2001)	34%	10%
Typhoon	Staab et al. (1996)	30%	37%
Cancer	Kangas & Bryant (2002)	53%	61%
MVA	Harvey & Bryant (1999b)	82%	29%
Brain injury	Harvey & Bryant (2000)	80%	72%

Note. ASD, acute stress disorder; PTSD, posttraumatic stress disorder; MVA, motor vehicle accident.

agnosis is performing reasonably well in predicting people who will develop PTSD. The lower rates of PTSD following ASD in some studies may be attributed to methodological factors in these studies. For example, both the O'Donnell et al. (2001) and the Schnyder et al. (2001) studies adopted strict exclusion criteria that may have limited the identification of ASD in these studies.

The utility of the ASD diagnosis is less promising, however, when one considers the proportion of people who eventually developed PTSD and who initially displayed ASD. Across studies, the minority of people who eventually developed PTSD initially met criteria for ASD. This convergence across studies suggests that whereas the majority of people who develop ASD are high risk for developing subsequent PTSD, there are many other people who will develop PTSD who do not initially meet ASD criteria. One probable reason for people who are high risk for PTSD not meeting the ASD criteria is the requirement that three dissociative symptoms be displayed. In one prospective study, 60% of people who met all ASD criteria except for the dissociation cluster met PTSD criteria 6 months later (Harvey & Bryant, 1998a), and 75% of these people still had PTSD 2 years later (Harvey & Bryant, 1999b). This pattern suggests that emphasizing dissociation as a key factor in predicting subsequent PTSD will result in many high-risk individuals being neglected.

It is important to note that there are significant differences across these studies in terms of populations, assessment tools, and inclusion criteria. In terms of inclusion criteria, various studies employed different exclusion criteria that variably included or excluded participants who had sustained a mild brain injury or used medications that mimicked dissociative reactions. These discrepancies have potentially influenced the extent to which ASD was identified and, accordingly, the reported relationship between ASD and subsequent PTSD. Similarly, there is considerable disparity in terms of how ASD has been assessed. Whereas some researchers have used tools that have been specifically developed to index ASD (Bryant & Harvey, 1998; Harvey & Bryant, 1998a), others derived ASD diagnoses on the basis of different measures that purportedly indexed symptoms that were comparable to ASD (Brewin et al., 1999; Staab et al., 1996). These procedural variations may account for some of the discrepant findings observed across the studies.

MECHANISMS OF ACUTE STRESS DISORDER

Although the ASD diagnosis itself has limited utility, its introduction has resulted in increasing knowledge about the mechanisms that may mediate the transition from acute stress response to chronic PTSD. These mechanisms are of interest because they indicate the processes that may underpin psychopathological trauma responses and also may point to processes that may need to be addressed during treatment. The major focus in recent years has been on cognitive and biological responses in the period shortly after trauma exposure.

In terms of cognitive responses, current models posit that psychopathological responses may be mediated by two core factors: (1) maladaptive appraisals of the trauma and its aftermath, and (2) disturbances in autobiographical memory that involve impaired retrieval (Ehlers & Clark, 2000). Consistent with this approach, there is evidence that people with ASD exaggerate both the probability of future negative events occurring and the adverse effects of these events (Warda & Bryant, 1998a). Moreover, ASD sufferers display cognitive biases for events related to external harm, somatic sensations, and social concerns (Smith & Bryant, 2000). There is also evidence that a catastrophic cognitive style in the period after trauma exposure predicts subsequent PTSD (Ehlers, Mayou, & Bryant, 1998; Engelhard, van den Hout, Arntz, & McNally, 2002). The tendency for ASD individuals to display catastrophic thinking is also supported by experimental findings that ASD participants respond to a hyperventilation task with more dysfunctional interpretations about their reactions than non-ASD participants (Nixon & Bryant, in press-a). Relatedly, the nature of attributions about the trauma shortly after the event apparently influences longer-term functioning. Prospective studies indicate that attributing responsibility to another person (Delahanty et al., 1997) and attributions of shame (Andrews, Brewin, Rose, & Kirk, 2000) in the acute phase are associated with later PTSD.

There is also evidence that people with ASD may manage trauma-related information differently from other trauma survivors. Specifically, individuals with ASD tend to avoid aversive information. One study employed a directed, forgetting paradigm that required ASD, non-ASD, and non-trauma-exposed control participants to read a series of trauma-related, positive, or neutral words, and after each presentation participants were instructed to either remember or forget the word (Moulds & Bryant, 2002). The finding that ASD participants recalled fewer trauma-related to-be-forgotten words than non-ASD participants suggests that they have an aptitude for forgetting aversive material. In a similar study that employed the list method form of directed forgetting, which indexes retrieval patterns, ASD participants displayed poorer recall of to-be-forgotten trauma words than non-ASD participants (Moulds & Bryant, in press). These findings suggest that people with ASD possess a cognitive style that avoids awareness of aversive or distressing information. This interpretation accords with findings that people with ASD use avoidant cognitive strategies to manage their trauma memories (Guthrie & Bryant, 2000; Warda & Bryant, 1998b). Avoidance of distressing information or memories may be associated with psychopathological responses because it may lead to impaired processing of trauma-related memories and affect. In terms of auto-biographical memory, one study has found that ASD participants report fewer specific positive memories than non-ASD participants, and this deficit contributes to subsequent PTSD severity (Harvey, Bryant, & Dang, 1998). This pattern may suggest that problems in retrieving positive memories about one's personal past may limit access to information that is useful in negative appraisals about the trauma and its consequences (Ehlers & Clark, 2000).

Biological perspectives have focused on fear conditioning and progressive neural sensitization in the weeks after trauma as possible explanations of the genesis of PTSD (Kolb, 1987; Pitman, Shalev, & Orr, 2000). It is possible that sensitization occurs as a result of repetitive activation by trauma reminders elevating sensitivity of limbic networks (Post, Weiss, & Smith, 1995), and that, as time progresses, these responses become increasingly conditioned to trauma-related stimuli (Le Doux, Iwata, Cicchetti, & Reis, 1988). In support of these proposals, there is evidence that people who eventually develop PTSD display elevated resting heart rates in the initial week after trauma (Bryant, Harvey, Guthrie, & Moulds, 2000; Shalev et al., 1998; see also Blanchard, Hickling, Galovski, & Veazey, 2002). In addition, it has been found that lower cortisol levels shortly after trauma predict subsequent PTSD (Delahanty, Raimonde, & Spoonster, 2000; McFarlane, Atchison, & Yehuda, 1997). Cortisol may act as an "antistress" hormone that regulates initial activation of cortisol to restore equilibrium, and lower cortisol levels may reflect an incapacity to lower arousal following trauma (Yehuda, 1997). The importance of increased arousal in the acute phase is also indicated by the prevalence of panic attacks in people ASD (Bryant & Panasetis, 2001; Nixon & Bryant, in press-b).

ASSESSMENT OF ACUTE STRESS DISORDER

There are currently three major measures for ASD. The first measure to be developed was the Stanford Acute Stress Reaction Questionnaire (SASRQ). The original version of the SASRQ (Cardeña, Classen, & Spiegel, 1991) was a self-report inventory that indexed dissociative (33 items), intrusive (11 items), somatic anxiety (17 items), hyperarousal (2 items), attention disturbance (3 items), and sleep disturbance (1 item) symptoms, and different versions of this measure have been employed by the authors across a range of studies (Cardeña & Spiegel, 1993; Classen et al., 1998; Freinkel et al., 1994; Koopman et al., 1994). The current version of the SASRQ (Cardeña, Koopman, Classen, Waelde, & Spiegel, 2000) is a self-report inventory that encompasses each of the ASD symptoms. Each item asks respondents to indicate the frequency of each symptom during and immediately following a trauma on a 6-point Likert scale (0 = "not experienced," 5 = "very often experienced") . The SASRQ possesses high internal consistency (Cronbach's alpha = .90 and .91 for dissociative and anxiety symptoms, respectively) and concurrent validity with scores on the Impact of Event Scale (r = .52 –.69; Koopman et al., 1994).

The Acute Stress Disorder Interview (ASDI; Bryant, Harvey, Dang, & Sackville, 1998) is a structured clinical interview that is based on DSM-IV criteria. The ASDI possesses good internal consistency (r = .90), test–retest reliability (r = .88), sensitivity (91%) and specificity (93%) relative to independent clinician diagnosis of ASD. The ASDI contains 19 dichotomously scored items that relate to the dissociative (Cluster B, five items), reexperiencing (Cluster C, four items), avoidance (Cluster D, four items), and arousal (Cluster E, six items) symptoms of ASD. Summing the affirmative responses to each symptom provides a total score indicative of acute stress severity (range 1–19). The Acute Stress Disorder Scale (ASDS; Bryant, Moulds, & Guthrie, 2000) is a self-report inventory based on the same items described in the ASDI. Each item on the ASDS is scored on a 5-point scale that reflects degrees of severity. Using a formula to identify ASD caseness, the ASDS possesses good sensitivity (95%) and specificity (83%) in relation to diagnoses based on the ASDI.

Development of these measures reflects some of the problems inherent in the ASD diagnosis. The construct of these measures assumes that there is some gold standard against which the measure can be validated. As discussed previously, the ASD diagnosis is based largely on theoretical constructs rather than evidence concerning the construct it describes. Development of measures typically relies on related measures or constructs to establish concurrent validity or construct validity (Haynes, Wilner, & Kubany, 1995). The absence of these measures in ASD results in measures being developed that attempt validation by comparing them against the same items that were driven by the DSM-IV construction of the diagnosis. This process can be criticized for a degree of circularity because there is no independent standard against which these measures can be judged. Test–retest reliability is also difficult to achieve because there is a potential confound between the reliability of an assessment tool across two different time points and the rapidly changing nature of acute stress reactions. Associated with the problem of the changing nature of acute stress reactions is the DSM-IV stipulation that ASD can be identified 2 days after trauma exposure. This time frame appears to lack any empirical justification. Evidence from a study of civilians involved in the Gulf War indicates that many people who suffered immediate stress symptoms in the initial days after trauma exposure subsequently made significant recoveries (Solomon et al., 1996). It is probable that attempting to diagnose individuals 2 days after a traumatic event will lead to incorrectly identifying transient stress reactions as pathological responses. Although there is little data to guide decision making about the optimal time to identify initial reactions that are predictive of subsequent psychopathology, it is likely that any diagnoses made within 1 week of a trauma are likely to increase the confusion between transient and longer-term stress reactions.

TREATING ACUTE STRESS DISORDER

The best-controlled studies of early intervention following trauma involve cognitive-behavioral therapy (CBT). The components that typically constitute CBT for PTSD include psychoeducation, anxiety management cognitive restructuring, and exposure. Psychoeducation usually includes education about common reactions to a traumatic event, the cognitive and behavioral mechanisms that mediate core PTSD reactions, and a rationale for the treatment. Anxiety management techniques provide individuals with coping skills to manage their fear, reduce arousal, and assist in managing distressing activities and trauma reminders. Anxiety management approaches often include stress inoculation training that follows Meichenbaum's (1975) program of psychoeducation, relaxation skills, thought stopping, and self-talk. Cognitive restructuring is based on models that emphasize the importance of appraisals in the aetiology and maintenance of PTSD (Ehlers & Clark, 2000; Janoff-Bulman, 1992). Cognitive restructuring involves teaching individuals to identify and evaluate the evidence for negative automatic thoughts, as well as helping patients to evaluate their beliefs about the trauma, the self, the world, and the future (Beck, Rush, Shaw, & Emery, 1979). Prolonged imaginal exposure requires the individual to vividly imagine the trauma for prolonged periods. The individual typically provides a narrative of their traumatic experience in a way that emphasizes all relevant details including sensory cues and affective responses. This exercise usually occurs for at least 50 minutes and is usually supplemented by daily homework exercises. Most exposure treatments supplement imaginal exposure with *in vivo* exposure that involves graded exposure to the feared, trauma-related stimuli. Although there is considerable debate about the change mechanisms associated with exposure (see Jaycox & Foa, 1996; Rothbaum & Mellman, 2001; Rothbaum & Schwartz, 2002), it is possible that therapy success is mediated by habituation of anxiety, integration of corrective information, modification of the belief that anxiety remains unless avoidance occurs, learning that the trauma is a discrete event that is not indicative of general threat, and self-mastery through management of exposure.

Although there were early trials of interventions that resembled CBT (Brom, Kleber, & Hofman, 1993; Viney, Clark, Bunn, & Benjamin, 1985), these were not well-controlled studies. In an early controlled attempt to prevent PTSD, Kilpatrick and Veronen (1983) randomly allocated 15 recent rape victims to repeated assessments, delayed assessment, or a brief behavioral intervention that was comprised of a 4–6-hour program that involved imaginal reliving of the trauma, education about psychological responses to trauma, cognitive restructuring, and anxiety management. Although this study found that the brief intervention was not more effective than the repeated assessments, its conclusions were limited by small sample sizes, the lack of rigorous application of exposure, and questions concerning the degree of pathology experienced after the rape (Kilpatrick & Calhoun, 1988). Foa and colleagues conducted a more rigorous study by providing brief CBT to sexual and nonsexual assault victims shortly after the assault (Foa, Hearst-Ikeda, & Perry, 1995). This study compared CBT, (including exposure, anxiety management, *in vivo* exposure, and cognitive restructuring) with matched participants who had received repeated assessments. Each participant received four treatment sessions and then underwent assessment by blind assessors at 2 months posttreatment and 5 months follow-up. Whereas 10% of the CBT group met criteria for PTSD at 2 months, 70% of the control group met criteria; there were no differences between groups at 5 months, although the CBT group was less depressed. Inferences from this study were limited, however, by the lack of random assignment.

A limitation of the aforementioned studies is that they included recently traumatized survivors who were unselected in terms of likelihood for developing subsequent disorder. Accordingly, it is possible that any observed effects may have occurred as a result of natural remission. Although the ASD diagnosis is flawed by the evidence that many people who do not meet criteria for the diagnosis can develop PTSD, there is reasonable support for the claim that people who do display ASD are at high risk for subsequent PTSD. That is, the likelihood that ASD will lead to PTSD provides a more stringent test for early intervention because these individuals' psychological distress is more likely to persist. This approach differs from other early intervention strategies that focus attention on all trauma survivors and that presume that all people are vulnerable to development of disorder (e.g., debriefing practices, see Litz, Chapter 5, this volume). Instead, this approach recognizes that the majority of people are resilient following trauma, and early intervention should focus only on those individuals who are most at risk of developing subsequent psychopathology.

In an initial study of ASD participants, Bryant and colleagues randomly allocated MVA or nonsexual assault survivors with ASD to either CBT or supportive counseling (Bryant, Harvey, Dang, Sackville, & Basten, 1998). Both interventions consisted of five 1½-hour, weekly, individual therapy sessions.

CBT included education about posttraumatic reactions, relaxation training, cognitive restructuring, and imaginal and *in vivo* exposure to the traumatic event. The supportive counseling condition included trauma education and more general problem-solving skills training in the context of an unconditionally supportive relationship. At the 6-month follow-up, there were fewer participants in the CBT group (20%) who met diagnostic criteria for PTSD compared to supportive counseling control participants (67%). In a subsequent study that dismantled the components of CBT, 45 civilian trauma survivors with ASD were randomly allocated to five sessions of either (1) CBT (prolonged exposure, cognitive therapy, and/or anxiety management), (2) prolonged exposure combined with cognitive therapy, or (3) supportive counseling (Bryant, Sackville, Dang, Moulds, & Guthrie, 1999). This study found that at 6-month follow-up, PTSD was observed in approximately 20% of both active treatment groups compared to 67% of those receiving supportive counseling. A follow-up of participants who completed these two treatment studies indicated that the treatment gains of those who received CBT were maintained 4 years after treatment (Bryant, Moulds, & Nixon, 2003).

Two recent studies by the same team have supported the utility of CBT for people with ASD. One study randomly allocated civilian trauma survivors ($n = 89$) with ASD to either CBT, CBT associated with hypnosis, or supportive counseling (Bryant, Moulds, Guthrie, & Nixon, in press). The hypnosis component was provided immediately prior to imaginal exposure in an attempt to facilitate emotional processing of the trauma memories. In terms of treatment completers, more participants in the supportive counseling condition (57%) met PTSD criteria at 6-month follow-up than those in the CBT (21%) or CBT + hypnosis (22%) condition. Interestingly, participants in the CBT + hypnosis condition reported greater reduction of reexperiencing symptoms at posttreatment than those in the CBT condition. This finding suggests that hypnosis may facilitate treatment gains in ASD participants. Finally, a recent study replicated the original Bryant, Harvey, Dang, Sackville, and Basten (1998) study with a sample of ASD participants ($n = 24$) who sustained mild traumatic brain injury following MVAs (Bryant, Moulds, Guthrie, & Nixon, 2003). This study investigated the efficacy of CBT in people who lost consciousness during the trauma as result of their traumatic injury. Consistent with the previous studies, fewer participants receiving CBT (8%) met criteria for PTSD at 6 months follow-up than those receiving supportive counseling (58%).

It is important to note that there are significant limitations to the current evidence for the effective use of CBT shortly after trauma exposure. First, although CBT does lead to significant reductions in recently traumatized people who complete treatment, a significant proportion of participants do drop out of treatment. For example, 20% of participants dropped out of both the Bryant et al. (1999) and Bryant et al. (in press) studies. That is, intent-to-treat analyses in these studies are not promising for the benefits of CBT (Bryant et al., 1999; Bryant et al., in press). There is a need to develop interventions that are efficacious and manageable for more recently traumatized people. Second, the majority of early intervention treatment studies for ASD have emerged from the one treatment center at the University of New South Wales. It is important that these findings are replicated in other sites before the generalizability of these protocols can be established.

FUTURE DIRECTIONS

Although the ASD diagnosis is flawed, its introduction has resulted in promising developments that can enhance our understanding and management of acute trauma reactions. It is probable that the ASD diagnosis will not be retained in DSM-V because the available evidence does not warrant its inclusion as a means of predicting chronic PTSD (Harvey & Bryant, 2002). Whether or not the ASD diagnosis is retained, the important goal for future research is to develop new evidence-based means of identifying acute trauma responses that will subsequently develop into chronic psychopathology. Considering the variable findings across existing studies, there is a need for multisite, large-scale prospective studies that will guide development of assessment tools that can reliably identify high-risk individuals who will require early interventions after trauma. Treatment of recently trauma-exposed people also requires considerable research. The major questions facing early intervention researchers are (1) the relative benefits of early versus later intervention and (2) the development of interventions that can be tolerated by more trauma survivors. Considering the many early intervention practices that currently occur without any empirical support, it is essential that future interventions are developed on the basis of sound theoretical models and rigorous scientific study.

REFERENCES

American Psychiatric Association. (1994). *Diagnostic and statistical manual of mental disorders* (4th ed.). Washington, DC: Author.

Andrews, B., Brewin, C. R., Rose, S., & Kirk, M. (2000). Predicting PTSD in victims of violent crime: The role of shame, anger and blame. *Journal of Abnormal Psychology, 109,* 69–73.

Beck, A. T., Rush, A. J., Shaw, B. F., & Emery, G. (1979). *Cognitive therapy of depression.* New York: Guilford Press.

Berah, E. F., Jones, H. J., & Valent, P. (1984). The experience of a mental health team involved in the early phase of a disaster. *Australian and New Zealand Journal of Psychiatry, 18*, 354–358.

Blanchard, E. B., Hickling, E. J., Barton, K. A., Taylor, A. E., Loos, W. R., & Jones Alexander, J. (1996). One-year prospective follow-up of motor vehicle accident victims. *Behaviour Research and Therapy, 34*, 775–786.

Blanchard, E. B., Hickling, E. J., Galovski, T., & Veazey, C. (2002). Emergency room vital signs and PTSD in a treatment seeking sample of motor vehicle accident survivors. *Journal of Traumatic Stress, 15*,(1) 199–204.

Brewin, C. R., Andrews, B., Rose, S., & Kirk, M. (1999). Acute stress disorder and posttraumatic stress disorder in victims of violent crime. *American Journal of Psychiatry, 156*, 360–366.

Brom, D., Kleber, R. J., & Hofman, M. (1993). Victims of traffic accidents: Incidence and prevention of post-traumatic stress disorder. *Journal of Clinical Psychology, 49*, 131–140.

Bryant, R. A. (2000). Acute stress disorder. *PTSD Research Quarterly, 11*, 1–7.

Bryant, R. A., & Harvey, A. G. (1996). Initial post-traumatic stress responses following motor vehicle accidents. *Journal of Traumatic Stress, 9*, 223–234.

Bryant, R. A., & Harvey, A. G. (1997). Acute stress disorder: A critical review of diagnostic issues. *Clinical Psychology Review, 17*, 757–773.

Bryant, R. A., & Harvey, A. G. (1998). Relationship of acute stress disorder and posttraumatic stress disorder following mild traumatic brain injury. *American Journal of Psychiatry, 155*, 625–629.

Bryant, R. A., & Harvey, A. G. (2000). New DSM-IV diagnosis of acute stress disorder [Letter to the Editor]. *American Journal of Psychiatry, 157*, 1889–1890.

Bryant, R. A., Harvey, A. G., Dang, S., & Sackville, T. (1998). Assessing acute stress disorder: Psychometric properties of a structured clinical interview. *Psychological Assessment, 10*, 215–220.

Bryant, R. A., Harvey, A. G., Dang, S. T., Sackville, T., & Basten, C. (1998). Treatment of acute stress disorder: A comparison of cognitive behavior therapy and supportive counseling. *Journal of Consulting and Clinical Psychology, 66*, 862–866.

Bryant, R. A., Harvey, A. G., Guthrie, R., & Moulds, M. (2000). A prospective study of acute psychophysiological arousal, acute stress disorder, and posttraumatic stress disorder. *Journal of Abnormal Psychology, 109*, 341–344.

Bryant, R. A., Moulds, M., & Guthrie, R. (2000). Acute stress disorder scale: A self-report measure of acute stress disorder. *Psychological Assessment, 12*, 61–68.

Bryant, R. A., Moulds, M. L., Guthrie, R., & Nixon, R. D. V. (2003). Treating acute stress disorder after mild brain injury. *American Journal of Psychiatry, 160*, 585–587.

Bryant, R. A., Moulds, M. L., Guthrie, R., & Nixon, R. D. V. (in press). The additive benefit of hypnotherapy and cognitive behavior therapy in treating acute stress disorder. *Journal of Consulting and Clinical Psychology.*

Bryant, R. A., Moulds, M. L., & Nixon, R. D. V. (2003). Cognitive behaviour therapy of acute stress disorder: A four-year follow-up. *Behaviour Research and Therapy, 41*, 489–494.

Bryant, R. A., & Panasetis, P. (2001). Panic symptoms during trauma and acute stress disorder. *Behaviour Research and Therapy, 39,* 961–966.

Bryant, R. A., Sackville, T., Dang, S. T., Moulds, M., & Guthrie, R. (1999). Treating acute stress disorder: An evaluation of cognitive behavior therapy and counselling techniques. *American Journal of Psychiatry, 156,* 1780–1786.

Butler, L. D. (2000). New DSM-IV diagnosis of acute stress disorder [Letter to the Editor]. *American Journal of Psychiatry, 157,* 1889.

Cardeña, E., Classen, C., & Spiegel, D. (1991). *Stanford Acute Stress Reaction Questionnaire.* Stanford, CA: Stanford University Medical School.

Cardeña. E., Koopman, C., Classen, C., Waelde, L. C., & Spiegel, D. (2000). Psychometric properties of the Stanford Acute Stress Reaction Questionnaire (SASRQ): A valid and reliable measure of acute stress. *Journal of Traumatic Stress, 13,* 719–734.

Cardeña, E., & Spiegel, D. (1993). Dissociative reactions to the San Francisco Bay Area earthquake of 1989. *American Journal of Psychiatry, 150,* 474–478.

Classen, C., Koopman, C., Hales, R., & Spiegel, D. (1998). Acute stress disorder as a predictor of posttraumatic stress symptoms. *American Journal of Psychiatry, 155,* 620–624.

Creamer, M., & Manning, C. (1998). Acute stress disorder following an industrial accident. *Australian Psychologist, 33,* 125–129.

Dancu, C. V., Riggs, D. S., Hearst-Ikeda, D., Shoyer, B. G., & Foa, E. B. (1996). Dissociative experiences and posttraumatic stress disorder among female victims of criminal assault and rape. *Journal of Traumatic Stress, 9,* 253–267.

Delahanty, D. L., Herberman, H. B., Craig, K. J., Hayward, M. C., Fullerton, C. S., Ursano, R. J., & Baum, A. (1997). Acute and chronic distress and posttraumatic stress disorder as a function of responsibility for serious motor vehicle accidents. *Journal of Consulting and Clinical Psychology, 65,* 560–567.

Delahanty, D. L., Raimonde, A. J., & Spoonster, E. (2000). Initial posttraumatic urinary cortisol levels predict subsequent PTSD symptoms in motor vehicle accident victims. *Biological Psychiatry, 48,* 940–947.

Ehlers, A., & Clark, D. (2000). A cognitive model of posttraumatic stress disorder. *Behaviour Research and Therapy, 38,* 319–345.

Ehlers, A., Mayou, R. A., & Bryant, B. (1998). Psychological predictors of chronic PTSD after motor vehicle accidents. *Journal of Abnormal Psychology, 107,* 508–519.

Engelhard, I. M., van den Hout, M. A., Arntz, A., & McNally, R. J. (2002). A longitudinal study of "intrusion-based reasoning" and posttraumatic stress disorder after exposure to a train disaster. *Behaviour Research and Therapy, 40,* 1415–1424.

Feinstein, A. (1989). Posttraumatic stress disorder: A descriptive study supporting DSM III-R criteria. *American Journal of Psychiatry, 146,* 665–666.

Freinkel, A., Koopman, C., & Spiegel, D. (1994). Dissociative symptoms in media witnesses of an execution. *American Journal of Psychiatry, 151,* 1335–1339.

Foa, E. B., Hearst-Ikeda, D., & Perry, K. J. (1995). Evaluation of a brief cognitive behavioral program for the prevention of chronic PTSD in recent assault victims. *Journal of Consulting and Clinical Psychology, 63,* 948–955.

Galea, S., Ahern, J., Resnick, H., Kilpatrick, D., & Vlahov, D. (2002, November). *Posttraumatic stress disorder and depression in New York City after 9/11*. Paper presented at the annual meeting of the International Society of Traumatic Stress Studies, Baltimore.

Galea, S., Resnick, H., Kilpatrick, D., Bucuvalas, M., Gold, J., & Vlahov, D. (2002). Psychological sequelae of the September 11 terrorist attacks in New York City. *New England Journal of Medicine, 346,* 982–987.

Green, B. L., Krupnick, J. L., Stockton, P., & Goodman, L. (2001). Psychological outcomes associated with traumatic loss in a sample of young women. *The American Behavioral Scientist, 44,* 817–837.

Guthrie, R., & Bryant, R. A. (2000). Attempted thought suppression over extended periods in acute stress disorder. *Behaviour Research and Therapy, 38,* 899–907

Harvey, A. G., & Bryant, R. A. (1998a). Relationship of acute stress disorder and posttraumatic stress disorder following motor vehicle accidents. *Journal of Consulting and Clinical Psychology, 66,* 507–512.

Harvey, A. G., & Bryant, R. A. (1998b). Acute stress disorder following mild traumatic brain injury. *Journal of Nervous and Mental Disease, 186,* 333–337.

Harvey, A. G., & Bryant, R. A. (1999a). Acute stress disorder across trauma populations. *Journal of Nervous and Mental Disease, 187,* 443–446.

Harvey, A. G., & Bryant, R. A. (1999b). A two-year prospective evaluation of the relationship between acute stress disorder and posttraumatic stress disorder. *Journal of Consulting and Clinical Psychology, 67,* 985–988.

Harvey, A. G., & Bryant, R. A. (2000). A two-year prospective evaluation of the relationship between acute stress disorder and posttraumatic stress disorder following mild traumatic brain injury. *American Journal of Psychiatry, 157,* 626–628.

Harvey, A. G., & Bryant, R. A. (2002). Acute stress disorder: A synthesis and critique. *Psychological Bulletin, 128,* 892–906.

Harvey, A. G., Bryant, R. A., & Dang, S. (1998). Autobiographical memory in acute stress disorder. *Journal of Consulting and Clinical Psychology, 66,* 500–506.

Haynes, S. N., Wilner, N., & Kubany, E. S. (1995). Content validity in psychological assessment: A functional approach to concepts and methods. *Psychological Assessment, 7,* 238–247.

Hillman, R. G. (1981). The psychopathology of being held hostage. *American Journal of Psychiatry, 138,* 1193–1197.

Holeva, V., Tarrier, N., & Wells, A. (2001). Prevalence and predictors of acute stress disorder and PTSD following road traffic accidents: Thought control strategies and social support. *Behavior Therapy, 32,* 65–83.

Janet, P. (1907). *The major symptoms of hysteria.* New York: Macmillan.

Janoff-Bulman, R. (1992). *Shattered assumptions: Towards a new psychology of trauma.* New York: Free Press.

Jaycox, L. H., & Foa, E. B. (1996). Obstacles in implementing exposure therapy for PTSD: Case discussions and practical solutions. *Clinical Psychology and Psychotherapy, 3,* 176–184.

Kangas, M., & Bryant, R. A. (2002). *Acute stress disorder and posttraumatic stress disor-*

der following cancer diagnosis. Paper presented at the annual meeting of the American Psychological Association, Chicago.

Keane, T. M., Kaufman, M., & Kimble, M. O. (2000). Peritraumaitc dissociative symptoms, acute stress disorder, and posttraumatic stress disorder: Causation, correlation, or epiphenomenona?. In L. Sanchez-Planell & C. Diez-Quevedo (Eds.), *Dissociative states* (pp. 21–43). Barcelona: Sprionger-Verlag.

Kilpatrick, D. G., & Calhoun, K. S. (1988). Early behavioral treatment for rape trauma: Efficacy or artifact? *Behavior Therapy, 19,* 421–427.

Kilpatrick, D. G., & Veronen, L. J. (1983). Treatment for rape-related problems: Crisis intervention is not enough. In L. H. Cohen, W. L., Claiborn, & C. A. Spector (Eds.), *Crisis intervention* (pp. 165–185). New York: Human Sciences Press.

Kolb, L. C. (1987). A neuropsychological hypothesis explaining post-traumatic stress disorder. *American Journal of Psychiatry, 144,* 989–995.

Koopman, C. (2000). New DSM-IV diagnosis of acute stress disorder [Letter to the Editor]. *American Journal of Psychiatry, 157,* 1888.

Koopman, C., Classen, C., Cardeña, E., & Spiegel, D. (1995). When disaster strikes, acute stress disorder may follow. *Journal of Traumatic Stress, 8,* 29–46.

Koopman, C., Classen, C., & Spiegel, D. (1994). Predictors of posttraumatic stress symptoms among survivors of the Oakland/Berkeley, Calif., firestorm. *American Journal of Psychiatry, 151,* 888–894.

Le Doux, J. E., Iwata, J., Cicchetti, P., & Reis, D. J. (1988). Different projections of the central amygdaloid nucleus mediate autonomic and behavioral correlates of conditioned fear. *Journal of Neuroscience, 8,* 2517–2529.

Madakasira, S., & O'Brien, K. F. (1987). Acute posttraumatic stress disorder in victims of a natural disaster. *Journal of Nervous and Mental Disease, 175,* 286–290.

Marmar, C. R., Weiss, D. S., Schlenger, W. E., Fairbank, J. A., Jordan, K., Kulka, R. A., & Hough, R. L. (1994). Peritraumatic dissociation and posttraumatic stress in male Vietnam theater veterans. *American Journal of Psychiatry, 151,* 902–907.

Marshall, G. N., & Schell, T. L. (2002). Reapraising the link between peritraumatic dissociation and PTSD symptom severity: Evidence from a longitudinal study of community violence survivors. *Journal of Abnormal Psychology, 111,* 626–636.

Marshall, R. D., Spitzer, R., & Liebowitz, M. R. (1999). Review and critique of the new DSM-IV diagnosis of acute stress disorder. *American Journal of Psychiatry, 156,* 1677–1685.

Marshall, R. D., Spitzer, R., & Liebowitz, M. R. (2000). New DSM-IV diagnosis of acute stress disorder. *American Journal of Psychiatry, 157,* 1890–1891.

McFarlane, A. C., Atchison, M., & Yehuda, R. (1997). The acute stress response following motor vehicle accidents and its relation to PTSD. In R. Yehuda & A. C. McFarlane (Eds.), *Psychobiology of posttraumatic stress disorder* (pp. 433–436). New York: New York Academy of Sciences.

Meichenbaum, D. (1975). Self-instructional methods. In F. H. Kanfer & A. P. Goldstein (Eds.), *Helping people change* (pp. 357–391). New York: Pergamon Press.

Moulds, L. M., & Bryant, R. A. (2002). Directed forgetting in acute stress disorder. *Journal of Abnormal Psychology, 111,* 175–179.

Moulds, M. L., & Bryant, R. A. (in press). Retrieval inhibition of traumatic stimuli in acute stress disorder. *Journal of Traumatic Stress.*

Nixon, R., & Bryant, R. A. (in press-a). Induced arousal and reexperiencing in acute stress disorder. *Journal of Anxiety Disorders.*

Nixon, R., & Bryant, R. A. (in press-b). Peritraumatic and persistent panic attacks in acute stress disorder. *Behaviour Research and Therapy.*

North, C. S., Smith, E. M., McCool, R. E., & Lightcap, P. E. (1989). Acute postdisaster coping and adjustment. *Journal of Traumatic Stress, 2,* 353–360.

Noyes, R., Hoenk, P.R., Kuperman, S., & Slymen, D.J. (1977). Depersonalization in accident victims and psychiatric patients. *Journal of Nervous and Mental Disease, 164,* 401–407.

Noyes, R., & Kletti, R. (1977). Depersonalizaton in response to life-threatening danger. *Comprehensive Psychiatry, 18,* 375–384.

O'Donnell, M. L., Creamer, M. C., Pattison, P., & Atkin, C. (2001). *Traumatic injury: Psychological consequences and their predictors.* Paper presented at the 17th annual meeting of the International Society of Traumatic Stress Studies, New Orleans.

Pitman, R. K., Shalev, A. Y., & Orr, S. P. (2000). Posttraumatic stress disorder: Emotion, conditioning and memory. In M. D. Corbetta & M. Gazzaniga (Eds.), *The new cognitive neurosciences* (2nd ed., pp. 1133–1147). New York: Plenum Press.

Post, R. M., Weiss, S. R. B., & Smith, M. (1995). Sensitization and kindling: Implication for the evolving neural substrates of posttraumatic stress disorder. In M. J. Friedman, D. S. Charney, & A. Y. Deutch (Eds.), *Neurobiological and clinical consequences of stress: From normal adaptation to posttraumatic stress disorder* (pp. 203–224). Philadelphia: Lippincott Raven.

Riggs, D. S., Rothbaum, B. O., & Foa, E. B. (1995). A prospective examination of symptoms of posttraumatic stress disorder in victims of non-sexual assault. *Journal of Interpersonal Violence, 10,* 201–214.

Rothbaum, B. O., Foa, E. B., Riggs, D. S., Murdock, T., & Walsh, W. (1992). A prospective examination of post-traumatic stress disorder in rape victims. *Journal of Traumatic Stress, 5,* 455–475.

Rothbaum, B. O., & Mellman, T. A. (2001). Dreams and exposure therapy for PTSD. *Journal of Traumatic Stress, 14,* 481–490.

Rothbaum, B. O., & Schwartz, A. C. (2002). Exposure therapy for posttraumatic stress disorder. *American Journal of Psychotherapy, 56,* 59–75.

Schnyder, U., Moergeli, H., Klaghofer, R., & Buddeberg, C. (2001). Incidence and prediction of posttraumatic stress disorder symptoms in severely injured accident victims. *American Journal of Psychiatry, 158,* 594–599.

Shalev, A. Y., Peri, T., Canetti, L., & Schreiber, S. (1996). Predictors of PTSD in injured trauma survivors: A prospective study. *American Journal of Psychiatry, 153,* 219–225.

Shalev, A. Y., Sahar, T., Freedman, S., Peri, T., Glick, N., Brandes, D., Orr, S. P., & Pitman, R. K. (1998). A prospective study of heart rate responses following trauma and the subsequent development of PTSD. *Archives of General Psychiatry, 55,* 553–559.

Simeon, D., & Guralnik, O. (2000). New DSM-IV diagnosis of acute stress disorder [Letter to the Editor]. *American Journal of Psychiatry, 157,* 1888–1889.

Sloan, P. (1988). Post-traumatic stress in survivors of an airplane crash-landing: A clinical and exploratory research intervention. *Journal of Traumatic Stress, 1,* 211–229.

Smith, K., & Bryant, R. A. (2000). The generality of cognitive bias in acute stress disorder. *Behaviour Research and Therapy, 38,* 709–715.

Solomon, Z., Laor, N., & McFarlane, A. C. (1996). Acute posttraumatic reactions in soldiers and civilians. In B. A. van der Kolk, A. C. McFarlane, & L. Weisaeth (Eds.), *Traumatic stress: The effects of overwhelming experience on mind, body, and society* (pp. 102–114). New York: Guilford Press.

Solomon, Z., & Mikulincer, M. (1992). Aftermaths of combat stress reactions: A three-year study. *British Journal of Clinical Psychology, 31,* 21–32.

Spiegel, D., Classen, C., & Cardeña, E. (2000). New DSM-IV diagnosis of acute stress disorder [Letter to the Editor]. *American Journal of Psychiatry, 157,* 1890–1891.

Staab, J. P., Grieger, T. A., Fullerton, C. S., & Ursano, R. J. (1996). Acute stress disorder, subsequent posttraumatic stress disorder and depression after a series of typhoons. *Anxiety, 2,* 219–225.

van der Kolk, B. A., & van der Hart, O. (1989). Pierre Janet and the breakdown of adaptation in psychological data. *American Journal of Psychiatry, 146,* 1530–1540.

Viney, L. L., Clark, A. M., Bunn, T. A., & Benjamin, Y. N. (1985). Crisis intervention counselling: An evaluation of long and short term effects. *Journal of Consulting and Clinical Psychology, 32,* 29–39.

Warda, G., & Bryant, R. A. (1998a). Cognitive bias in acute stress disorder. *Behaviour Research and Therapy, 36,* 1177–1183.

Warda, G., & Bryant, R. A. (1998b). Thought control strategies in acute stress disorder. *Behaviour Research and Therapy, 36,* 1171–1175.

World Health Organization. (1992). *The ICD-10 classification of mental and behavioural disorder: Diagnostic criteria for research* (10th rev.). Geneva, Switzerland: Author.

Yehuda, R. (1997). Sensitization of the hypothalamic–pituitary–adrenal axis in post-traumatic stress disorder. *Annals of the New York Academy of Sciences, 821,* 57–75.

3

Risk and Resilience Factors in the Etiology of Chronic Posttraumatic Stress Disorder

DANIEL W. KING
DAWNE S. VOGT
LYNDA A. KING

$\mathbf{A}$s noted several places in this volume, a number of important large-scale studies have documented that experiencing a traumatic event is not uncommon in our modern society (e.g., Breslau, Davis, Andreski, & Peterson, 1991; Davidson, Hughes, Blazer, & George, 1991; Kessler, Sonnega, Bromet, Hughes, & Nelson, 1995; Norris, 1992; Resnick, Kilpatrick, Dansky, Saunders, & Best, 1993). Moreover, posttraumatic stress disorder (PTSD) is a significant mental health problem, with U.S. prevalence estimates of lifetime PTSD approximating 8%, more than 10% for women, and about 5% for men (Kessler et al., 1995). On the other hand, the preponderance of trauma victims—though possibly quite symptomatic in the early postexposure period—tend to recover and adjust with the passage of time. Therefore, other factors must contribute to the likelihood that exposure to traumatic events and circumstances will have long-term mental health consequences. These factors may include features of the traumatic event itself, preexisting demographic and other individual differences characteristics of the trauma victim, and aspects of the post-exposure recovery environment, among others. Collectively, these are often referred to as *risk and resilience factors.* Other terms that are commonly used are *vulnerability or hazard and protective or preventive factors,* respectively.

It is important at the outset to clarify the terms "risk factor" and "resilience factor." In the context of negative mental health consequences of trauma exposure, we use the term "risk factor" to label those characteristics of the event, the individual, or the environment that are associated with an increase in PTSD. We use the term "resilience factor" to label those characteristics of the event, the individual, or the environment that are associated with a decrease in PTSD. We view this as simply a linguistic convenience because, in effect, the opposite pole of a risk factor (e.g., low socioeconomic status) could be judged a resilience factor (e.g., high socioeconomic status). Likewise, the opposite pole of a resilience factor (e.g., the presence of strong social support in the recovery environment) could be judged a risk factor (e.g., the absence of a structural or functional social support system following the trauma).

In this chapter, we seek to integrate substantive evidence concerning risk and resilience for PTSD with the special methodological issues that must be confronted in understanding the etiology of PTSD. In the first section to follow, we provide a brief overview of factors that have been shown to covary, either positively or negatively, with PTSD symptomatology. In the next section, we propose four methodological recommendations to assist researchers to validly assert the place of particular risk and resilience factors in the network of causal associations leading to PTSD. We close with a summary commentary on implications for prevention, treatment, and policy.

OVERVIEW OF RISK AND RESILIENCE LITERATURE

The recognition that PTSD is by no means a universal response to trauma has inspired a growing body of literature aimed at documenting risk and resilience factors for PTSD following trauma exposure. The majority of early research in this area focused on factors related to how combat veterans, and Vietnam veterans in particular, responded to war-related trauma (e.g., Egendorf, Kadushin, Laufer, Rothbart, & Sloan, 1981; Figley, 1978; Foy, Sipprelle, Rueger, & Carroll, 1984; Penk et al., 1981; Strange, 1974). Later, researchers began to study the factors that contribute to posttrauma dysfunction in response to other types of traumatic experiences, including natural and technological disasters (e.g., Baum, Cohen, & Hall, 1993; Green, Lindy, Grace, & Leonard, 1992), sexual assault (e.g., Foa, Molnar, & Cashman, 1995; Resnick, Kilpatrick, & Lipovsky, 1991), domestic violence (e.g., Astin, Ogland-Hand, Coleman, &

Foy, 1995; Kemp, Rawlings, & Green, 1991), crime (e.g., Kilpatrick et al., 1989), serious motor vehicle accidents (e.g., Blanchard, Hickling, Taylor, & Loos, 1995), death of a close family member or friend (e.g., Norris, 1992), life-threatening medical conditions (e.g., Green, Epstein, Krupnick, & Rowland, 1997), and acts of terrorism (e.g., Galea et al., 2002; North et al., 1999).

In the remainder of this section, we present a selective review of the literature on psychosocial risk and resilience factors for PTSD, drawing attention to several areas in which additional research is needed. For comprehensive reviews of these factors, the reader is referred to Brewin, Andrews, and Valentine's (2000) recent meta-analysis of this literature, Yehuda's (1999) edited work on the topic, as well as the earlier works of Gibbs (1989) and Green (1994). Although we recognize that there may be a constitutional/hereditary component of PTSD, it is not the focus of this chapter.

As discussed previously, psychosocial risk factors can be categorized into features of the traumatic event itself, preexisting attributes of the trauma victim, and posttrauma circumstances. We summarize research on each of these categories in turn, after which we provide a conceptual integration that highlights the role of available resources and coping strategies as mechanisms through which many of these factors may be implicated.

Features of the Traumatic Event

The largest portion of research has focused on features of the traumatic event itself. Perhaps the most widely studied risk factor is the severity of the traumatic event. There is ample evidence for a dose–response relationship between the severity of the stressor and posttraumatic stress symptomatology (e.g., Fairbank, Keane, & Malloy, 1983; Foy, Carroll, & Donahoe, 1987; March, 1993; Rodriguez, Vande-Kemp, & Foy, 1998). Brewin et al.'s (2000) meta-analysis of risk factors for PTSD revealed a significant effect of trauma severity among both military populations, where the traumatic experience was combat, and civilian populations, in which a variety of other traumatic experiences were represented. In fact, trauma severity was found to be one of the strongest risk factors for PTSD, particularly among military samples.

A number of other important aspects of trauma have been identified as well (Green, 1993), and research has increasingly focused on how these contribute to PTSD. For example, traumas that involve injury have been found to be more highly predictive of PTSD than those that do not (Acierno, Resnick, Kilpatrick, Saunders, & Best, 1999; Green, 1990, 1993; Green, Grace, & Gleser, 1985; March, 1993). Traumas that are more malicious and grotesque are associated with a much greater risk for posttraumatic adjustment problems (e.g., Gallers, Foy, Donahoe, & Goldfarb, 1988; Green et al., 1985; Kessler et al., 1995;

Laufer, Gallops, & Frey-Wouters, 1984). Whether one is actively involved in a traumatic event (as either perpetrator or victim) or merely a witness to a traumatic event affects the likelihood of PTSD (Fontana & Rosenheck, 1999; Green, 1990, 1993; March, 1993); being directly involved in a traumatic event is more likely to lead to a dysfunctional response than being an observer of a traumatic event (Breslau & Davis, 1987; Laufer et al., 1984; Lund, Foy, Sipprelle, & Strachan, 1984). Other aspects of the traumatic experience have been studied as well. For example, King, King, Gudanowski, and Vreven (1995) and Solomon, Mikulincer, and Hobfoll (1987) found that both objective and subjective aspects of war-zone exposure were associated with stress symptomatology. In addition, King et al. (1995) and Litz, King, King, Orsillo, and Friedman (1997) documented the importance of lower-magnitude stressors in association with PTSD symptom severity for Vietnam veterans and Somalia peacekeepers, respectively.

Pretrauma Characteristics

Researchers have increasingly attended to the role of prior trauma exposure in understanding how people respond to subsequent trauma exposure. A number of studies suggest that prior trauma may sensitize an individual to later traumatic experiences, making recovery more difficult (Andrykowski & Cordova, 1998; King, King, Foy, & Gudanowski, 1996; King, King, Foy, Keane, & Fairbank, 1999; Koopman, Classen, & Speigel, 1994; Moran & Britton, 1994; Peretz, Baider, Ever-Hadani, & De-Nour, 1994; van der Kolk & Greenberg, 1987), while other findings indicate that prior trauma might serve to inoculate individuals, thus reducing the impact of the trauma (Bolin, 1985; Burgess & Holmstrom, 1979; Cohen, 1953; Norris & Murrell, 1988; Quarantelli, 1985; Warheit, 1985). Some researchers have suggested that these mixed findings can be reconciled by a consideration of the similarity of previous and current traumatic events; when stressors resemble each other, there may be an inoculation effect, and when they are different, a sensitization effect might result (e.g., Follette, Polusny, Bechtle, & Naugle, 1996; Norris & Murrell, 1988). However, a recent study failed to fully support this hypothesis among a sample of workers at the site of a major air disaster (Dougall, Herberman, Inslicht, Baum, & Delahanty, 2000), finding support for sensitization effects when stressors differ but not for inoculation effects when stressors are similar. Clearly, additional research is needed to better understand the circumstances under which prior trauma sensitizes or inoculates individuals to the effects of subsequent trauma.

Related to the realm of prior traumatic or stressful experiences are family and early childhood variables that may serve as risk or resilience factors for PTSD. Along these lines, researchers have found associations between self-reports of earlier childhood abuse and PTSD following exposure to subsequent trauma (Andrews, Brewin, Rose, & Kirk, 2000; Bremner, Southwick, Johnson, Yehuda, & Charney, 1993). There is also evidence for the impact of family psychiatric history, as well as early separation from parents, on PTSD (Breslau et al., 1991; Bromet, Sonnega, & Kessler, 1998; Emery, Emery, Sharma, Quiana, & Jassani, 1991). Other adverse childhood experiences associated with PTSD include family instability and poor family functioning (Fontana & Rosenheck, 1994; King et al., 1996; King et al., 1999). Importantly, findings generally appear to suggest that pretrauma family factors may be stronger risk factors for people exposed to military trauma than for civilian populations (Brewin et al., 2000). However, as Brewin et al. (2000) noted, military samples are more likely than civilian samples to include individuals with chronic PTSD, and, thus, it may not be that these risk factors are better predictors of PTSD following military trauma per se but that they are stronger predictors of chronic PTSD than acute stress symptomatology.

Another preexisting factor that may contribute to the development of PTSD following trauma exposure is one's own previous psychiatric history. Individuals who have suffered from various prior or ongoing psychiatric disorders may be more likely to develop other forms of psychopathology (Green, Grace, Lindy, Gleser, & Leonard, 1990; O'Toole, Marshall, Schureck, & Dobson, 1998; Resnick, Kilpatrick, Best, & Kramer, 1992; Schnurr, Friedman, & Rosenberg, 1993). The findings of Schnurr et al. (1993) are particularly compelling, given that the scores derived for preexisting psychopathology were based on data collected before military service rather than collected retrospectively after trauma exposure. Relatedly, early conduct problems as exhibited by antisocial tendencies have been indirectly linked with later PTSD following a traumatic event (King et al., 1996).

Other preexisting demographic and individual factors that have been associated with the development of PTSD include socioeconomic status, education, race, gender, age, and intelligence. In general, findings suggest that lower socioeconomic status, less education, minority racial status, female gender, younger age at trauma, and lower intelligence all serve as risk factors for the development of PTSD following trauma exposure (Brewin et al., 2000). However, these associations are generally quite small. Moreover, the impact of many of these factors may depend on the type of trauma. For example, although findings for socioeconomic status and education were similar across trauma types in Brewin et al.'s (2000) meta-analysis, gender was a risk factor for PTSD following most types of trauma but was not a risk factor for PTSD among military samples. However, gender may be somewhat confounded with combat exposure in many of these studies due to their reliance on samples of

Vietnam veterans, in which most women had only peripheral exposure to combat. A recent study by Wolfe, Erickson, Sharkansky, King, and King (1999) found that gender was a risk factor for PTSD following combat exposure in the Gulf War. Likewise, Brewin et al. (2000) found that younger age served as a risk factor for the development of PTSD following combat exposure but not other forms of trauma. Minority racial status exhibited a weak association with PTSD following combat exposure but was unrelated to PTSD following other types of trauma. Though there was evidence for the impact of low intelligence as a risk factor for PTSD among military samples (e.g., Macklin et al., 1988), no studies on intelligence as a risk factor for PTSD following other types of trauma met the criteria for inclusion in Brewin et al.'s (2000) meta-analysis. Thus, conclusions cannot be drawn regarding the association between intelligence and response to other types of trauma.

Additional research is clearly needed to understand why some demographic/background characteristics serve as risk or resilience factors for some types of trauma and not others. Moreover, as will be discussed in greater detail shortly, research is needed to identify why these factors may serve as risk factors or, more precisely, what the risk mechanisms are through which these demographic/background characteristics have their effect on PTSD.

Posttrauma Recovery Environment

Two primary aspects of the posttrauma recovery environment have received research attention: the social support that is available to trauma victims as they attempt to recover and exposure to additional life stressors. Findings indicate that social support may mediate or moderate the impact of trauma; those with higher levels of social support are likely to suffer less from PTSD than those with lower levels of social support (e.g., Egendorf et al., 1981; Keane, Scott, Chavoya, Lamparski, & Fairbank, 1985; King et al., 1999; Solomon & Mikulincer, 1990; Solomon, Mikulincer, & Avitzur, 1988; Solomon, Mikulincer, & Flum, 1989). Indeed, lack of social support proved to be one of the strongest risk factors for PTSD in Brewin et al.'s (2000) meta-analysis of the literature, and this finding applied equally well to both military and civilian samples.

Additional life stressors after exposure to the index trauma also demonstrate a strong association with posttraumatic distress (Brewin et al., 2000). As King, King, Fairbank, Keane, and Adams (1998), Green (1994), and Resnick et al. (1991) noted, PTSD may be the consequence of a series of highly stressful life events, extending both back into one's personal history (thus, the attention to prior trauma) and forward in time to the present (thus, the attention to additional life stressors).

Risk Mechanisms

Importantly, the risk and resilience factors described earlier may have their impact on PTSD through many different mechanisms (Rutter, 2000a, 2000b). Two issues that deserve special attention are the resources available to an individual exposed to a traumatic event and the coping strategies drawn on as one attempts to deal with a traumatic event and its associated sequelae. Many factors may carry risk through their impact on one's access to resources that can be mobilized for successful adaptation (Hobfall, 1991). For example, many of the demographic and individual factors reviewed previously may have implications for the availability of resources. It may be that individuals who are from lower socioeconomic backgrounds, those who have less education, racial minorities, women, younger individuals, and those who are less intelligent have less access to resources that will facilitate recovery from trauma (see further analysis in the section to follow). Likewise, social support in the period following trauma exposure may signify the availability of both concrete resources, such as financial support, and emotional resources, someone to whom one can turn for empathy and guidance.

Relatedly, factors may carry risk through their impact on coping with the event and its aftermath. For example, the more severe the event, the more threatening the experience may be to an individual's assumption of the world as predictable, controllable, and benevolent, and the more likely may be feelings of "intense fear, helplessness, or horror" (American Psychiatric Association, 1994, p. 428) that challenge one's ability to make sense of and recover from the experience. Coping is an ongoing process and is relevant to many aspects of trauma exposure and recovery: coping with actual trauma-related stressful events and circumstances (e.g., Sharkansky et al., 2000; Sutker, Davis, Uddo, & Ditta, 1995; Suvak, Vogt, Savarese, King, & King, 2002); coping with stress reactions at the time of their occurrence (e.g., Solomon et al., 1989); coping with posttrauma symptomatology (e.g., Fairbank, Hansen, & Fitterling, 1991); and coping with additional postexposure life stressors (e.g., Solomon et al., 1988). Not only is the choice of coping strategies salient, but the effectiveness of coping efforts may have significance for later adaptation. As discussed previously, findings regarding whether prior trauma serves an inoculating or sensitizing role in subsequent response to trauma have been mixed. It may be that this association depends on how successfully one has coped with the prior trauma. Successful coping may lead to positive beliefs about one's ability to cope with adversity (Rutter, 1981), which, in turn, could result in more effective coping with subsequent trauma.

There is also some evidence that certain people may be better able to cope with stressors across the life course. Preexisting hardiness, conceptualized as a stable intrapersonal resource that facilitates effective coping, may play a protective role in posttrauma adjustment (King et al., 1998; King et al., 1999). In other words, individuals who are hardier to begin with may be more resilient to the effects of trauma. Then, again, there may some traumatic events that overwhelm the coping capabilities of even the hardiest individual. Clearly, additional research attention must be paid to both the risk and resilience factors associated with PTSD and the mechanisms through which these relationships arise.

SEEKING VALID INFERENCE ABOUT RISK AND RESILIENCE: RECOMMENDATIONS TO TRAUMA RESEARCHERS

Understanding how the aforementioned risk and resilience factors influence PTSD necessitates clear thinking about causality and the validity of causal inferences that we draw from empirical work. Although there are variations on the theme of causality, most methodologists impose at least three criteria for valid inference:

1. *Covariation* between the putative causal agent and the effect or outcome: Changes in the cause (e.g., level of postexposure social support) must be accompanied by changes in the outcome (PTSD symptom severity).
2. *Temporal precedence* of the putative cause to the outcome: The causal agent (e.g., the exposure) must precede the outcome (PTSD) in time.
3. No *"third variables"*: All other spurious or alternative explanations for the association (e.g., a prior exposure to an extreme stressor) must be ruled out or deemed improbable.

The gold standard for achieving these criteria is the true experiment in which study participants are randomly assigned to one of a number of researcher-manipulated conditions, the manipulation is performed, and then the outcome is measured. If there are differences between conditions on the outcome, the covariation criterion is met. The design, manipulation followed by assessment, insures temporal precedence. Random assignment reduces the probability that some preexisting factor might explain the findings, as random assignment is intended to eliminate the systematic influence of alternative variables on the outcome.

As noted by King and King (1991) however, research on trauma-related dysfunction can never be truly experimental because the investigator has no control, random or otherwise, to assign individuals to the "treatment"—the traumatic experience. Furthermore, in the study of etiology, one cannot randomly assign individuals to the types of experiential (e.g., early childhood adversity), personal (e.g., hardiness), or environmental (e.g., a large network of social support structures) attributes that comprise the typical repertoire of risk and resilience factors described in the previous section. Hence, the study of risk and resilience for PTSD mandates an awareness of threats to the validity of causal inference that are endemic to quasi-experimental designs.

Without doubt, the preponderance of PTSD risk and resilience research has been and continues to be passive observational and cross-sectional, usually with retrospective self-reports of features of the traumatic experience itself, as well as retrospective accounts of the victim's pretrauma life and any postexposure events and circumstances that may have occurred up until the time of the investigation. Although such designs may be successful in establishing covariation between a putative risk or resilience factor and PTSD, temporal precedence may be unclear and we are left with ambiguity concerning the direction of cause and effect. King and King (1991) and King et al. (1999) discussed a number of issues that might contribute to such ambiguity. These include demand characteristics of the research setting, researcher-imposed expectancies, response biases such as social desirability or acquiescence, but especially poor recall and associated reconstruction of memory coupled with the tendency for one's contemporary mental state to influence accounts of prior experiences or conditions. For example, one who is highly symptomatic and distraught might judge the extent and degree of trauma exposure to have been quite extreme in some attempt to create balance or congruity in self-conceptions. In like manner, assessments of one's early family life and childhood might be filtered through the lens of current posttraumatic distress, to validate negative appraisals of the self (e.g., Bachman, 1988; Swann, 1983): Does the risk factor (e.g., distressing childhood environment) belong to the causal network responsible for the postexposure condition (PTSD), or does the trauma victim's postexposure condition (PTSD) influence the retrospective report of status on a risk factor (e.g., distressing childhood environment)?

Ambiguity about the direction of cause and effect will continue to be nearly ubiquitous in research on risk and resilience for PTSD. In general, we cannot know in advance who will be exposed, nor can we anticipate and acquire scores on pertinent measures of risk and resilience prior to that exposure. (Some noteworthy exceptions include studies by Card, 1987; Macklin et al., 1998; Schnurr et al., 1993) Yet, careful attention to contemporary methodological theory and techniques can help us confront the challenges to understanding etiology in trauma research. We offer a series of recommendations aimed at enhancing the ability to make valid causal inferences about risk and resilience for PTSD.

1. Recognize the Importance of Precise Risk Terminology and Thoughtfully Delineated Risk Mechanisms

We base this recommendation largely on the thoughtful work of Kraemer and colleagues (e.g., Kraemer et al., 1997, 1999; Kraemer, Stice, Kazdin, Offord, & Kupfer, 2001) and Rutter and colleagues (e.g., Rutter, 2000a, 2000b; Rutter & Sroufe, 2000). Several years ago, Kraemer et al. (1997) proposed a taxonomy that provides a highly useful conceptual framework to organize and catalog the many risk and resilience factors identified within PTSD research. Arguing that precise risk terminology is critical for valid causal inference, scientific communication, and appropriate clinical and policy applications, they proposed a decision tree (p. 341) whereby variables appearing to relate to an outcome of interest (*correlates* and therefore potential risk factors for PTSD) can be classified into one of several mutually exclusive categories, each of which carries special meaning with regard to the operation of that factor in the etiological network. When a correlate is observed, a first decision is whether temporal precedence exists (i.e., Is the factor under consideration antecedent to PTSD?). An affirmative response connotes the potential for a *risk* (or *resilience*) *factor*. A negative response would suggest that the correlate is not a risk factor but rather a *concomitant* or *consequence* of PTSD. A good example might be comorbid depression that is observed following exposure to trauma: There is a body of literature (e.g., Breslau, Davis, Peterson, & Schultz, 1997; Erickson, Wolfe, King, King, & Sharkansky, 2001; Skodol et al., 1996) examining the interplay between PTSD and depression and attempting to determine temporal precedence. If we observe that postexposure depressive symptomatology covaries with PTSD symptomatology, evidence that depression is antecedent to the onset of PTSD would make it a likely risk factor candidate (prior psychiatric history). Evidence that depression merely accompanies PTSD but did not actually precede PTSD would place it in the concomitant or consequence category.

Kraemer et al. (1997) elucidated several categories of risk factors. A risk factor that does not vary within an individual over time is termed a "fixed marker." Examples here would be age at exposure to the index trauma, gender, race, ethnicity, and other preexisting, permanent, and unchanging characteristics of individuals that have been shown to be associated with PTSD. A "variable risk factor," conversely, is one that either changes for the individual naturally (e.g., additional life stressors following the index event) or can be manipulated in some way (e.g., the infusion of social support resources into communities following a disaster). Moreover, at the point at which a variable risk factor can be shown to be manipulable (changing social support by providing resources) and, when manipulated, a demonstrated change in the outcome is achieved (decreased prevalence of PTSD), that risk factor is designated a "causal risk factor."

This taxonomy has implications for those who study trauma. It is important to state, as did Kraemer et al. (1997), that use of the term "causal risk factor" does not imply that the researcher necessarily understands the causal mechanism. In other words, the third variable problem remains. The provision of support resources to victims of a large-scale disaster may result in a reduction in PTSD caseness, but do we really understand the mechanism? It could involve the reduction of additional stressful life events or the enhancement of self-esteem or sense of mastery or some combination of these and other factors. But establishing a risk factor as a causal risk factor gives the researcher a glimpse of possible mechanisms and clues for additional scientific inquiry. Along the same lines, the distinction between a variable risk factor and a causal risk factor may be merely a function of the state of the science at a given point in time. One goal of PTSD research, then, should be to isolate or identify which risk factors are causal risk factors and hence assist in triangulating on the real causal mechanism in the absence of a true experimental design.

In a similar spirit to improve our understanding of risk and resilience in PTSD, we turn to Rutter's (2000a, 2000b) observations regarding *risk indicators* and especially *risk mechanisms*. The former are akin to Kraemer et al.'s (1997) fixed markers, factors that index but do not influence outcomes. The latter appear to be elaborations of the processes by which Kraemer et al.'s causal risk factors are translated into change in outcomes. According to Rutter, an understanding of mechanisms demands that we clearly recognize what risk factors are associated with what variables. In particular, risk factors for exposure to a traumatic event may not be the same factors that explain the mechanism by which exposure leads to PTSD. In some of our own work (e.g., King et al., 1996; King et al., 1999), albeit with cross-sectional and retrospective data, we documented an association between childhood antisocial behavior and combat exposure, but the direct link between childhood antisocial behavior and PTSD was trivial. A prominent intervening variable, or risk mediator, was perceived threat in the war zone. Thus, prior psychopathology (antisocial behavior) operated according to one set of mechanisms in predicting trauma exposure (perhaps via risk taking or thrill seeking) and via another set of mechanisms in predicting PTSD (fear of death or bodily harm).

2. Apply Multivariate Methods to Aid Understanding of Complex Causal Mechanisms

Accumulating knowledge about bivariate associations between each of an abundance of possible risk and resilience factors and a health outcome of interest falls far short of the goal of specifying causal processes, because simple relationships are not particularly informative of the underlying mechanisms that govern etiology (Kraemer et al., 2001). Causal mechanisms are typically quite complicated, and, especially because we are confined to passive observational quasiexperimental designs, multivariate statistical methods become a critical tool. Recall the third criterion for causality: the no "third variables" requirement. One elaboration of this criterion is in terms of spurious effects by variables outside the observed association that are, in some simple to complex way, responsible for that association and thus may reveal the mechanisms by which the presumptive cause affects the outcome.

Previous analyses using the National Vietnam Veterans Readjustment Study (NVVRS) database offer good examples of how uncovering spurious effects may inform possible causal mechanisms. Consider a *mediational paradigm* (Baron & Kenny, 1986). Using NVVRS data, King et al. (1995) identified and operationalized four dimensions of war-zone experiences (exposure to traditional combat events and circumstances, exposure to atrocities and incidents of extraordinarily abusive violence, perceived threat or fear of death or bodily harm, and exposure to the lower-level discomforts and irritations of the malevolent war-zone environment) and subsequently related these to PTSD symptom severity. Although the bivariate relationship between combat exposure and PTSD symptom severity was quite strong—as it should be—a more revealing and theoretically useful finding was the role of perceived threat as a powerful mediator of this relationship. In the presence of the perceived threat variable, the association between combat exposure and PTSD symptom severity was rendered trivial. Hence, a possible mechanism explaining the association between trauma and PTSD may be the intervening variable of fear of death or bodily harm, with the effect of combat on PTSD being indirect through perceived threat. To some extent, this pattern substantiates the importance of PTSD's Criterion A2. As another illustration with NVVRS data, King et al. (1996) attempted to evaluate a network of premilitary background variables and their indirect and direct associations with PTSD. They pointed to exposure to heavy combat as a possible mechanism for an observed bivariate association between childhood antisocial behavior and involvement in atrocities and abusive violence in Vietnam. That is, the link between childhood antisocial behavior and involvement in atrocities was indirect and via the combat variable; this result might suggest that veterans with prewar behavior problems were not necessarily predisposed to atrocious acts in the war zone, but that the association between these two variables is mediated by or in the context of heavy combat.

In both of the foregoing cases, had not the third variable been introduced into the model, evidence of a potential process by which a risk factor presumably affects another variable would have been lost. Of course, given that the data were cross-sectional and retrospective, the direction of influence is still problematic, and the specification of the mechanism remains probabilistic and subject to future investigation. Although King et al. (1995) and King et al. (1996) specified and evaluated a mediational model, with perceived threat and combat exposure, respectively, acting as intermediary variables, two other equally plausible models are possible. One alternative is for the third or spurious variable to covary with the antecedent risk factor and have a direct influence on the outcome. A second equally plausible model would have the spurious variable as a "cause" of both the risk factor and outcome. The lesson here is that statistical methods alone are not sufficient to confirm a causal process. Sound statistical methods must be accompanied by solid design and supported by theory.

Multivariate methods are also available to answer questions regarding possible *synergistic or joint effects* among risk and resilience factors, traditionally framed within the context of moderator or interaction analyses (Baron & Kenny, 1986). As a case in point, the literature on coping as a resilience factor in the face of trauma is large and somewhat inconclusive, especially with regard to the value of approach-based or problem-focused coping, engaging in behaviors aimed at active intervention or direct confrontation to resolve the stressful situation. Some studies have found approach-based or problem-focused coping to be beneficial in their negative association with trauma sequelae, whereas others have found rather minimal associations (see Sharkansky et al., 2000; Suvak et al., 2002). Yet, a third variable that might govern the coping-outcome relationship is the general context in which the coping takes place (e.g., Folkman, Schaefer, & Lazarus, 1979; Forsythe & Compas, 1987; Park, Folkman, & Bostrom, 2001): To what extent does the success or failure of the coping strategy depend on features of the stressor that evoke the coping process? One characteristic that comes to mind is a risk factor: the severity of the stressor. In particular, does the coping-outcome relationship vary with the intensity of the exposure, such that understanding the causal mechanism requires both a consideration of the level of expression of coping behaviors and the amount of trauma exposure?

For example, Suvak et al. (2002) hypothesized and demonstrated the synergistic influence of problem-focused coping and degree of trauma exposure in the prediction of long-term educational and occupational achievement among Vietnam veterans. Specifically, the strength of the association between the use of problem-focused coping strategies in the war zone and the outcome varied curvilinearly as a function of the level of combat. Consistent with expectations, at low levels of combat, where there was no need to engage in problem-focused coping, the relationship was negligible. With increasing levels of exposure to combat, and concomitant greater need for coping, the relationship strengthened in the proposed direction: the more problem-focused coping, the more achievement. And, as exposure to combat became extreme, at a level where problem-focused coping may become less efficacious or even fruitless, the association between problem-focused coping and achievement again weakened. Thus, problem-focused coping may be effective at moderate levels of trauma exposure, but at low levels, it may be unnecessary, and at high levels, it may be irrelevant; hence the curvilinear interaction or quadratic moderator effect. Although Suvak et al.'s outcome was long-term achievement, we have found a similar significant quadratic but inverse problem-focused coping interaction with the outcome of PTSD symptom severity.

Mediator and moderator effects employing continuous outcomes such as PTSD symptom severity are almost always evaluated by means of ordinary least-squares regression-based statistical methods and probably most frequently by some type of multiple regression. (Variations on logistic regression, including polytomous and ordinal logistic regression, with maximum likelihood estimation would apply when the outcome is a categorical variable, such as PTSD diagnosis.) Even more complex systems of relationships can be mapped and assessed through use of a series of simultaneous ordinary least-squares regression equations, to reflect a chain of hypothesized causal mechanisms from more distal risk and resilience factors through more proximal factors and terminating in PTSD. Specification and appraisal of such a network of associations is a *path analysis*. The reader is directed to a comprehensive compilation of applied multiple regression procedures, including an introduction to path analysis, in the new Cohen, Cohen, West, and Aiken (2002) text.

An even more elegant elaboration of multiple regression and path analysis for testing mechanisms of risk and resilience is the class of statistical procedures called *structural equation modeling*. Although structural equation modeling often appears challenging to execute, under certain conditions it can offer distinct advantages over regression-based path analysis. First, when properly implemented, structural equation modeling yields associations among perfectly reliable variables; as a consequence, all parameter estimates are unbiased, a condition that cannot be guaranteed with ordinary least-squares regression and path analysis with measures of varying and less-than-perfect reliabilities. Second, in structural equation modeling, all the information in the data set is used in the estimation of all parameters; thus, parameter estimates are efficient, with standard errors as small as they can be, given the data. Third, structural equation modeling provides estimates of the overall goodness of fit of the multivariate model to the data and allows for the selection of the best in a series of competing models. As in multiple regression analysis, techniques for assessing mediation and moderation are available (see, e.g., Cortina, Chen, & Dunlap, 2001; Jaccard & Wan, 1996; Joreskog & Yang, 1996, for guides to evaluating interaction effects in structural equation modeling).

We recapitulate the warning, however, that elegant statistics, even "causal modeling," do not overcome the fundamental deficiency of a cross-sectional design that might include retrospective accounts of exposure or pretrauma status. In such a research situation, path analysis and especially structural equation modeling can be informative and suggestive of risk mechanisms, but direction of causality is still ambiguous. Bollen (1989), Hayduk (1989, 1996), Loehlin (1998), Kline (1998), and Schumacher and Lomax (1996), among others, provide excellent introductory treatments of structural equation modeling.

3. Consider a Reconceptualization of Outcome as Process

Without doubt, longitudinal research designs are better suited than cross-sectional designs to clarify temporal precedence and thus directionality of associations among key variables. Moreover, longitudinal designs are critical to understanding the course of a posttrauma condition, either naturalistically over time or as a function of intervention or treatment. Initial calls for longitudinal studies of trauma consequences were penned by Green, Lindy, and Grace (1985), Denny, Rabinowitz, and Penk (1987) and Keane, Wolfe, and Taylor (1987), who recommended particular attention to tracking the efficacy of alternative therapeutic interventions. King and King (1991) expanded on these suggestions by endorsing a developmental perspective on trauma research and the incorporation of then-available longitudinal designs and analytic strategies, which could elucidate both temporal precedence and the phenomenology of chronicity or recovery and response to treatment.

Indeed, a number of prominent trauma research teams (Blanchard et al., 1996; Bolton, Litz, Glenn, Orsillo, & Roemer 2002; Foa & Riggs, 1995; Green et al., 1990; Marmar et al., 1999; McFarlane, 1988, 1992; Rothbaum, Foa, Riggs, Murdock, & Walsh, 1992; Shalev, Freedman, et al., 1998; Shalev, Sahar, et al., 1998; Solomon, Benbenishty, & Mikulincer, 1991; Southwick et al., 1995; Ursano, Fullerton, Kao, & Bhartiya, 1995; Wolfe et al., 1999) have increasingly incorporated prospective designs in their work. Most have employed ordinary least-squares regression-based analytical methods in which a respondent's status on prior-measured variables is used to predict standing on subsequent PTSD. The predictor may be the dependent variable assessed at a previous time point, for example, PTSD in the first days following an exposure predicting PTSD at one or more subsequent assessments. The predictor may be one or more risk (e.g., severity of exposure) or resilience (e.g., hardiness) factors measured on an earlier occasion. Or, the predictor may be the presence or absence of, or one or more core features of, a strategic intervention (e.g., early debriefing). In this case, another likely predictor is respondent's status on the outcome prior to treatment (e.g., a baseline PTSD score). The logic here is that the "partialed" effect of the treatment (in the presence of the baseline score) on the outcome measured on any one of a series of follow-up assessments represents a posttreatment change in status.

Using standard autoregressive statistical models, regression coefficients tell us how a person's standing in relation to the mean of an independent variable assessed on one occasion (say, PTSD at 1 week postexposure) mirrors that person's standing in relation to the mean of the dependent variable assessed on a later occasion (PTSD at 1 month or PTSD at 3 months postexposure). This representation is important but rather static in that there is a prediction of where an individual will end up on the variable of interest (e.g., relatively high or relatively low) but not how that individual got there as a function of time since exposure and various risk and resilience factors. A relevant question is, "Over time, postexposure, whose symptoms will remain nonclinical, whose will diminish, whose will continue to be elevated, and whose might even increase?" Hence, an individual-differences characteristic, an index of an individual's *change in symptoms* over the full time course or across selected time intervals—a statistic describing trajectory, or increasing or decreasing trends in symptom severity, not simply a *score* at some time point—becomes the pertinent dependent variable. Given the shift in outcome from static score to dynamic change, there is likely a concomitant need to readdress risk and resilience factors. This interindividual-differences-in-intraindividual-change perspective was endorsed by Rutter (2000a), who noted that stronger causal inference is possible when change in a risk or resilience factor is accompanied by within-individual change in an outcome over time.

As with developmental and aging research, which uses age or time since birth as a fundamental component of this within-individual change methodology (McArdle, Ferrer-Caja, Hamagami, & Woodcock, 2002), research on the sequelae to traumatic events has a start date, the point of exposure, from which the manifestation of an individual's symptoms can be mapped and profiled as a function of time. This distinguishing aspect of trauma-based mental health research makes it ideal for the application of methods designed to explicate interindividual differences in intraindividual change and thus to gain knowledge of what points in time-since-exposure symptom trajectories may be critical to understanding influences on chronicity and recovery and most accommodating to intervention. These modern approaches include accelerated longitudinal or cohort-sequential designs (Bell, 1954; McArdle & Bell, 2000), latent growth curve modeling applied to continuous data (e.g., McArdle & Epstein, 1987; Meredith & Tisak, 1984, 1990; Willett & Sayer, 1996) and to categorical data (Muthen, 1996), random coefficients regression (Raudenbush & Bryk, 2002; McArdle et al., 2002), and dynamic latent difference score analysis (Hamagami & McArdle, 2001; McArdle, 2001; McArdle & Hamagami, 2001).

Willett (1988), Ragosa (1995), and Lawrence and Hancock (1998) provide excellent introductions to the concept of interindividual differences in intra-individual change.

4. Index and Appraise Effect Sizes of Risk and Resilience Factors

In recent years, research in the behavioral, social, public health, and biomedical sciences has been experiencing a paradigm shift with regard to the reporting and interpretation of empirical findings. Reliance on what is known as null-hypothesis-significance-testing logic has been proclaimed an impediment to the advancement of scientific knowledge, and a growing number of prominent methodologists have called for its actual ban in the research literature (e.g., Hunter, 1997; Kirk, 1996, 2003; Schmidt, 1996, Thompson, 2002). Journals in public health and epidemiology have taken a lead in disallowing the reporting of significance tests in published articles, and the American Psychological Association commissioned its Task Force on Statistical Inference to study the issue and make recommendations for reporting strategies in its scientific publications.

The primary criticism of null hypothesis significance testing is that it misrepresents the probability of an incorrect decision. Although it is true that if, indeed, the null hypothesis is correct and there is no effect or association, the probability of a Type 1 error or alpha is an accurate probability of an incorrect decision. But, critics note that under most conditions, the alternative hypothesis is correct and there is some level of effect or association. As a consequence, the error is not in falsely rejecting the null hypothesis but rather in falsely rejecting the alternative hypothesis of an effect or association (where probability equals 1 − power). In other words, reaching a conclusion of nonsignificance under the condition of the alternative hypothesis is incorrect. Associated with this technical argument are several misguided beliefs held by researchers who employ null hypothesis significance testing:

1. That a statistically significant association at a given probability level (an alpha of .05 or .01) means that the probability of replicating the finding in future analyses is 1 − alpha. In actuality, this is false; the probability of replication is the power, which is unrelated to alpha but is related to the true effect size.
2. That the p value according to the calculated test statistic is an index of the size and importance of the effect or association. In actuality, the p value is a function of the sample size or degrees of freedom and should never be used to interpret how "highly significant" a finding is.

3. That nonsignificance is equivalent to no effect or association. In actuality, nonsignificance does not translate to an effect of zero or no association.

Schmidt (1996) provides an excellent elaboration of these falsely held beliefs and related issues.

In lieu of significance testing, the emerging recommendation is to report effect sizes with accompanying confidence intervals, a practice that is particularly appealing in research on risk and resilience factors for PTSD and other health outcomes. Two arguments are offered in support of this recommendation. First, the reporting of effect sizes for risk and resilience factors allows for a consideration of the relative strengths of the effects and not simply a dichotomous yes–no decision, which might dismiss an effect that is small yet informative. Even a weak effect or an effect with a calculated confidence interval that includes zero can have theoretical and possibly practical meaning. Second, the reporting of effect sizes and confidence intervals encourages a meta-analytic point of view in which the researcher's attention is drawn to the accumulation of findings in an effort to arrive at more precise and encompassing estimates of relative effect size across a collection of studies, perhaps a collection of populations. To date, there have been few meta-analytic studies on trauma and its effects (see those by Kaylor, King, & King, 1987; Rubonis & Bickman, 1991; Weaver & Clum, 1995); Brewin et al.'s (2000) work is especially important in the risk and resilience arena, and the very recent meta-analysis by Ozer, Best, Lipsey, and Weiss (2003) is likewise an extraordinarily valuable resource. More quantitative syntheses of this type are encouraged. There are a good number of texts on effect sizes, confidence intervals, and meta-analytic techniques, including those by Cooper and Hedges (1994), Harlow, Mulaik, and Steiger (1997), Hunter and Schmidt (1990), Lipsey and Wilson (2001), and Oakes (1986). A recent special section in *Educational and Psychological Measurement* contains a series of articles on the computation of effect sizes and their confidence intervals for different statistical procedures, along with suggested computer scripts (e.g., Cumming & Finch, 2001; Fidler & Thompson, 2001; Smithson, 2001).

IMPLICATIONS FOR PREVENTION, TREATMENT, AND POLICY

Historically, clinicians and policymakers have taken a "one-size-fits-all" approach to the provision of programs and services to individuals exposed to traumatic events (Litz, Gray, Bryant, & Adler, 2002). This is unfortunate because not everyone who is exposed to trauma is at equal risk for experiencing posttraumatic symptomatology and response to exposure certainly varies.

Only recently have practitioners and planners begun to attend to the literature on risk and resilience factors for PTSD (Everly, 2000) and to apply these findings to clinical and policy decision making concerning management of risk (Kraemer et al., 1997). Although this trend is encouraging, a lack of understanding about the causal inferences that can be drawn from studies of risk and resilience can considerably reduce the usefulness of this information for prevention, treatment, and policy (Litz et al., 2002), and valuable resources may be squandered on interventions that fail to have the desired impact.

Kraemer et al.'s (1997) risk taxonomy is quite valuable in a service planning and delivery context. Programs that target factors that cannot readily be affirmed as antecedents to the outcome, referred to as concomitants or consequences by Kraemer et al., are unlikely to achieve a reduction in PTSD. Yet given the cross-sectional nature of much of the risk and resilience literature, as well as the fact that concomitants or consequences of PTSD are likely to demonstrate stronger associations with PTSD than variables that meet the criteria for causal risk factors, early intervention practitioners attend to posttraumatic symptoms and functional impairments to the detriment of other factors, such as fixed markers and causal risk factors, that may have more promise for informing intervention efforts (Kraemer et al., 1997).

Risk factors that are considered fixed markers are useful for targeting a population that is most vulnerable and should receive services, especially when assets are limited. They are likewise useful in identifying groups that deserve priority screening. Whereas fixed markers have their primary role in the identification of individuals to target for programs and services, to the extent that the mechanism through which fixed markers have their impact on PTSD can be identified, this information can also be used to inform service delivery. For example, the finding that the association between race or ethnicity and PTSD is mediated through the impact of the former on the availability of resources that can facilitate recovery might inform programs aimed at providing those resources that are found to be critical to recovery.

Causal risk factors are most revealing when a program of prevention or intervention is planned, with of course the intention that manipulation via the program will produce changes in outcome (Kraemer et al., 1997). Rutter (2000a, 2000b) likewise endorsed the planning of prevention and intervention research based on sound knowledge of the processes that underlie causal links between risk factors and outcomes; mechanism-based treatments are not only more likely to succeed but are more etiologically informative. Interestingly, PTSD presents an unusual case for the Kraemer et al. risk taxonomy in that there is more often than not an identifiable time of exposure to an event or circumstance such that many individual characteristics of the victim *at the time of exposure* are fixed markers. Thus, although current age and current marital status may be variable risk factors—with persons in different age groups demonstrating varying levels of mental distress—age or marital status at time of exposure is a fixed marker.

Of course, the impact of causal risk factors on PTSD may be moderated or mediated by other variables, and knowledge of these associations can inform practice. For example, the previously described finding that some coping strategies are only effective under certain circumstances (e.g., moderate trauma exposure vs. high or low exposure; Suvak et al., 2002) cautions against preventive programs that encourage a particular coping strategy regardless of contextual factors. Relatedly, much of the evidence on the impact of risk and resilience factors on PTSD suggests that these factors operate differently for different trauma populations (Brewin et al., 2000). Therefore, those who deliver services or those responsible for policy decisions about prevention or intervention must be well informed about the repertoire of risk and resilience factors that may operate differentially, depending on context or trauma population. In addition, knowledge regarding indirect associations between risk and resilience factors and PTSD (i.e., mediator effects) can inform prevention and intervention efforts. Some risk factors may demonstrate indirect associations with PTSD or have their effect on PTSD through other factors in the chain of causation.

The recognition that most associations between risk factors and PTSD are quite complex brings us to yet another issue with regard to the literature on risk and resilience for PTSD. Sometimes, what appears to be a simple association between a particular risk factor and PTSD may be complicated by a third variable. Rutter (2000b) offers an excellent example: The simple recognition that parental divorce is associated with negative outcomes for children could lead practitioners and policymakers to conclude that a reduction in divorce is necessary to avoid these negative outcomes. A very different approach would be elicited by the knowledge that the causal mechanism through which divorce affects outcomes is by its indirect effects through parent–child relationships and parenting practices.

In addition, as Kraemer et al. (1997) noted, different features of the time course of a psychiatric entity (time of onset and trends toward recovery, remission, or relapse) may be predicted by different sets of risk and resilience factors, an observation that fits well with our call for a reconceptualization of outcome as process. Thus, as a case in point, interventions need to be geared to the particular stress phenomenon that is being targeted (e.g., chronic PTSD in response to combat-related trauma vs. acute stress symptomatology expressed in the immediate aftermath of an act of terrorism).

Finally, the reporting of effect sizes, or risk factor *potency* (Kraemer et al., 1997, 1999), and the accumulation of effect size statistics over studies are likewise meaningful for clinical and policy decisions. Without this information, it is impossible to differentiate between those associations that represent clinically meaningful relationships and those that are so small as to be practically meaningless. Risk factors that have little potency may be of negligible value to clinical, policy, and research application (Kraemer et al., 1997), and limited resources may be misspent when intervention efforts are geared toward risk factors that have little practical impact on PTSD. Of course, the importance of a particular effect size may be up for debate, and researchers may determine that a fairly small effect is of practical significance. What is key here is that practitioners move beyond simply attending to statistical significance to a recognition that effects differ in magnitude and that those of a higher magnitude may be better candidates for intervention.

In conclusion, practitioners are urged to undertake prevention, treatment, and policy efforts with knowledge about the validity of causal inference and its implications for the conclusions that can be drawn from the existing literature on risk and resilience for PTSD. More generally, the recognition that causal mechanisms are quite complicated cautions against universal or rigidly applied interventions. Interventions should be informed by knowledge pertaining to how factors operate in the etiological network, as well as the recognition that these factors may operate differently for different trauma populations, or even subpopulations within trauma populations (e.g., women versus men; minority versus nonminority). Attention to these issues can result in more effective prevention, treatment, and policy efforts and ultimately can lead to a reduction in the negative consequences of exposure to traumatic events.

ACKNOWLEDGMENTS

Preparation of this chapter was supported by funding from the Department of Defense (United States Army Medical Research and Materiel Command) in collaboration with the Department of Veterans Affairs (Grant PG Project DoD-87, "Measurement and Validation of Psychosocial Risk and Resilience Factors Associated with Physical and Mental Health and Health-Related Quality of Life in Persian Gulf Veterans," Daniel W. King and Lynda A. King, Co-principal Investigators).

REFERENCES

Acierno, R., Resnick, H., Kilpatrick, D. G., Saunders, B., & Best, C. L. (1999). Risk factors for rape, physical assault, and posttraumatic stress disorder in women: Examination of differential multivariate relationships. *Journal of Anxiety Disorders, 13*(6), 541–563.

American Psychiatric Association. (1994). *Diagnostic and statistical manual of mental disorders* (4th ed.). Washington, DC: Author.

Andrews, B., Brewin, C. R., Rose, S., & Kirk, M. (2000). Predicting PTSD symptoms in victims of violent crime: The role of shame, anger, and childhood abuse. *Journal of Abnormal Psychology, 109*(1), 69–73.

Andrykowski, M. A., & Cordova, M. J. (1998). Factors associated with PTSD symptoms following treatment for breast cancer: Test of the Anderson model. *Journal of Traumatic Stress, 11,* 189–203.

Astin, M. C., Ogland-Hand, S. M., Coleman, E. M., & Foy, D. W. (1995). Posttraumatic stress disorder and childhood abuse in battered women: Comparisons with maritally distressed women. *Journal of Consulting and Clinical Psychology, 63*(2), 308–312.

Bachman, C. W. (1988). The self: A dialectical approach. In L. Berkowitz (Ed.), *Advances in experimental social psychology* (Vol. 21, pp. 229–260). New York: Academic Press.

Baron, R. M., & Kenny, D. A. (1986). The moderator–mediator variable distinction in social psychological research: Conceptual, strategic, and statistical considerations. *Journal of Personality and Social Psychology, 51,* 1173–1182.

Baum, A., Cohen, L., & Hall, M. (1993). Control and intrusive memories as possible determinants of chronic stress. *Psychosomatic Medicine, 55*(3), 274–286.

Bell, R. Q. (1954). An experimental test of the accelerated longitudinal approach. *Child Development, 25,* 281–286.

Blanchard, E. B., Hickling, E. J., Barton, K. A., Taylor, A. E., Loos, W. R., & Jones-Alexander, J. (1996). One-year prospective follow-up of motor vehicle accident victims. *Behavior Research and Therapy, 34,* 775–786.

Blanchard, E. B., Hickling, E. J., Taylor, A. E., & Loos, W. (1995). Psychiatric morbidity associated with motor vehicle accidents. *Journal of Nervous and Mental Disease, 183*(8), 495–504.

Bollen, K. A. (1989). *Structural equations with latent variables.* New York: Wiley.

Bolin, R. (1985). Disaster characteristics and psychosocial impacts. In B. Sowder (Ed.), *Disasters and mental health: Selected contemporary perspectives* (pp. 3–28). Rockville, MD: National Institute of Mental Health.

Bolton, E., Litz, B. T., Glenn, D. M., Orsillo, S., & Roemer, L. (2002). The impact of homecoming reception on the adaptation of peacekeepers following deployment. *Military Psychology, 14,* 241–251.

Bremner, J. D., Southwick, S. M., Johnson, D. R., Yehuda, R., & Charney, D. S. (1993). Childhood physical abuse and combat-related posttraumatic stress disorder in Vietnam veterans. *American Journal of Psychiatry, 150,* 235–239.

Breslau, N., & Davis, G. C. (1987). Posttraumatic stress disorder: The stressor criterion. *Journal of Nervous and Mental Disease, 175,* 255–264.

Breslau, N., Davis, G. C., Andreski, P., & Peterson, E. (1991). Traumatic events and posttraumatic stress disorder in an urban population of young adults. *Archives of General Psychiatry, 48,* 216–222.

Breslau, N., Davis, G. C., Peterson, E. L., & Schultz, L. (1997). Psychiatric sequelae of posttraumatic stress disorder in women. *Archives of General Psychology, 12,* 359–370.

Brewin, C. R., Andrews, B., & Valentine, J. D. (2000). Meta-analysis of risk factors for posttraumatic stress disorder in trauma-exposed adults. *Journal of Consulting and Clinical Psychology, 68*(5), 748–766.

Bromet, E., Sonnega, A., & Kessler, R. C. (1998). Risk factors for DSM-III-R posttraumatic stress disorder: Findings from the National Comorbidity Survey. *American Journal of Epidemiology, 147,* 353–361.

Burgess, A. W., & Holmstrom, L. L. (1979). *Rape: Crisis and recovery.* Bowine, MD: Robert J. Brady.

Card, J. (1987). Epidemiology of PTSD in a national cohort of Vietnam veterans. *Journal of Clinical Psychology, 43,* 6–17.

Cohen, E. A. (1953). *Human behavior in the concentration camp.* New York: Grosset & Dunlap.

Cohen, J., Cohen, P., West, S. G., & Aiken, L. S. (2002). *Applied multiple regression/correlation analysis for the behavioral sciences* (3rd ed.). Mahwah, NJ: Erlbaum.

Cooper, H., & Hedges, L. V. (Eds.). (1994). *The handbook of research synthesis.* New York: Russell Sage.

Cortina, J. M., Chen, G., & Dunlap, W. P. (2001). Testing interaction effects in LISREL: Examination and illustration of available procedures. *Organizational Research Methods, 4*(4), 324–360.

Cumming, G., & Finch, S. (2001). A primer on the understanding, use, and calculation of confidence intervals that are based on central and noncentral distributions. *Educational and Psychological Measurement, 61*(4), 532–574.

Davidson, J., Hughes, D., Blazer, D., & George, L. (1991). Post-traumatic stress disorder in the community: An epidemiological study. *Psychological Medicine, 21,* 713–721.

Denny, N., Robinowitz, R., & Penk, W. (1987). Conducting applied research on Vietnam combat-related post-traumatic stress disorder. *Journal of Clinical Psychology, 43,* 56–66.

Dougall, A. L., Herberman, H. B., Inslicht, S. S., Baum, A., & Delahanty, D. L. (2000). Similarity of prior trauma exposure as a determinant of chronic stress responding to an airline disaster. *Journal of Consulting and Clinical Psychology, 68*(2), 290–295.

Egendorf, A., Kadushin, C., Laufer, R. S., Rothbart, G., & Sloan, L. (1981). *Legacies of Vietnam: Comparative adjustment of veterans and their peers.* New York: Center for Policy Research.

Emery, V. O., Emery, P. E., Sharma, D. K., Quiana, N. A., & Jassani, A. K. (1991). Predisposing variables in PTSD patients. *Journal of Traumatic Stress, 4,* 325–343.

Erickson, D. J., Wolfe, J., King, D. W., King, L. A., & Sharkansky, E. J. (2001). Posttraumatic stress disorder and depression symptomatology in a sample of Gulf war veterans: A prospective analysis. *Journal of Consulting and Clinical Psychology, 69*(1), 41–49.

Everly, G. S. (2000). Five principles of crisis intervention: Reducing the risk of premature crisis intervention. *International Journal of Emergency Mental Health, 2*(1), 1–4.

Fairbank, J. A., Hansen, D. J., & Fitterling, J. M. (1991). Patterns of appraisal and coping across different stressor conditions among former prisoners of war with and without posttraumatic stress disorder. *Journal of Consulting and Clinical Psychology, 59,* 274–281.

Fairbank, J. A., Keane, T. M., & Malloy, P. F. (1983). Some preliminary data on the psychological characteristics of Vietnam veterans with posttraumatic stress disorder. *Journal of Consulting and Clinical Psychology, 51,* 912–919.

Fidler, F., & Thompson, B. (2001). Computing correct confidence intervals for ANOVA fixed-and random-effects effect sizes. *Educational and Psychological Measurement, 61,* 575–604.

Figley, C. R. (1978). Symptoms of delayed combat-stress among a college sample of Vietnam veterans. *Military Medicine, 143,* 107–110.

Foa, E. B., Molnar, C., & Cashman, L. (1995). Change in rape narratives during exposure therapy for posttraumatic stress disorder. *Journal of Traumatic Stress, 8*(4), 675–690.

Foa, E. B., & Riggs, D. S. (1995). Posttraumatic stress disorder following assault: Theoretical considerations and empirical findings. *Current Directions in Psychological Science, 4,* 61–65.

Folkman, S., Schaefer, C., & Lazarus, R. S. (1979). Cognitive processes as mediators of stress and coping. In V. Hamilton & D. M. Warburton (Eds.), *Human stress and cognition* (pp. 265–298). Chichester, UK: Wiley.

Follette, V. M., Polusny, M. A., Bechtle, A. E., & Naugle, A. E. (1996). Cumulative trauma: The impact of child sexual abuse, adult sexual assault, and spouse abuse. *Journal of Traumatic Stress, 9,* 25–35.

Fontana, A., & Rosenheck, R. (1994). Posttraumatic stress disorder among Vietnam theater veterans: A causal model of etiology in a community sample. *Journal of Nervous and Mental Disease, 182*(12), 677–684.

Fontana, A., & Rosenheck, R. (1999). A model of war zone stressors and posttraumatic stress disorder. *Journal of Traumatic Stress, 12*(1), 111–126.

Forsythe, C. J., & Compas, B. E. (1987). Interaction of cognitive appraisals of stressful events and coping: Testing the goodness of fit hypothesis. *Cognitive Therapy and Research, 11,* 473–485.

Foy, D. W., Carroll, E. M., & Donahoe, C. P. (1987). Etiological factors in the development of PTSD in clinical samples of Vietnam combat veterans. *Journal of Clinical Psychology, 43*(1), 17–27.

Foy, D. W., Sipprelle, R. C., Rueger, D. B., & Carroll, E. M. (1984). Etiology of PTSD in Vietnam veterans: Analysis of premilitary, military, and combat exposure influences. *Journal of Consulting and Clinical Psychology, 52,* 79–87.

Galea, S., Ahern, J., Resnick, H., Kilpatrick, D., Bucuvalas, M., Gold, J., & Vlahow, D. (2002). Psychological sequelae of the September 11 terrorist attacks in New York City. *New England Journal of Medicine, 346*(13), 982–987.

Gallers, J., Foy, D. W., Donahoe, C. P., & Goldfarb, J. (1988). Post-traumatic stress disorder in Vietnam combat veterans: Effects of traumatic violence exposure and military adjustment. *Journal of Traumatic Stress, 1,* 181–192.

Gibbs, M. S. (1989). Factors in the victim that mediate between disaster and psychopathology: A review. *Journal of Traumatic Stress, 2*(4), 489–514.

Green, B. L. (1990). Defining trauma: Terminology and generic stressor dimensions. *Journal of Applied Social Psychology, 20,* 1632–1642.

Green, B. L. (1993). Identifying survivors at risk. In J. P. Wilson, & B. Raphael (Eds.), *International handbook of traumatic stress syndromes* (pp. 135–144). New York: Plenum Press.

Green, B. L. (1994). Psychological research in traumatic stress: An update. *Journal of Traumatic Stress, 7*(3), 341–362.

Green, B. L., Epstein, S. A., Krupnick, J. L., & Rowland, J. H. (1997). Trauma and medical illness: Assessing trauma-related disorders in medical settings. In J. P. Wilson & T. M. Keane (Eds.), *Assessing psychological trauma and PTSD* (pp. 160–191). New York: Guilford Press.

Green, B. L., Grace, M. C., & Gleser, G. C. (1985). Identifying survivors at risk: Long-term impairment following the Beverly Hills supper club fire. *Journal of Consulting and Clinical Psychology, 53*(5), 672–678.

Green, B. L., Grace, M. C., Lindy, J. D., Gleser, G. C., & Leonard, A. (1990). Risk factors for PTSD and other diagnoses in the general sample of Vietnam veterans. *American Journal of Psychiatry, 147,* 729–733.

Green, B. L., Lindy, J. D., & Grace, M. C. (1985). Post-traumatic stress disorder: Toward DSM-IV. *Journal of Nervous and Mental Disorders, 173,* 406–411.

Green, B. L., Lindy, M. D., Grace, M. C., & Leonard, A. C. (1992). Chronic posttraumatic stress disorder and diagnostic comorbidity in a disaster sample. *Journal of Nervous and Mental Disease, 180*(12), 760–766.

Hamagami, F., & McArdle, J. J. (2001). Advanced studies of individual differences linear dynamic models for longitudinal data analysis. In G. Marcoulides & R. Schumacker (Eds.), *New developments and techniques in structural equation modeling* (pp. 203–246). Hillside, NJ: Erlbaum.

Harlow, L. A., Mulaik, S. A., & Steiger, J. H. (Eds.). *What if there were no significance tests?* Mahwah, NJ: Erlbaum.

Hayduk, L. A. (1989). *Structural equation modeling with LISREL: Essentials and advances.* Baltimore: Johns Hopkins University.

Hayduk, L. A. (1996). *LISREL: Issues, debates, and strategies.* Baltimore: Johns Hopkins University.

Hobfoll, S. E. (1991). Traumatic stress: A theory based on rapid loss of resources. *Anxiety Research, 4*(3), 187–197.

Hunter, J. E. (1997). Needed: A ban on the significance test. *Psychological Science, 8*(1), 3–7.

Hunter, J. E., & Schmidt, F. L. (1990). *Methods of meta-analysis: Correcting error and bias in research findings.* Newbury Park, CA: Sage.

Jaccard, J., & Wan, C. K. (1996). *LISREL approaches to interaction effects in multiple regression* (Vol. 7). Thousand Oaks, CA: Sage.

Joreskog, K. G., & Yang, F. (1996). Nonlinear structural equation models: The Kenny-Judd model with interaction effects. In G. A. Marcoulides & R. E. Schumacker (Eds.), *Advanced structural equation modeling: Issues and techniques* (pp. 57–88). Mahwah, NJ: Erlbaum.

Kaylor, J., King, D. W., & King, L. A. (1987). Psychological effects of military service in Vietnam: A meta-analysis. *Psychological Bulletin, 102,* 257–271.

Keane, T. M., Scott, W. O., Chavoya, G. A., Lamparski, D. M., & Fairbank, J. A. (1985). Social support in Vietnam veterans with posttraumatic stress disorder: A comparative analysis. *Journal of Consulting and Clinical Psychology, 53,* 95–102.

Keane, T. M., Wolfe, J., & Taylor, K. (1987). Post-traumatic stress disorder: Evidence for diagnostic validity and methods of psychological assessment. *Journal of Clinical Psychology, 43,* 32–43.

Kemp, A., Rawlings, E. I., & Green, B. L. (1991). Post-traumatic stress disorder (PTSD) in battered women: A shelter sample. *Journal of Traumatic Stress, 4*(1), 137–148.

Kessler, R. C., Sonnega, A., Bromet, E., Hughes, M., & Nelson, C. B. (1995). Posttraumatic stress disorder in the National Comorbidity Survey. *Archives of General Psychiatry, 52,* 1048–1060.

Kilpatrick, D. G., Saunders, B. E., Amick-McMullan, A., Best, C. L., Veronen, L. J., & Resnick, H. S. (1989). Victim and crime factors associated with the development of crime-related post-traumatic stress disorder. *Behavior Therapy, 20*(2), 199–214.

King, D. W., & King, L. A. (1991). Validity issues in research on Vietnam veteran adjustment. *Psychological Bulletin, 109,* 107–124.

King, D. W., King, L. A., Foy, D. W., & Gudanowski, D. M. (1996). Prewar factors in combat-related posttraumatic stress disorder: Structural equation modeling with a national sample of female and male Vietnam veterans. *Journal of Consulting and Clinical Psychology, 64,* 520–531.

King, D. W., King, L. A., Foy, D. W., Keane, T. M., & Fairbank, J. A. (1999). Posttraumatic stress disorder in a national sample of female and male Vietnam veterans: Risk factors, war-zone stressors, and resilience-recovery variables. *Journal of Abnormal Psychology, 108*(1), 164–170.

King, D. W., King, L. A., Gudanowski, D. M., & Vreven, D. L. (1995). Alternative representations of war zone stressors: Relationships to posttraumatic stress disorder in male and female Vietnam veterans. *Journal of Abnormal Psychology, 104*(1), 184–196.

King, L. A., King, D. W., Fairbank, J. A., Keane, T. M., & Adams, G. A. (1998). Resilience-recovery factors in post-traumatic stress disorder among female and male Vietnam veterans: Hardiness, postwar social support, and additional stressful life events. *Journal of Personality and Social Psychology, 74*(2), 420–434.

Kirk, R. E. (1996). Practical significance: A concept whose time has come. *Educational and Psychological Measurement, 56*(5), 746–759.

Kirk, R. E. (2003). The importance of effect magnitude. In S. F. Davis (Ed.), *Handbook of research methods in experimental psychology* (pp. 83–105). Oxford, UK: Blackwell.

Kline, R. B. (1998). *Principles and practice of structural equation modeling.* New York: Guilford Press.

Koopman, C., Classen, C., & Spiegel, D. (1994). Predictors of posttraumatic stress symptoms among survivors of the Oakland/Berkeley California firestorm. *American Journal of Psychiatry, 151,* 888–894.

Kraemer, H. C., Kazdin, A. E., Offord, D. R., Kessler, R. C., Jensen, P. S., & Kupfer, D. J. (1997). Coming to terms with the terms of risk. *Archives of General Psychiatry, 54,* 337–343.

Kraemer, H. C., Kazdin, A. E., Offord, D. R., Kessler, R. C., Jensen, P. S., & Kupfer, D. J. (1999). Measuring the potency of risk factors for clinical or policy significance. *Psychological Methods, 4*(3), 257–271.

Kraemer, H. C., Stice, E., Kazdin, A., Offord, D., & Kupfer, D. (2001). How do risk factors work together? Mediators, moderators, and independent, overlapping, and proxy risk factors. *American Journal of Psychiatry, 158,* 848–856.

Laufer, R. S., Gallops, M. S., & Frey-Wouters, E. (1984). War stress and trauma: The Vietnam veteran experience. *Journal of Health and Social Behavior, 25,* 65–85.

Lawrence, F. R., & Hancock, G. R. (1998). Methods, plainly speaking: Assessing change over time using latent growth modeling. *Measurement and Evaluation in Counseling and Development, 30,* 211–224.

Lipsey, M. W., & Wilson, D. B. (Eds.). (2001). *Practical meta-analysis* (Applied Social Research Methods Series, Vol. 49). Thousand Oaks, CA: Sage.

Litz, B. T., Gray, M. J., Bryant, R. A., & Adler, A. B. (2002). Early intervention for trauma: Current status and future directions. *Clinical Psychology: Science and Practice, 9*(2), 112–134.

Litz, B. T., King, L. A., King, D. W., Orsillo, S. M., & Friedman, M. J. (1997). Warriors as peacekeepers: Features of the Somalia experience and PTSD. *Journal of Consulting and Clinical Psychology, 65*(6), 1001–1010.

Loehlin, J. C. (1998). *Latent variable models: An introduction to factor, path, and structural analysis* (3rd ed.). Mahwah, NJ: Erlbaum.

Lund, M., Foy, D., Sipprelle, C., & Strachan, A. (1984). The combat exposure scale: A systematic assessment of trauma in the Vietnam war. *Journal of Clinical Psychology, 40,* 1323–1328.

Macklin, M. L., Metzger, L. J., Litz, B. T., McNally, R. J., Lasko, N. B., Orr, S. P., & Pitman, R. K. (1998). Lower precombat intelligence is a risk factor for posttraumatic stress disorder. *Journal of Consulting and Clinical Psychology, 66*(2), 323–326.

March, J. S. (1993). What constitutes a stressor? The "Criterion A" issue. In J. R. T. Davidson & E. B. Foa (Eds.), *Posttraumatic stress disorder: DSM-IV and beyond* (pp. 37–54). Washington, DC: American Psychiatric Association.

Marmar, C. R., Weiss, D. S., Metzler, T. J., Delucci, K. L., Best, S. R., & Wentworth, K. A. (1999). Longitudinal course and predictors of continuing distress following critical incident exposure in emergency services personnel. *Journal of Nervous and Mental Disease, 187,* 15–22.

McArdle, J. J. (2001). A latent difference score approach to longitudinal dynamic structural analyses. In R. Cudeck, S. du Toit, & D. Sorbom (Eds.), *Structural equation modeling: Present and future* (pp. 342–380). Lincolnwood, IL: Scientific Software International.

McArdle, J. J., & Bell, R. W. (2000). An introduction to latent growth models for developmental data analysis. In T. D. Little, K. U. Schnabel, & J. Baumert (Eds.), *Modeling longitudinal and multilevel data: Practical issues, applied approaches, and specific examples* (pp. 69–107). Mahwah, NJ: Erlbaum.

McArdle, J. J., & Epstein, D. (1987). Latent growth curves within developmental structural equation models. *Child Development, 58,* 110–133.

McArdle, J. J., Ferrer-Caja, E., Hamagami, F., & Woodcock, R. (2002). Comparative longitudinal structural analyses of the growth and decline of multiple intellectual abilities over the life span. *Developmental Psychology, 38*(1), 115–142.

McArdle J., & Hamagami, F. (2001). Latent difference score structural models for linear dynamic analyses with incomplete longitudinal data. In L. Collins (Ed.), *New methods for the analysis of change: Decade of behavior* (pp. 139–175). Washington, DC: American Psychological Association.

McFarlane, A. C. (1988). The longitudinal course of posttraumatic morbidity: The range of outcomes and their predictors. *Journal of Nervous and Mental Disease, 176,* 30–40.

McFarlane, A. C. (1992). Avoidance and intrusion in post-traumatic stress disorder. *Journal of Nervous and Mental Disorder, 180*(7), 439–445.

Meredith, W., & Tisak, J. (1984). *"Tuckerizing" curves.* Paper presented at the annual meeting of the Psychometric Society, Santa Barbara, CA.

Meredith, W., & Tisak, J. (1990). Latent curve analysis. *Psychometrika, 55*(1), 107–122.

Moran, C., & Britton, N. R. (1994). Emergency work experience and reactions to traumatic incidents. *Journal of Traumatic Stress, 7,* 575–585.

Muthén, B. (1996). Growth modeling with binary responses. In A.V. Eye & C. Clogg (Eds.), *Categorical variables in developmental research: Methods of analysis* (pp. 37–54). San Diego: Academic Press.

Norris, F. H. (1992). Epidemiology of trauma: Frequency and impact of different potentially traumatic events on different demographic groups. *Journal of Consulting and Clinical Psychology, 60*(3), 409–418.

Norris, F. H., & Murrell, S. A. (1988). Prior experience as a moderator of disaster impact on anxiety symptoms in older adults. *American Journal of Community Psychology, 16,* 665–683.

North, C. S., Nixon, S. J., Shariat, S., Mallonee, S., McMillen, J. C., Spitznagel, E. L., & Smith, E. M. (1999). Psychiatric disorders among survivors of the Oklahoma City bombing. *Journal of the American Medical Association, 282*(8), 755–762.

Oakes, M. (1986). *Statistical inference: A commentary for the social and behavioral sciences.* New York: Wiley.

O'Toole, B. I., Marshall, R. P., Schureck, R. J., & Dobson, M. (1998). Posttraumatic stress disorder and comorbidity in Australian Vietnam veterans: Risk factors, chronicity and combat. *Australian and New Zealand Journal of Psychiatry, 32,* 32–42.

Ozer, E. J., Best, S. R., Lipsey, T. L., & Weiss, D. S. (2003). Predictors of posttraumatic stress disorder and symptoms in adults: A meta-analysis. *Psychological Bulletin, 129,* 52–73.

Park, C. L., Folkman, S., & Bostrom, A. (2001). Appraisals of controllability and coping in caregivers and HIV+ men: Testing for goodness-of-fit hypothesis. *Journal of Consulting and Clinical Psychology, 69,* 481–488.

Penk, W. E., Robinowitz, B., Roberts, W. R., Patterson, E. T., Dolan, M. P., & Atkins, H. G. (1981). Adjustment differences among male substance abusers varying in degree of combat experience in Vietnam. *Journal of Consulting and Clinical Psychology, 49*, 426–437.

Peretz, T., Baider, L., Ever-Hadani, P., & De-Nour, A. K. (1994). Psychological distress in female cancer patients with Holocaust experience. *General Hospital Psychiatry, 16*, 413–418.

Quarantelli, E. L. (1985). What is disaster?: The need for clarification in definition and conceptualization in research. In B. J. Sowder (Ed.), *Disasters and mental health: Selected contemporary perspectives* (pp. 41–73). Rockville, MD: National Institute of Mental Health.

Ragosa, D. (1995). Myths and methods: "Myths about longitudinal research" plus supplemental questions. In J. M. Gottman (Ed.), *The analysis of change* (pp. 3–66). Mahwah, NJ: Erlbaum.

Raudenbush, S. W., & Bryk, A. S. (2002). *Hierarchical linear models: Application and data analysis methods.* Thousand Oaks, CA: Sage.

Resnick, H. S., Kilpatrick, D. G., Best, C. L., & Kramer, T. L. (1992). Vulnerability-stress factors in development of posttraumatic stress disorder. *Journal of Nervous and Mental Disease, 180*, 424–430.

Resnick, H. S., Kilpatrick, D. G., Dansky, B., Saunders, B., & Best, C. (1993). Prevalence of civilian trauma and posttraumatic stress disorder in a representative national sample of women. *Journal of Consulting and Clinical Psychology, 61*, 984–991.

Resnick, H. S., Kilpatrick, D. G., & Lipovsky, J. A. (1991). Assessment of rape-related posttraumatic stress disorder: Stressor and symptom dimensions. *Psychological Assessment, 3*, 561–572.

Rodriguez, N., Vande-Kemp, H., & Foy, D. W. (1998). Posttraumatic stress disorder in survivors of childhood sexual and physical abuse: A critical review of the empirical research. *Journal of Child Sexual Abuse, 7*(2), 17–45.

Rothbaum, B. O., Foa, E. B., Riggs, D., Murdock, T., & Walsh, W. (1992). A prospective examination of post-traumatic stress disorder in rape victims. *Journal of Traumatic Stress, 5*, 455–475.

Rubonis, A. V., & Bickman, L. (1991). Psychological impairment in the wake of disaster: The disaster-psychopathology relationship. *Psychological Bulletin, 109*, 384–399.

Rutter, M. (1981). Stress, coping and development: Some issues and some questions. *Journal of Child Psychology and Psychiatry, 22*, 323–356.

Rutter, M. (2000a). Psychosocial influences: Critiques, findings, and research needs. *Development and Psychopathology, 12*, 375–405.

Rutter, M. (2000b, July–August). Resilience in the face of adversity. *World Congress on Medicine and Health* [On-line]. Available: http://www.mh-hannover.de/aktuelles/projectte/mmm/englishversion/fs_programme/speech/Rutter_V.html.

Rutter, M., & Sroufe, A. (2000). Developmental psychopathology: Concepts and challenges. *Development and Psychopathology, 12*, 265–296.

Schmidt, F. L. (1996). Statistical significance testing and cumulative knowledge in psychology: Implications for training of researchers. *Psychological Methods, 1*(2), 115–129.

Schnurr, P. P., Friedman, M. J., & Rosenberg, S. D. (1993). Premilitary MMPI scores as predictors of combat-related PTSD symptoms. *American Journal of Psychiatry, 150,* 479–483.

Schumacker, R. E., & Lomax, R. G. (1996). *A beginner's guide to structural equation modeling.* Mahwah, NJ: Erlbaum.

Shalev, A. Y., Freedman, S., Peri, T., Brandes, D., Sahar, T., Orr, S. P., & Pitman, R. K. (1998). Prospective study of posttraumatic stress disorder and depression following trauma. *American Journal of Psychiatry, 155,* 630–637.

Shalev, A. Y., Sahar, T., Freedman, S., Peri, T., Glick, N., Brandes, D., Orr, S. P., & Pitman, R.K. (1998). A prospective study of heart rate response following trauma and the subsequent development of posttraumatic stress disorder. *Archive of General Psychiatry, 55,* 553–559.

Sharkansky, E. J., King, D. W., King, L. A., Wolfe, J., Erickson, D. J., & Stokes, L. R. (2000). Coping with Gulf War combat stress: Mediating and moderating effects. *Journal of Abnormal Psychology, 109*(2), 188–197.

Skodol, A. E., Schwartz, S., Dohrenwend, B. P., Levav, I., Shrout, P. E., & Reiff, M. (1996). PTSD symptoms and comorbid mental disorders in Israeli war veterans. *British Journal of Psychiatry, 169,* 217–225.

Smithson, M. (2001). Correct confidence intervals for various regression effect sizes and parameters: The importance of noncentral distributions in computing intervals. *Educational and Psychological Measurement, 61,* 605–632.

Solomon, Z., Benbenishty, R., & Mikulincer, M. (1991). The contribution of wartime, pre-war, and post-war factors to self-efficacy: A longitudinal study of combat stress reaction. *Journal of Traumatic Stress, 4,* 345–361.

Solomon, Z., & Mikulincer, M. (1990). Life events and combat-related posttraumatic stress disorder: The intervening role of locus of control and social support. *Military Psychology, 2,* 241–256.

Solomon, Z., Mikulincer, M., & Avitzur, E. (1988). Coping, locus of control, social support, and combat-related posttraumatic stress disorder: A prospective study. *Journal of Personality and Social Psychology, 55,* 279–285.

Solomon, Z., Mikulincer, M., & Flum, H. (1989). The implications of life events and social integration in the course of combat-related post-traumatic stress disorder. *Social Psychiatry and Psychiatric Epidemiology, 24,* 41–48.

Solomon, Z., Mikulincer, M., & Hobfoll, S. E. (1987). Objective versus subjective measurement of stress and social support: Combat-related reactions. *Journal of Consulting and Clinical Psychology, 55*(4), 577–583.

Southwick, S. M., Morgan, C. A., Darnell, A., Bremner, D., Nicolaou, A. L., Nagy, L. M., & Charney, D. S. (1995). Trauma-related symptoms in veterans of Operation Desert Storm: A two-year follow-up. *American Journal of Psychiatry, 152,* 1150–1155.

Strange, R. E. (1974). Psychiatric perspectives of the Vietnam veteran. *Military Medicine, 139,* 96–98.

Sutker, P. B., Davis, J. M., Uddo, M., & Ditta, S. R. (1995). War zone stress, personal resources, and PTSD in Persian Gulf War Returnees. *Journal of Abnormal Psychology, 104,* 344–352.

Suvak, M. K., Vogt, D. S., Savarese, V. W., King, L. A., & King, D. W. (2002). Relationship of war-zone coping strategies to long-term general life adjustment among Vietnam veterans: Combat exposure as a moderator variable. *Personality and Social Psychology Bulletin, 28*(7), 974–985.

Swann, W. B. (1983). Self-verification: Bring social reality into harmony with the self. In J. Sulfs, & A. G. Greenwald (Eds.), *Psychological perspectives on the self* (Vol. 2, pp. 33–66). Hillsdale, NJ: Erlbaum.

Thompson, B. (2002). What future quantitative social science research could look like: Confidence intervals for effect sizes. *Educational Researcher, 31*(3), 25–32.

Ursano, R. J., Fullerton, C. S., Kao, T. C., & Bhartiya, V. R. (1995). Longitudinal assessment of posttraumatic stress disorder and depression after exposure to traumatic death. *Journal of Nervous and Mental Disease, 183*(1), 36–42.

van der Kolk, B. A., & Greenberg, M. S. (1987). The psychobiology of the trauma response: Hyperarousal, constriction, and addiction to traumatic reexposure. In B. A. van der Kolk (Ed.), *Psychological trauma* (pp. 63–87). Washington, DC: American Psychiatric Association.

Warheit, G. T. (1985). A prepositional paradigm for estimating the impact of disasters on mental health. In B. J. Sowder (Ed.), *Disasters and mental health: Selected contemporary perspectives* (pp. 196–214). Rockville, MD: National Institute of Mental Health.

Weaver, T. L., & Clum, G. A. (1995). Psychological distress associated with interpersonal violence: A meta-analysis. *Clinical Psychology Review, 15*, 115–140.

Willett, J. B. (1988). Questions and answers in the measurement of change. In E. Rothkopf (Ed.), *Review of research in education 1988–89* (pp. 345–422). Washington, DC: American Educational Research.

Willett, J. B., & Sayer, A. G. (1996). Cross-domain analyses of change over time: Combining growth modeling and covariance structure analysis. In G. A. Marcoulides, & R. E. Schumacker (Eds.), *Advanced structural equation modeling: Issues and techniques* (pp. 125–157). Mahwah, NJ: Erlbaum.

Wolfe, J., Erickson, D. J., Sharkansky, E. J., King, D. W., & King, L. A. (1999). Course and predictors of posttraumatic stress disorder among Gulf War veterans: A prospective analysis. *Journal of Consulting and Clinical Psychology, 67*(4), 520–528.

Yehuda, R. (Ed.). (1999). *Risk factors for posttraumatic stress disorder.* Washington DC: American Psychiatric Association.

4

Conceptual and Definitional Issues in Complicated Grief

MATT J. GRAY
HOLLY G. PRIGERSON
BRETT T. LITZ

E ncounters with potentially traumatizing events are unfortunately common as evidenced by estimates that slightly over half of all U.S. citizens will experience such an event at some point during their life (Kessler, Sonnega, Bromet, & Nelson, 1995). Although life-threatening events are undeniably harrowing and elicit intense fear and acute psychological distress, the overwhelming majority of individuals exposed to such events do not develop chronic psychopathology (Breslau et al., 1998). Nevertheless, the ubiquity of traumatic exposure translates into a substantial number of individuals who will develop significant posttraumatic psychopathology, despite the relatively small percentage of trauma victims who develop chronic difficulties. For instance, even the most conservative estimates of the lifetime prevalence of posttraumatic stress disorder (PTSD) indicate that nearly 3 million U.S. citizens will develop the disorder at some point during their life (American Psychiatric Association, 1994). Because the majority of traumatic life events are life-threatening situations, mental health researchers and providers have understandably focused on disorders such PTSD and acute stress disorder, which are primarily characterized by pathological fear and anxiety. However, many severely distressing adverse life events involve the sudden, unexpected death of a close friend or relative instead of, or in addition to, personal life threat or endangerment. Notably, incidents of terrorism and mass violence typically yield a tremendous loss of life. For every survivor of such an atrocity, there is an untold number of suddenly bereaved individuals struggling with the death of a loved one who did not survive. Moreover, for every individual personally endangered by his or her proximity to such an event, there are countless individuals worldwide who are directly affected by the death of one of the victims. For example, the estimates for individuals bereaved as a result of the terrorist attacks on 9-11-01 in the United States alone is 6 million (Schlenger et al., 2002).

Although the mental health community has laudably stepped up its efforts to care for victims suffering from debilitating conditions that result from direct trauma, such as fear and anxiety, the emotional and psychological needs of the traumatically bereaved have been comparatively neglected. As of the writing of this chapter, a quick PsycINFO search revealed that articles addressing PTSD in the aftermath of incidents of mass violence or terrorism have outpaced articles addressing grief and bereavement issues following such events by a 3-to-1 ratio, despite the tremendous number of bereaved individuals who are left in the wake of such events. Although incidents of mass violence command a great deal of media attention, they account for a small portion of individuals experiencing complicated grief reactions. Much more prevalent but smaller-scale events such as motor vehicle accidents account for the great majority of traumas characterized by the death of a loved one. Further, despite this text's focus on early intervention following trauma and traumatic loss, it should be acknowledged that complicated grief reactions can ensue following deaths that are the result of natural causes as well. Complicated grief (CG), in its present conceptualization, does not disaggregate unique consequences which may be associated with deaths owing to frankly traumatic events such as homicide, natural disaster, or incidents of mass violence. It is abundantly clear at present that individuals experiencing the loss of a close friend or relative through any means—traumatic or nontraumatic—can develop chronic, unremitting, or otherwise severe grief reactions. What is unclear at present is whether the death of a loved one owing to particularly horrific causes (e.g., the World Trade Center attacks) is associated with unique complications in addition to or instead of PTSD or CG as it is presently conceptualized.

Limited knowledge exists on the differences between pathological grief reactions stemming from traumatic events relative to grief reactions stemming from deaths owing to natural causes. The few studies that have examined whether the traumatic nature of the death has an important influence on the risk for CG and the severity of the CG response have actually yielded negative results (e.g., Prigerson et al., 2002). Although, more studies are needed before firm conclusions can be drawn about the role played by the nature of the death in vulnerability to CG, extant knowledge suggests that CG is equally likely to result from losses that are natural versus those that are unnatural. Consequently, findings pertaining to CG studied largely as the result of natural causes are expected to generalize to CG following from unnatural causes.

This chapter describes the constellation of symptoms that comprise the distinct clinical disorder of CG generally and distinguishes it from PTSD and major depressive disorder (MDD). As more empirical research bearing on the unique sequelae of loss by traumatic means accumulates (e.g., homicide), it is likely that different acute clinical management and treatment implications will emerge as well. At present, however, our observations are necessarily confined to complicated grief reactions generally as the CG literature is still in its infancy. We enumerate and describe etiological influences and risk factors for CG and also highlight adverse clinical outcomes associated with complicated grief reactions. Finally, we briefly describe treatment implications and review promising interventions for CG.

COMPLICATED GRIEF VERSUS UNCOMPLICATED GRIEF

Although researchers have long recognized that some individuals experience debilitating, unremitting distress following the death of a loved one, disagreement about defining features of a pathological grief reaction has prevented its establishment as a formal diagnostic entity in the nosology of mental disorders. Moreover, a historical focus on major depressive reactions following the death of a loved one has arguably resulted in an underestimate of individuals experiencing pathological grief reactions (Horowitz et al., 1997). As will be reviewed shortly, many bereaved individuals can experience chronic and debilitating grief-related distress without meeting diagnostic criteria for MDD. Recently, two separate groups of researchers have proposed diagnostic criteria for CG (Horowitz et al., 1997; Prigerson, Shear, et al., 1999). The relatively strong convergence in their independently proposed criteria is encouraging as it highlights the growing consensus in the field about the defining features of the disorder and, accordingly, increases the likelihood that unremitting psychological and emotional distress resulting from bereavement will be identified and treated.

As a result of a consensus conference convened to develop criteria for pathological grief reactions, Prigerson, Shear, et al. (1999) proposed that traumatic grief includes two core symptom categories. First, a person must be experiencing significant separation distress (Criterion A), as evidenced by at least three of the following four symptoms (experienced "often" or "always"): intrusive preoccupation or thoughts of the deceased, yearning for the deceased, searching for the deceased, or loneliness. Second, the person must be experiencing significant symptoms of traumatic distress in response to the death as evidenced by endorsement of at least 6 of the following 11 symptoms (occurring "often" or "always"): avoidance, futility about the future, numbness or detachment, feeling shocked or dazed, disbelief about the death, emptiness, feeling unfulfilled without the deceased, feeling that part of the self has died, shattered world view (e.g., lost sense of trust, security, or control), assuming symptoms or harmful behaviors of the deceased, or bitterness. At that time, the panel recommended that this constellation of symptoms needed to persist for at least 2 months after the death. This criterion has since been changed to a minimum duration of 6 months (Prigerson & Jacobs, 2001). Although it is recognized that this period may encroach on "normal" bereavement-related distress which may ultimately remit on its own, it provides an opportunity for identification and intervention for individuals experiencing pronounced difficulties a few months after the loss and who are at significantly heightened risk of physical and psychological morbidity in the coming years (Prigerson et al., 1997). Furthermore, recent longitudinal studies indicate that although there may be slight CG symptom remission beyond 6 months, symptoms have generally stabilized by this point (Prigerson et al., 1997). Finally, Criterion D requires that these disturbances cause significant impairment of social, occupational, or other important areas of functioning. It should be noted that the formal label of this proposed disorder has changed from traumatic grief to CG in recognition of the fact that sustained, pathological grief reactions can ensue following deaths resulting from natural causes (i.e., these clinical problems need not be triggered by a violent or accidental death).

Using common symptoms gleaned from interviews with bereaved individuals over the course of their adaptation to loss, Horowitz et al. (1997) also proposed criteria for a diagnosis of CG. As opposed to Prigerson et al.'s 6-month criterion, Horowitz et al. proposed that at least 14 months must elapse following the death of the loved one before a diagnosis of CG can be given. Although this time frame likely minimizes false positives, it may make it difficult to identify and treat severe grief reactions that might be effectively ameliorated earlier (Jacobs, Mazure, & Prigerson, 2000). With respect to the diagnostic criteria proposed by Horowitz and colleagues, any three of the following symptoms reported with sufficient intensity to interfere with daily functioning warrants a diagnosis of CG: intrusive memories or fantasies related to the lost relationship, strong pangs of severe emotion related to the deceased, strong yearnings for the deceased, feelings of loneliness or emptiness, strong efforts to avoid people, activities or places that remind one of the deceased, disrupted sleep, or loss of interest in social, recreational, or occupational activities. Although further empirical research is needed to resolve the inconsistencies in the two sets of proposed diagnostic criteria (e.g., time elapsed following the death for the diagnosis to be given), the similarities provide evidence for the convergent validity of the CG construct.

Complicated grief is distinguished from "normal" or uncomplicated grief primarily by the presence of unremitting and incapacitating distress that interferes markedly with functioning. The loss of a significant other is inordinately distressing for virtually everyone. Most individuals experiencing such an event, however, experience an initial state of shock followed by acute emotional or somatic discomfort and social withdrawal but ultimately learn to accept the loss and resume prebereavement levels of functioning (Bowlby, 1963; Parkes & Brown, 1972). That is, they can eventually regain a sense of meaning and purpose, feel that the future holds potential for fulfillment, enjoy leisure and social activities, and generally function without significant impairment or acute distress. In contrast, those exhibiting complicated courses of bereavement do not exhibit a waning of symptoms over time but instead remain withdrawn, isolated, and severely emotionally distressed for several months or years following the loss. As will be reviewed shortly, this inordinate, sustained distress is associated with myriad adverse physical and psychological outcomes that do not typically ensue following normative bereavement processes. Moreover, as noted later, other diagnostic entities which have often been used to account for pathological grief responses often fail to adequately identify a substantial proportion of individuals experiencing significant grief-related psychopathology.

DISTINGUISHING COMPLICATED GRIEF FROM MAJOR DEPRESSIVE DISORDER

Although depressed affect is a universal response to the death of a loved one, and although CG and MDD are certainly not mutually exclusive possibilities, it would be a mistake to assume that severe grief reactions can be fully subsumed under the rubric of depression. First, in two separate studies of individuals who had recently suffered the death of a spouse, factor-analytic analyses revealed that symptoms of CG loaded highly on the first-order factor (i.e., the CG factor) but loaded quite poorly on anxiety and depression factors

(Prigerson et al., 1995; Prigerson et al., 1996). Accordingly, it is not simply the case that individuals experiencing pronounced symptoms of CG invariably experience concomitant severe depression. Moreover, in contrast to MDD, symptoms of CG have not been shown to respond to interpersonal psychotherapy alone or in combination with antidepressant medications (Pasternak et al., 1991; Reynolds et al., 1999). In addition, CG and MDD appear to entail distinct neuroendocrine responses (Jacobs, 1987) and sleep-state electroencephelograhy (McDermott, Prigerson, & Reynolds, 1997). Finally, and perhaps most important, in a sample of widowed individuals from the community, nearly half of the participants who endorsed clinically significant levels of CG did not meet diagnostic criteria for MDD (Prigerson et al., 1995; Prigerson, Bridge, et al., 1999; Silverman, Johnson, & Prigerson, 2001). Clearly, an exclusive focus on MDD criteria following bereavement experiences would result in a significant portion of severely distressed individuals going unidentified and untreated.

DISTINGUISHING COMPLICATED GRIEF
FROM ADJUSTMENT DISORDER

As noted in DSM-IV (American Psychiatric Association, 1994), the hallmark feature of an adjustment disorder is significant emotional distress or behavioral symptoms in response to a readily identifiable psychosocial stressor. This would seem to be an appropriate depiction of complicated bereavement responses, but a diagnosis of adjustment disorder may not be given more than 6 months after the termination of the stressor. Both sets of independently proposed criteria for CG (Horowitz et al., 1997; Prigerson, Shear, et al., 1999) require that the symptoms persist for at least 6 months, thereby precluding a diagnosis of adjustment disorder. Within the first few months following the death of a loved one, the defining features of CG are not uncommon and are best conceptualized as normal responses to significant loss. It is only when the symptoms persist and contribute to sustained dysfunction that the course of bereavement can be considered complicated. Furthermore, the criteria for diagnosing adjustment disorder specifically prohibit this diagnosis in response to bereavement (American Psychiatric Association, 1994). Finally, criteria for adjustment disorder are notably imprecise and do not specifically reference the unique constellation of symptoms enumerated earlier (Prigerson, Shear, et al., 1999). Thus, although a diagnosis of adjustment disorder would connote that the bereaved individual was experiencing marked distress following the death of a loved one, the lack of specificity fails to provide direction for treatment planning.

DISTINGUISHING COMPLICATED GRIEF
FROM POSTTRAUMATIC STRESS DISORDER

Although CG can ensue following loss from natural causes, it can also result from traumatic deaths, such as those resulting from motor vehicle accidents, homicides, suicides, and mass violence or terrorism (Prigerson et al., 2002). Although traumatic incidents that lead to loss of life routinely produce pronounced distress, and emotional and cognitive disorganization characteristic of acute stress disorder and loss by traumatic means is one of the most significant risk factors for chronic PTSD (Breslau et al., 1998), bereavement by traumatic means can lead to complicated bereavement as well. In theory, early intervention that neglects the unique psychosocial consequences of bereavement by focusing solely on acute stress disorder (ASD) can result in unaddressed, sustained, and unremitting grief-related distress. Because it is especially commonplace to diagnose survivors of such events with ASD/PTSD without necessarily considering unique features of the grief response, it is important to fully delineate the distinguishing features of the two disorders and their implications for early intervention and treatment.

Since the inclusion of PTSD in the psychiatric nosology (starting with DSM-III), loss by traumatic means (e.g., homicide) has been considered a traumatic stressor that could cause ASD/PTSD. However, PTSD fails to sufficiently capture the unique experiences of those who suffer from chronic grief as a result of violent loss of an important attachment figure. Nevertheless, Green (2000) and Green et al. (2001) argued cogently that loss by traumatic means should be treated as a traumatic stressor, and that the resulting chronic condition that arises in a small percentage of cases should be classified as PTSD. In this conceptualization, violent and unexpected loss results in severe feelings of personal vulnerability and forces the individual to confront the prospect of death, creating intense anxiety, which arguably is the psychological aftereffect common to all traumatic stressors.

In an attempt to study the effects of traumatic loss relative to non–loss-related trauma, Green et al. (2001) systematically studied the mental health outcomes in individuals with a single traumatic bereavement, those with a single non–loss-related trauma, and those with no traumatic experience. These researchers found that 16% of those who had experienced a loss by traumatic means met the criteria for PTSD and 22% met the lifetime criteria for a trauma-related disorder. The prevalence of major depression was no higher in the traumatic loss group, compared to the other two groups, which underscores the fact that the postloss syndrome is not simply depression or anhedonia. The most stigmatized deaths and those associated with malicious intent tended to produce higher rates of stress disorder. In fact, loss by traumatic means led to more severe intrusive symptoms and greater functional impairment in comparison to a group of individuals who suffered physical assault, which suggests that loss by traumatic means may be more pernicious than direct trauma. Unfortunately, Green et al. (2001) failed to take into account the nature and extent of the attachment relationship in those who lost loved ones to violence. In addition, they failed to directly contrast PTSD as an outcome variable with symptoms of CG.

Although PTSD and CG can co-occur, CG is conceptually distinct from PTSD. Fundamental differences in defining features of the disorders have important treatment implications which may go unheeded if one hastily assigns a PTSD diagnosis without considering unique features of grief-related pathology.

With respect to the Criterion B (reexperiencing symptoms) of PTSD for instance, similarities between CG and PTSD are evident. Notably, both disorders may involve intrusive, distressing thoughts or memories related to the event in the case of PTSD or the deceased in the case of CG. However, reexperiencing symptoms of PTSD invariably results in heightened anxiety and distress. In contrast, "reexperiencing" types of symptoms of CG is not necessarily distressing or anxiety provoking. In fact, the bereaved individual actively yearns and searches for the deceased, and contact with reminders of the deceased is actually a source of comfort as opposed to a source of anxiety to be avoided (Rees, 1971). Although reminders of the deceased understandably trigger negative affective states because they are painful reminders of loss, they may also be a source of solace (Prigerson et al., 2000). Thus, in contrast to PTSD, "reexperiencing" symptoms can elicit ambivalent responses and reminders are sometimes actively sought instead of uniformly avoided. Despite the fact that reminders of the deceased can be comforting for those with CG reactions, excessive ruminations about the deceased may increase suicidal ideation as the bereaved may seek to be reunited with the deceased (Prigerson et al., 2000).

The avoidance and numbing symptom cluster of the PTSD construct (Criterion C) also overlaps with CG criteria, but yet again important differences are evident. In a recent empirical test of the performance of CG, item response theory (IRT) was used to evaluate the relationship of individual CG symptoms to a unidimensional construct of CG (Prigerson et al., 2000). Results indicated that "numbness" and "shattered world view" were most strongly related to the CG attribute. "Numbing" symptoms are a hallmark feature of PTSD, and fundamental alterations in one's belief system (i.e., a shattered world view) are common sequelae (McCann, Sakheim, & Abrahamson, 1988). However, numbness and detachment in instances of CG typically represent a withdrawal from social activity and other interpersonal relationships as opposed to a volitional or unconscious attempt to dissociate from the event itself.

Perhaps, more central to distinguishing CG from PTSD is the symptom of avoidance. Although initially proposed consensus criteria for CG include avoidance, recent empirical evidence calls into question the importance of this symptom in identifying severe or protracted grief reactions. Specifically, the same IRT analysis described earlier revealed that avoidance demonstrated the poorest relationship to the CG construct and did not efficiently classify individuals with and without CG. Others have found that avoidance symptoms exhibit poor sensitivity in identifying CG (Horowitz et al., 1997) and may be infrequently endorsed among individuals experiencing sudden, unexpected deaths of loved ones (e.g., Spooren, Henderick, & Jannes, 2000). In contrast, avoidance is not only a defining feature of PTSD but is widely believed to be the most prominent factor in maintaining the disorder and, accordingly, most cognitive-behavioral interventions for PTSD explicitly target avoidance symptoms and behaviors (Resick & Calhoun, 2001). To the extent that avoidance is not central to CG, it would suggest that exposure-based treatments may be misguided in that they target fears that are not at the core of the disorder.

Criterion D for PTSD (hyperarousal) represents the greatest point of departure between PTSD and CG. Symptoms of increased arousal are seldom endorsed by those meeting criteria for CG. When "hypervigilance" does occur, it appears to be the result of the bereaved individual scanning the environment for reminders of the deceased and is therefore not akin to scanning the environment for danger or threat as is the case with PTSD (Raphael & Martinek, 1997). Unlike the case for PTSD, in which hypervigilance is a reaction to the fear that an horrific event will reoccur, in CG hypervigilance relates to a wish to be reunited and to regain contact with the missed person who had been lost.

Although there is no doubt that loss of an important attachment figure by violent means is potentially traumatizing and could result in symptoms of PTSD, there is also sufficient empirical evidence and compelling alternative conceptual frameworks to argue against a restrictive and narrow conceptualization of loss by traumatic means as psychological trauma. The "loss as trauma" framework proposed by Green (2000) fails to sufficiently acknowledge the unique biological, psychological, and social behavior implications of bereavement, which will color posttraumatic adaptation to loss by violence. In addition, within the field of traumatic stress, there is general consensus that certain types of traumatic events in certain contexts or developmental periods lead to unique posttraumatic outcomes. For example, although interpersonal trauma (incest, sexual assault, physical assault by caregivers and attachment figures, etc.) is defined in the same way as noninterpersonal trauma (e.g., motor vehicle accident) in the diagnostic framework, interpersonal trauma leads to a dramatically different repertoire of posttraumatic deficits and liabilities, while sharing the same summary label of "PTSD" (e.g., Herman, 1992; Zlotnick, Zakriski, Shea, & Costello, 1996). In a similar vein, we argue that pathological grief responses can color the trauma of loss and develop in the absence of PTSD. There is certainly some degree of overlap between diagnostic criteria for CG and PTSD, but differences abound. This is most evident in studies that concurrently evaluate CG and PTSD in individuals experiencing recent deaths of loved ones.

In a study of friends of high school suicide victims assessed 6 years after the death, less than half of individuals exhibiting syndromal levels of CG also met diagnostic criteria for PTSD (Prigerson, Bridge, et al., 1999). Similarly, in a larger sample of recently widowed individuals, 66% of those meeting criteria for CG did not meet criteria for PTSD and over one-third of those individuals failed to meet diagnostic criteria for MDD or PTSD (Silverman et al., 2001). Thus, although there are some similarities among diagnostic criteria for these disorders, an exclusive focus on bereavement-related depression or PTSD would result in a significant proportion of individuals experiencing protracted, CG responses going undetected.

PSYCHOLOGICAL AND PHYSICAL MORBIDITY ASSOCIATED WITH COMPLICATED GRIEF

The distress associated with CG is certainly debilitating in its own right, but CG is also associated with substantive long-term psychological and physical impairments. Using follow-up data obtained from 76 young adults who had experienced the suicide of a close friend, Prigerson, Bridge, et al. (1999) found that participants who endorsed syndromal levels of CG were five times more likely to report suicidal ideation relative to individuals not experiencing elevated levels of complicated CG. CG was a significant predictor of suicidal ideation even after depressive symptoms were controlled in hierarchical regression analyses, indicating that CG is an independent risk factor for suicidal ideation.

CG has also been shown to be associated with an array of quality-of-life impairments. Silverman and colleagues (2000) evaluated a sample of 67 recently widowed individuals using a diagnostic interview for CG, structured interviews for PTSD and major depressive episodes, and a paper-and-pencil measure designed to evaluate functioning in eight domains: physical functioning, social functioning, limitations in activities of daily living, mental health, energy, pain, change in health within the past year, and general perceptions of current health. CG was a significant predictor of impairments in social functioning, mental health, and energy level. These effects were significant after controlling for age, sex, time elapsed since the loss, and major depressive episode and PTSD diagnoses. The fact that these impairments are uniquely associated with CG above and beyond the effects of MDD and PTSD underscores the importance of considering symptoms and complications unique to the grief context.

In a longitudinal study of 150 widows and widowers, CG symptoms 6 months after the death of the spouse were significantly associated with adverse physical health (e.g., cancer, cardiac problems, and high blood pressure) and mental and behavioral health problems (e.g., suicidal ideation, changes in eating habits) at 13- and 25-month follow-up assessments (Prigerson et al., 1997). Once again, these associations remained significant after controlling for age, sex, and prior pathology. It may not be bereavement per se which places individuals at risk for adverse physical and emotional outcomes, but CG reactions may heighten one's risk for a number of subsequent physical and psychological outcomes.

Another recent study compared syndromal levels of CG, depression, and anxiety among widows and widowers in predicting mental and physical health outcomes (Chen et al., 1999). Syndromal levels of CG predicted adverse physical health events (e.g., myocardial infarctions and cancer) at 25 months for widows but not for widowers. High symptom levels of anxiety following the death of a spouse predicted suicidal ideation at 25 months among widowers. Whether the associations with deleterious mental and physical health outcomes are the result of a direct causal link or whether this relationship is mediated by poorer self-care, social withdrawal, or other maladaptive coping strategies remains to be explicated by future empirical studies.

ETIOLOGICAL INFLUENCES AND RISK FACTORS FOR COMPLICATED GRIEF

Given that CG can only be identified after many months have passed after loss, the crucial question that arises with respect to early intervention is: Who is most at risk for CG? In this context, a number of risk factors for the development of protracted grief reactions have been identified. Van Doorn, Kasl, Beery, Jacobs, and Prigerson (1998) investigated relationship characteristics which have been theorized to influence the course of bereavement. Specifically, they examined insecure attachment styles and relationships that may be characterized as very "security enhancing" (i.e., relationships typified by dependency on the partner, enhanced feelings of security, and active emotional support). These researchers found that security-enhancing marriages (evaluated preloss) are significantly associated with CG and only modestly associated with depressive symptoms. CG was also significantly associated with a composite attachment style index (formed by aggregating excessive dependency, compulsive caregiving, and defensive separation attachment styles). In sum, a security-enhancing marital relationship and an insecure attachment style are independently predictive of CG symptoms. Not surprisingly, loss of close familial relationships (e.g., parent–child and spousal) is the best predictor of CG reactions (Cleiren, Diekstra, Kerkhof, and van der Wal, 1994; Prigerson et al., 2002).

There is accumulating evidence to suggest that adverse early life experiences such as parental loss and abuse in childhood may be associated with vulnerability to later-life bereavement difficulties (Prigerson et al., 1997; Silverman et al., 2001). Although speculative, such adversity may be operative by influencing the development of insecure attachment styles. Attachment disturbances may cause or exacerbate fears of abandonment, impulsivity, or difficulties with affect modulation which may become active when one is faced with the loss of a security-enhancing relationship (Prigerson et al., 1997). These reactions can ultimately result in a complicated, enduring pathological grief reaction.

Finally, there is some evidence to suggest that gender may be associated with differential susceptibility to CG following the death of a loved one. In a recent study of mental and physical health outcomes following the death of a spouse, widows had significantly higher symptoms of depression, anxiety, and CG relative to widowers (Chen et al., 1999).

TREATMENT FOR COMPLICATED GRIEF

Despite the fact that CG represents a relatively recent conceptualization of disordered functioning following bereavement, observations of severe or enduring pathological grief reactions have been noted in the clinical literature for decades (e.g, Freud, 1917/1953; Lindemann, 1944). Accordingly, there have been numerous therapeutic interventions spawned by clinicians from diverse theoretical perspectives to treat pathological grief reactions. As a general rule, the bulk of these interventions reported in the literature have not been evaluated in the context of controlled clinical trials; thus it is difficult to evaluate their efficacy. Nevertheless, some controlled trials of bereavement-specific interventions have been published, and a brief review of seemingly beneficial yet diverse interventions may be fruitful in identifying common "curative" elements.

Brief psychodynamic therapies have been used to treat recently bereaved individuals and have demonstrated significant symptom reductions over time (Horowitz, Marmar, Weiss, De Witt, & Rosenbaum, 1984; Marmar, Horowitz, Weiss, Wilner, & Kaltreider, 1988). However, active treatment conditions in these investigations did not exhibit symptom improvement that was appreciably greater than controls. Accordingly, it is not clear that treatment facilitated symptom improvement above and beyond that which may be expected as a function of the passage of time.

Behavior therapies for CG reactions have tended to focus on systematic exposure to avoided bereavement-related cues and reminders. These "guided mourning" interventions have generally been associated with significant reductions in "emotional distress" (not CG symptoms, per se) following bereavement. Once again, however, the data are somewhat mixed, with some investigations showing active treatment groups to improve significantly relative to controls (e.g., Mawson, Marks, Ramm, & Stern, 1981) and some showing comparable symptom reductions among treatment and control conditions (e.g., Sireling, Cohen, & Marks, 1988). In a study comparing an exposure-based behavioral intervention, hypnosis, and a brief psychodynamic therapy, all groups improved significantly relative to no-treatment controls (Kleber & Brom, 1987), suggesting that therapeutic contact for those experiencing psychological distress secondary to bereavement is superior to improvement that may be expected with the passage of time, though, again, these studies did not examine the effects of the treatments on the symptoms of CG explicitly. In contrast to many other investigations, a substantial proportion of participants in this study had experienced the loss of a loved one due to traumatic or otherwise unexpected causes, and all individuals were deemed to be experiencing "pathological grief." Accordingly, participants in this investigation were less likely to be experiencing uncomplicated courses of grief, and it may be that the majority of participants were experiencing psychological distress, including PTSD symptoms, that was unlikely to remit on its own over time.

Behavioral interventions' focus on exposure to avoided bereavement may not be fully instrumental in accounting for postbereavement improvement in light of recent research indicating that avoidance may not be especially common or influential in the development of CG (Horowitz et al., 1997; Spooren et al., 2000). Dismantling research would provide a test of the utility of this particular component relative to other components in behavioral treatment packages for bereavement. It may be that although CG is not generally characterized by marked avoidance, certain individuals (e.g., those who lost a loved one to an act of violence) experience greater levels of avoidance and that exposure-based interventions are more efficacious for this subset of individuals experiencing CG reactions by helping to reduce co-occurring PTSD symptomatology. Perhaps studies that have documented superior treatment gains using exposure-based methods have targeted samples endorsing higher levels of avoidance. This possibility remains to be empirically investigated.

Although therapy generally appears to be helpful in the amelioration of bereavement-related distress, no particular form of intervention has been shown to be superior. There are two (not necessarily mutually exclusive) implications that may be gleaned from this fact. First, it has been suggested that the nonspecific factors common to virtually all forms of psychotherapy are responsible for alleviating psychological distress stemming from bereavement (Raphael, Middleton, Martinek, & Misso, 1993), and that specific techniques may be less important. It may be that the compassionate, genuine, empathic relationship with the therapist is particularly important given that the source of the distress is the loss of a security-enhancing relationship. The therapist may help to fill this void to some small extent which may be partially responsible for treatment gains. Second, it seems quite reasonable to suppose that the optimal intervention for CG has yet to be developed. Because interventions to date have generally focused on symptoms of other disorders which may ensue following the death of a loved one as opposed to specifically targeting unique features of CG, it is possible that most trials of bereavement interventions have used less than optimal interventions and that future treatments tailored specifically to symptoms of CG will prove to be more efficacious (Jacobs & Prigerson, 2000).

What constitutes a CG-specific intervention? Recently, Shear et al. (2001) published pilot data for an intervention designed specifically to target symptoms of CG. The intervention was applied only to individuals experiencing significant symptoms of CG and consisted of 16 weekly sessions of individual therapy. The intervention included imaginal and *in vivo* exposure to cues and situations that the bereaved individual had been avoiding. Interpersonal therapy methods were also used to facilitate social reengagement and processing the meaning of the loss. In addition, patients provided a history of the relationship, provided an account of the circumstances surrounding the death, and described present relationships. A psychoeducational component was included to familiarize patients with symptoms of CG. Individually tailored hierarchies of avoided situations were obtained and imaginal and *in vivo* exposure exercises were conducted. The imaginal exercises were tape-recorded and patients were instructed to listen to these daily between sessions as homework assignments. Both the completer group (13 of 21 who began therapy) and the intent-to-treat participants exhibited significant reductions in symptoms of CG, depression, and anxiety. Although the sample was small, the methods were eclectic and in the process of development and standardization, and it was not a controlled clinical trial, the authors noted that several patients demonstrated improvement when they had not benefited from the receipt of prior interventions.

Interventions should target those individuals who experience severe or protracted grief responses rather than bereavement generally. We wish to emphasize that we are not advocating interventions for all people surviving the death of a significant other because we recognize that the vast majority of bereavement individuals adapt effectively over time without the need for professional intervention. The majority of individuals experiencing the loss of a loved one will not experience CG, and severe acute distress that they may be experiencing following the death will typically abate over time without treatment. Previous studies that failed to document significant treatment gains in therapy conditions, relative to controls, may indeed have employed effective interventions, but if the control group exhibited significant spontaneous remission due to the normal course of bereavement (i.e., if the intervention was applied to any or all recently bereaved individuals instead of intervening only with those experiencing particularly severe or enduring grief reactions), it would be difficult to document a clinically significant treatment gain. Indeed, a recent meta-analysis of bereavement interventions (Neimeyer, 2000) revealed that bereavement interventions have been associated with very modest effects ($d = .13$). However, the average effect size of interventions which specifically targeted complicated bereavement reactions was three times as large ($d = .39$, which may be regarded as a medium effect size). Accordingly, it appears that treatment effects may be diluted if interventions are applied to any and all bereaved individuals, as most of these individuals would experience a significant remission of symptoms in the absence of treatment. Intervening only with individuals unlikely to exhibit such remission spontaneously would likely make it easier to document gains for truly effective treatments and would also be a more judicious use of limited clinical resources.

In terms of traumatic loss, the challenge for the future is to find ways of identifying individuals most at risk for CG and to provide a secondary prevention intervention specifically designed to reduce the risk for chronic CG. However, much more research is needed to identify individuals who will have the most difficulty adjusting to unpredictable and unexplainable loss on their own, over time. As is the case in the trauma field, in the absence of more conclusive risk factor research and randomized controlled trials of early interventions for CG in those most at risk, the most prudent and rational approach is to provide psychological first aid to anyone who suffers a tragic loss (especially a loss by means of malicious violence) and to provide information about the signs and symptoms of CG for victims and support persons to appeal to in the coming months, postloss. The recommendation would be that as soon as symptoms of grief become unmanageable and as soon as there are significant problems reestablishing preloss levels of functioning, the person should be evaluated for treatment to prevent chronic CG. The intervention would be an amalgam of standard therapies, cognitive-behavioral approaches, and interpersonal treatment.

CONCLUSIONS

Although mental health professionals have long recognized that some bereaved individuals can have particularly severe or enduring complications following the death of a loved one, researchers and clinicians have tended to focus rather narrowly on grief reactions which mimic other disorders (i.e., MDD and PTSD) while failing to attend to unique bereavement-specific reactions. Although grieving individuals may endorse symptoms of MDD or PTSD, it has become apparent that CG is distinct from both disorders and that a substantial proportion of individuals experiencing complicated courses of bereavement fail to meet criteria for PTSD or MDD. Accordingly, an exclusive focus on these symptoms following a death may fail to identify numerous highly distressed individuals. Similarly, mental health professionals have become increasingly responsive to the psychological and emotional needs of victims of large-scale disasters and other traumatic events involving the loss of life. However, such attention has often focused exclusively on PTSD (as evidenced by outcomes measured in early intervention studies) and comparatively little attention has been paid to grief and bereavement issues that may result from such tremendous loss of life. Certainly, severe emotional distress following such events should not be pathologized. Profound grief following a trauma resulting in the death of a loved one is inevitable and is indisputably a normal human reaction to a horrific event. Most individuals will experience a gradual remission of symptoms and will be able to resume adaptive (if not pre-bereavement) functioning using their existing social supports and coping strategies. Many individuals, however, will experience unremitting symptoms of CG in the absence of formal intervention, and this is especially true for events involving tremendous loss of life such as incidents of mass violence, plane crashes, and so forth.

In the immediate aftermath of such an event, mental health professionals may promote adaptive recovery by educating victims about normal and CG reactions, providing information about common maladaptive coping strategies, encouraging utilization of existing social supports, and informing victims about mental health services that are available if victims feel that they need more support. Moreover, although formal assessment in the immediate wake of such events is likely futile given that most survivors will be experiencing significant emotional distress as a normal human reaction to trauma, it may be possible in the future to screen for risk factors for CG in order to identify individuals who are likely to experience protracted grief reactions. At present, formal interventions for CG should include the treatment components reviewed previously, although the next decade will likely witness significant advances in the development of formalized treatment for CG. Additional complications in the course of bereavement or additional treatment implications as a function of the circumstances of death (e.g., traumatic vs. natural causes) may become apparent with additional empirical research. Regardless, traumatic events, which entail loss of life, should not narrow a clinician's focus exclusively to PTSD. If a traumatic event is compounded by the loss of life, it is imperative that mental health professionals attend to the unique needs of the bereaved and consider equally distressing but oft-neglected CG reactions.

REFERENCES

American Psychiatric Association. (1994). *Diagnostic and statistical manual of mental disorders* (4th ed.). Washington, DC: Author.

Bowlby, J. (1963). Pathological mourning and childhood mourning. *Journal of the American Psychoanalytic Association, 11,* 500–541.

Breslau, N., Kessler, R., Chilcoat, H., Schultz, L., Davis, G., & Andreski, P. (1998). Trauma and posttraumatic stress disorder in the community: The 1996 Detroit area survey of trauma. *Archives of General Psychiatry, 55,* 626–632.

Chen, J. H., Bierhals, A. J., Prigerson, H. G., Kasl, S. V., Mazure, C. M., & Jacobs, S. (1999). Gender differences in the effects of bereavement-related psychological distress in health outcomes. *Psychological Medicine, 29,* 367–380.

Cleiren, M., Diekstra, R., Kerkhof, A., & van der Wal, J. (1994). Mode of death and kinship in bereavement: Focusing on the "who" rather than the "how." *Crisis, 15,* 22–36.

Freud, S. (1953). Mourning and melancholia. *The standard edition of the complete psychological works of Sigmund Freud* (Vol. 14) (James Strachey, ed., in collaboration with Anna Freud). London: Hogarth. (Original work published 1917)

Green, B. (2000). Traumatic loss: Conceptual and empirical links between trauma and bereavement. *Journal of Personal and Interpersonal Loss, 5,* 1–17.

Green, B., Krupnick, J., Stockton, P., Goodman, L. Corcoran, C., & Petty, R. (2001). Psychological outcomes associated with a traumatic loss in a sample of young women. *American Behavioral Scientist, 44,* 817–837.

Herman, J. (1992). Complex PTSD: A syndrome in survivors of prolonged and repeated trauma. *Journal of Traumatic Stress, 5,* 377–391.

Horowitz, M., Marmar, C., Weiss, D., DeWitt, K., & Rosenbaum, R. (1984). Brief psychotherapy of bereavement reactions: The relationship of process to outcome. *Archives of General Psychiatry, 41,* 418–438.

Horowitz, M. J., Siegel, B., Holen, A., Bonanno, G. A., Milbrath, C., & Stinson, C. H. (1997). Diagnostic criteria for complicated grief disorder. *American Journal of Psychiatry, 154,* 904–910.

Jacobs, S. (1987). Psychoendocrine aspects of bereavement. In S. Zisook (Ed.), *Biopsychosocial aspects of bereavement.* Washington, DC: American Psychiatric Association Press.

Jacobs, S., Mazure, C., & Prigerson, H. (2000). Diagnostic criteria for traumatic grief. *Death Studies, 24,* 185–200.

Jacobs, S., & Prigerson, H. (2000). Psychotherapy of traumatic grief: A review of evidence for psychotherapeutic treatments. *Death Studies, 24,* 479–496.

Kessler, R., Sonnega, A., Bromet, E., & Nelson, C. (1995). Posttraumatic stress disorder in the National Comorbidity Survey. *Archives of General Psychiatry, 52,* 1048–1060.

Kleber, R., & Brom, D. (1987). Psychotherapy and pathological grief: Controlled outcome study. *Israeli Journal of Psychiatry and Related Sciences, 24,* 99–109.

Lindemann, E. (1944). Symptomatology and management of acute grief. *American Journal of Psychiatry, 101,* 141–148.

Marmar, C., Horowitz, M., Weiss, D., Wilner, N., & Kaltreider, N. (1988). A controlled trial of brief psychotherapy and mutual help group treatment of conjugal bereavement. *American Journal of Psychiatry, 145,* 203–209.

Mawson, D., Marks, I., Ramm, L., & Stern, R. (1981). Guided mourning for morbid grief: A controlled study. *British Journal of Psychiatry, 138,* 185–193.

McCann, I., Sakheim, D., & Abrahamson, D. (1988). Trauma and victimization: A model of psychological adaptation. *The Counseling Psychologist, 16,* 531–594.

McDermott, O., Prigerson, H., & Reynolds, C. (1997). EEG sleep in complicated grief and bereavement-related depression: A preliminary report. *Biological Psychiatry, 41,* 710–716.

Neimeyer, R. (2000). Searching for the meaning of grief: Grief therapy and the process of reconstruction. *Death Studies, 24,* 541–558.

Parkes, C. M., & Brown, R. (1972). Health after bereavement: A controlled study of young Boston widows and widowers. *Psychosomatic Medicine, 34,* 449–461.

Pasternak, R. E., Reynolds, C. F., Schlernitzauer, M., Hoch, C. C., Buysse, D. J., Houck, P. R., & Perel, J. M. (1991). Acute open-trial nortriptyline therapy of bereavement-related depression in late life. *Journal of Clinical Psychiatry, 52,* 307–310.

Prigerson, H., Ahmed, I., Silverman, G., Saxena, A., Maciejewski, P., Jacobs, S., Kasl, S., & Hamirani, M. (2002). Rates and risks of complicated grief among psychiatric clinic patients in Karachi, Pakistan. *Death Studies, 26,* 781–792.

Prigerson, H. G., Bierhals, A. J., Kasl, S. V., Reynolds, C. F. III, Shear, M. K., Day, N., Beery, L. C., Newsom, J. T., & Jacobs, S. (1997). Traumatic grief as a risk factor for mental and physical morbidity. *American Journal of Psychiatry, 154,* 616–623.

Prigerson, H. G., Bierhals, A. J., Kasl, S. V., Reynolds, C. F. III, Shear, M. K., Newsom, J. T., & Jacobs, S. (1996). Complicated grief as a disorder distinct from bereavement-related depression and anxiety: A replication study. *American Journal of Psychiatry, 153,* 1484–1486.

Prigerson, H. G., Bridge, J., Maciejewski, P. K., Beery, L. C., Rosenheck, R. A., Jacobs, S. C., Bierhals, A. J., Kupfer, D. J., & Brent, D. A. (1999). Influence of traumatic grief on suicidal ideation among young adults. *American Journal of Psychiatry, 156,* 1994–1995.

Prigerson, H. G., Frank, E., Kasl, S. V., Reynolds, C. F. III, Anderson, B., Zubenko, G. S., Houck, P. R., George, C. J., & Kupfer, D. J. (1995). Complicated grief and bereavement-related depression as distinct disorders: Preliminary validation in elderly bereaved spouses. *American Journal of Psychiatry, 152,* 22–30.

Prigerson, H. G., & Jacobs, S. C. (2001). Caring for bereaved patients: "All the doctors just suddenly go." *Journal of the American Medical Association, 286,* 1369–1376.

Prigerson, H. G., Shear, M. K., Jacobs, S., Kasl, S. V., Maciejewski, P. K., Silverman, G. K., Narayan, M., & Bremner, J. (2000). Grief and its relationship to PTSD. In D. Nutt, J. R. T. Davidson, & J. Zohar (Eds.), *Posttraumatic stress disorders: Diagnosis, management and treatment* (pp. 163–186). New York: Martin Dunitz.

Prigerson, H. G., Shear, M. K., Jacobs, S. C., Reynolds, C. F. III, Maciejewski, P. K., Davidson, J. R., Rosenheck, R., Pilkonis, P. A., Wortman, C. B., Williams, J. B., Widiger, T. A., Frank, E., Kupfer, D. J., & Zisook, S. (1999). Consensus criteria for traumatic grief: A preliminary empirical test. *British Journal of Psychiatry, 174,* 67–73.

Raphael, B., & Martinek, N. (1997). Assessing traumatic bereavement and posttraumatic stress disorder. In J. P. Wilson & T. M. Keane (Eds.), *Assessing psychological trauma and PTSD* (pp. 373–395). New York: Guilford Press.

Raphael, B., Middleton, W., Martinek, N., & Misso, V. (1993). Counseling and therapy of the bereaved. In M. S. Stroebe, W. Stroebe, & R. D. Hansson (Eds.), *Handbook of bereavement: Theory, research, and intervention* (pp. 587–612). Cambridge, UK: Cambridge University Press.

Rees, W. D. (1971). The hallucinations of widowhood. *British Medical Journal, 4,* 37–41.

Resick, P. A., & Calhoun, K. S. (2001). Posttraumatic stress disorder. In D. H. Barlow (Ed.), *Clinical handbook of psychological disorders* (3rd ed., pp. 60–113). New York: Guilford Press.

Reynolds, C. F., Miller, M. D., Pasternak, R. E., Frank, E., Perel, J. M., Cornes, C., Houck, P. R., Mazumdar, S., Dew, M. A., & Kupfer, D. J. (1999). Treatment of bereavement-related Major Depressive Episodes in later life: A controlled study of acute and continuation treatment with nortriptyline and interpersonal psychotherapy. *American Journal of Psychiatry, 152,* 202–208.

Schlenger, S., Caddell, J., Ebert, L., Jordan, B., Rourke, K., Wilson, D., Thalji, L., Dennis, J., Fairbank, J., & Kulka, R. (2002). Psychological reactions to terrorist attacks: Findings from the National Study of Americans' Reactions to September 11. *Journal of the American Medical Association, 288,* 581–588.

Shear, M. K., Frank, E., Foa, E., Cherry, C., Reynolds, C. F., Vander Bilt, J., & Masters, S. (2001). *American Journal of Psychiatry, 158,* 1506–1508.

Silverman, G. K., Jacobs, S. C., Kasl, S. V., Shear, M. K., Maciejewski, P. K., Noaghiul, F. S.,

& Prigerson, H. G. (2000). Quality of life impairments associated with diagnostic criteria for traumatic grief. *Psychological Medicine, 30,* 857–862.

Silverman, G., Johnson, J., & Prigerson, H. (2001). Preliminary explorations of the effects of prior trauma and loss on risk for psychiatric disorders in recently widowed people. *Israeli Journal of Psychiatry Related Sciences, 38,* 202–215.

Sireling, L., Cohen, D., & Marks, I. (1988). Guided mourning for morbid grief: A replication. *Behavior Therapy, 19,* 121–132.

Spooren, D., Henderick, H., & Jannes, C. (2000). A retrospective study of parents bereaved from a child in a traffic accident: Service satisfaction, available support and psychiatric sequelae. *Omega, 42,* 171–185.

Van Doorn, C., Kasl, S. V., Beery, L. C., Jacobs, S. C., & Prigerson, H. G. (1998). The influence of marital quality and attachment styles on traumatic grief and depressive symptoms. *Journal of Nervous and Mental Disease, 186,* 566–573.

Zlotnick, C., Zakriski, A., Shea, M., & Costello, E. (1996). The long-term sequelae of sexual abuse: Support for a complex posttraumatic stress disorder. *Journal of Traumatic Stress, 9,* 195–205.

II

Empirical Research
on Early Interventions
for Trauma and Traumatic Loss

5

Early Intervention for Trauma in Adults

A Framework for First Aid and Secondary Prevention

BRETT T. LITZ
MATT J. GRAY

In this chapter, we describe early intervention strategies for adults exposed to trauma and critically examine the empirical research on secondary prevention of chronic posttraumatic stress disorder (PTSD). We clarify conceptually the temporal parameters of posttrauma service delivery, discuss the importance of palliative and supportive first aid in the immediate aftermath of trauma, and underscore the need to separate first-aid services from formal secondary prevention interventions. We then describe psychological debriefing in detail and the controversies surrounding the use of critical incident stress debriefing (CISD). This description is followed by a discussion of the application of cognitive-behavioral therapy as a secondary prevention strategy. Throughout the chapter, we describe a number of specific issues that need further research and clarification.

We argue that the field of early intervention needs to be far more integrated and connected to advances in the scientific study of psychological trauma and advances in research on the treatment of PTSD. In the past, however, early intervention for trauma has been the specialized purview of clinicians who have studied, or trained in, the traditions of crisis intervention and grief counseling (e.g., Mitchell, 1983; Roberts, 1991). These approaches to early intervention have been widely applied in the past because of their compelling face validity, sensitivity, and awareness of organizational goals; the certification provided to professional care providers; and because, on average, survivors of trauma appreciate getting some kind of assistance, even if it does not improve their recovery (Litz, Gray, Bryant, & Adler, 2002). In addition, the need to provide some sort of supportive, palliative care in the face of disaster and trauma has far outweighed interest in, and concerns about, evidence supporting the efficacy of crisis intervention strategies. On the other side of the coin, early interventions have only recently been the subject of rigorous clinical research and there has been scant attention paid to conducting research on chronic PTSD that could translate to the early intervention context.

We argue that if designed as a vehicle to reduce risk for chronic posttraumatic psychopathology (secondary prevention), early intervention practices that do not have a sound evidentiary base should not promoted. However, at present, there are more empirical questions about early intervention that have gone unaddressed or unanswered than there is evidence to definitively support various methods. Because there is no question that most people adapt to trauma on their own, over time, the danger is that the field of early intervention reverts insidiously to assumptions and actions that may prove destructive in the long run. For example, it would be inappropriate to conclude that as most people adjust to extreme trauma on their own, everyone should be left alone until those most vulnerable to chronic posttraumatic problems seek care on down the line. We also do not want to deny the suffering of those who develop posttraumatic difficulties by blaming them for some personal inadequacy, which would be horrendously stigmatizing and decrease help seeking. On the other hand, it is inappropriate and untenable to prescribe formal secondary prevention services to everyone exposed to trauma. To work toward redressing this quandary, we describe a set of palliative and information-sharing strategies that are appropriate for all who survive trauma and a set of interventions designed to prevent chronic PTSD in those most at risk.

To contextualize strategies for early intervention, we first summarize the history of early intervention for trauma and the treatment of posttraumatic stress. This will provide a backdrop to appreciate the genesis and attractiveness of early intervention for trauma.

A BRIEF HISTORY OF EARLY INTERVENTION FOR TRAUMA

Modern early intervention for trauma and the treatment of PTSD have direct roots in practices initiated during and immediately after World War I and World War II especially. Soldiers in both of these wars who were traumatized or exhausted were told that their reactions were normal and that they would be able to return to combat. They were given immediate respite and rest as close to their unit as possible (see Salmon, 1919, for the original concepts). This directly parallels modern notions of crisis intervention and psychological debriefing, especially the provision of early interventions to emergency services personnel who reenter dangerous circumstances (e.g., firefighters; Flannery & Everly, 2000), as well as the modern soldiers engaging in combat (Solomon & Benbenishty, 1986). It was a common assumption in military psychiatry that soldiers who were incapacitated in battle or during redeployment were impaired because they had repressed their memories of the horrors they witnessed in battle. To treat such a condition, psychiatrists would prompt soldiers to disclose the emotional details of their combat memories (e.g., Grinker & Spiegel, 1945; Kardiner, 1941). This was, at times, facilitated by the use of sodium amobarbitol, a barbiturate, which produced a relaxed and hynogogic state that prompted uninhibited and spontaneous sharing of traumatic memories (see Karon & Widener, 1997). In a related fashion, Dollard and Miller (1950) were the first to systematically describe (and apply) a treatment for posttraumatic pathology that employed principles of human learning and conditioning, which presaged modern cognitive-behavioral treatments for PTSD and several components of psychological debriefing. They had traumatized World War II veterans disclose their painful memories of combat, repeatedly, which produced systematic reductions in negative affect and avoidance.

Also during the World War II era, the concept of debriefing was developed and implemented by Marshall (1950; see Shalev, 1994), which is standard operating procedure in the armed forces and various law enforcement agencies to this day (e.g. Williams, 1990). Debriefing, which is a precursor to modern psychological debriefing, entailed having all soldiers in a unit gather in a group, as soon as possible after an incident (e.g., loss of a comrade in a battle), to discuss the event in great detail. During a debriefing, rank was set aside and all opinions were respected. Emotional reactions from soldiers were recognized and validated. The "debriefer" or leader created an empathic and congenial atmosphere to facilitate communication and openness. Debriefing was seen as a method of creating a historical record, learning lessons from battle, building trust, group cohesion, and morale, as well as motivating troops to return to hazardous duty.

The central tenets of CISD, influenced by Marshall's original concepts, are groups of individuals with similar exposure to danger/tragedy experienced as a result of occupational demands (e.g., police officers), getting together soon after a traumatic event to give a systematic and detailed account of experiences and feelings surrounding the event (see Mitchell & Everly, 1996). However, the concept of operational debriefing is designed to meet organizational goals (to gather facts about mission execution, maintain combat readiness, etc.) and does not serve a mental health function (e.g., to assist soldiers to cope with trauma and reduce risk for chronic posttraumatic pathology). During this time, debriefings performed to improve mental health normalized and accepted reactions to trauma in order to motivate soldiers to face their fears and dread and to instill the expectation that, regardless of the quality or severity of psychological reaction, return to combat was expected. It has been argued that in work cultures (e.g., firefighters), CISD may be attractive because it provides operational debriefing (e.g., Litz et al., 2002). CISD may meet organizational mandates because the normality of any response to trauma and the expectation that return to work is expected are emphasized. In addition, CISD provides services which are completely integrated into the work culture (e.g., mandated by management and approved by immediate supervisors, peer cointervention). However, contrary to intended goals, CISD does not necessarily affect long-term adaptation to trauma.

THE SCOPE AND IMPACT OF TRAUMA: WHY IS EARLY INTERVENTION SO IMPORTANT?

In the last decade, there has been a tremendous proliferation of research on the acute and chronic impact of all types of trauma across the lifespan. Epidemiological studies revealed that the risk for exposure to trauma in the general population of the United States is very high. In a community survey of young adults enrolled in a health maintenance organization (HMO) in the Midwest, Breslau, Davis, Andreski, and Peterson (1991) found that more than one-third of respondents had experienced at least one traumatic event. In a survey of exposure to trauma in four different cities in the Southeast, Norris (1992) found that two-thirds of participants had experienced at least one trauma at some time during their life and that one-fifth had been exposed to trauma in the past year. In a nationwide study, Resnick, Kilpatrick, Dansky, Saunders, and Best (1993) found that women reported a wide range of criminal victimization experiences, such as being sexually and physically assaulted, and close to 70% of respondents had experienced one or more victimizations across the lifespan. In the National Comorbidity Study, Kessler and colleagues, found that

60.7% of men and 51.2% of women reported exposure to at least one traumatic event across their lifetime (Kessler, Sonnega, Bromet, Hughes, & Nelson, 1995).

Not all traumas are equally likely across the lifespan, which suggests that preparation and planning for early intervention needs to take into account relative risk of exposure for various populations. For example, Breslau et al. (1998) found that 37% of respondents reported a physical assault of some kind (such as rape, torture, or military combat), 59% experienced some other traumatic personal injury or severely stressful experience (e.g., motor vehicle accident, disaster, life-threatening illness, or witnessing a traumatic event), 60% experienced the sudden, unexpected death of a loved one, and 62% lived through a traumatic experience suffered by a loved one (e.g., family member assaulted or spouse seriously injured in an accident).

If everyone exposed to trauma was equally at risk for developing PTSD and other impairments in functioning as a result of trauma, then early intervention for trauma would be a straightforward process. In the ideal case, everyone would be advised to receive an early preventive intervention that was proven to prevent chronic PTSD. However, epidemiological studies of posttraumatic adjustment have revealed that the large majority of victims of trauma are remarkably resilient, and only a small percentage are at risk for developing chronic PTSD. After a variable interval of disrupted functioning, most individuals exposed to trauma do not develop chronic posttraumatic mental health problems (e.g., Rothbaum, Foa, Riggs, Murdock, & Walsh, 1992). Breslau et al. (1991) found that 11% of Detroit-area HMO enrollees had PTSD. Resnick et al. (1993) found that 12% of women exposed to physical and sexual assaults reported a lifetime history of PTSD. In the National Comorbidity Study, 8% of respondents had a lifetime history of PTSD (Kessler et al., 1995). Some traumatic experiences pose considerably higher risk for PTSD than others. For example, physical assaults and other forms of interpersonal violence as well as violence to significant others that resulted in loss are associated with substantially higher risk for PTSD (e.g., Breslau et al., 1998).

Generally, the psychological risks from exposure to trauma are proportional to the magnitude or severity of exposure, and the degree of life threat and malicious intent involved (e.g., Green, 1994). For example, people who lived below Canal Street in New York City were three times as likely to have PTSD 1 to 2 months after the attack on the World Trade Center, relative to individuals who lived in northern Manhattan (Galea et al., 2002). The extent to which individuals witness grotesque human suffering and the extent of loss of personal resources are additional event-related characteristics that moderate risk for chronic PTSD (e.g., Green, Grace, Lindy, Gleser, & Leonard, 1990; McCarroll, Urasano, & Fullerton, 1994). Finally, the degree of preparation and predictability of events affects outcome—emergency services personnel fair better than direct victims of trauma, as do combat soldiers when compared to refugees and other victims of war.

A number of individual vulnerabilities have also been shown to moderate risk for PTSD. For example, individuals who have a history of psychiatric problems (in particular, depression), poor coping resources or capacities, and past history of trauma and mistreatment are at increased risk (e.g., Breslau et al., 1998; Freedman, Brandes, Peri, & Shalev, 1999; North et al., 1999; Shalev, Peri, Canetti, & Schreiber, 1996). Individuals who show intense and frequent symptoms of acute stress disorder (particularly, severe hyperarousal; Shalev, Freedman, Peri, Brandes, & Sahar, 1997) in the weeks following trauma are particularly at risk for chronic PTSD (e.g., Harvey & Bryant, 1999), although the mechanisms responsible for this are uncertain. In addition, the quality and breadth of supports in the recovery context and beyond can affect risk for PTSD. This research suggests that the people who need early intervention most are the ones who are isolated and cannot get the respite they may need, have few secure and reliable outlets for unburdening their experiences, and receive little or no validation in the weeks, months, and years following exposure to trauma (e.g., Foy, Sipprelle, Rueger, & Carroll, 1984; Keane, Scott, Chavoya, Lamparski, & Fairbank, 1985; Martin, Rosen, Durand, Knudson, & Stretch, 2000; Pennebaker & O'Heeron, 1984).

Thus, posttraumatic mental health problems are caused by a complex set of interrelated factors (e.g., King, King, Fairbank, Keane, & Adams, 1998). Effective early intervention for those victims who will have more than a brief disruption in functioning would be greatly facilitated by screening those who are at risk for chronic PTSD. However, attention to risk factors has been ignored by the majority of practitioners and planners (until recently, e.g., Everly, 2000). Typically in the history of psychological debriefing, it was believed that everyone exposed to trauma required early intervention, because, if unaddressed (not shared and emotionally processed), trauma would cause PTSD (Mitchell & Everly, 1996). To be fair, it is difficult, in most traumatic contexts, to implement a screening program. However, given the state of the field, logistical and practical problems with screening need to be worked out operationally (see Wright, Huffman, Adler, & Castro, 2002).

Although PTSD is the modal pathological response to trauma, it is often comorbid with depression, other anxiety disorders, and substance abuse (Breslau et al., 1991; Kulka et al., 1988). Thus, early intervention may serve to reduce the risk for a host of mental health problems (although this hypothesis needs to be assessed in clinical trials). Because research has shown that different traumas, experienced at different developmental periods, present dissimilar psychosocial sequelae, early interventions also need to be tailored to the unique exigencies and risks of different trauma contexts. For example, natural and technological disasters usually destroy resources used to sustain well-being (e.g., housing; Norris et al., 2002). Interpersonal trauma such as sexual assault can result in generalized negative beliefs about trust and safety, which can be debilitating (e.g., Koss, 1993).

There is increasing recognition that early intervention is critical because chronic PTSD is pernicious and disabling across the lifespan (e.g., Green, Lindy, et al., 1990; Kulka et al., 1988). Most patients with chronic PTSD do not seek or receive services for their condition, as a result of other pressing priorities, the availability and knowledge of treatment resources, income disparities, stigma, and shame (e.g., Kessler et al., 1995). Although 38% of individuals with PTSD are likely to be receiving mental health treatment at a given point in time, this group remains chronic and resistant to treatment (Kessler et al., 1995). Finally, it should be noted that the individual and societal costs associated with PTSD are very high. A history of PTSD is associated with risk of suicide attempts, failures in educational achievement, marital instability, and downward spirals in social and occupational functioning (e.g., Kessler et al., 1995; Kulka et al., 1988). This remains the most important argument for early preventive interventions for trauma.

TEMPORAL PARAMETERS IN THE PROCESS OF TRAUMA RECOVERY

There is no consensus about the optimal time frame for providing different types of early mental health interventions for trauma. Although it is safe to say that early intervention for trauma is indicated, the field is uncertain with respect to the complex synergy of issues of timing (when), intervention options (what), and selection (with whom). First and foremost, we feel it is important to distinguish the period of acute adaptation from that period in which the immediate psychological and biological impact of trauma is still manifest. We propose to call the first interval the *immediate impact phase*, in contrast with the *acute phase*, in which individuals are better prepared to receive secondary prevention interventions. We argue that it is inappropriate to consider formal secondary prevention interventions during the immediate impact phase of response to trauma. For secondary prevention interventions to be effective, the recipient needs to be an active participant in a process of learning, reframing, and implementing a plan of action, as occupational, interpersonal, and self-care demands emerge over time (Litz et al., 2002; Shalev, 2002). The immediate impact phase is not a time in which a person can listen carefully, absorb new information, and appreciate the nuances and the demands ahead of them to promote recovery. The immediate impact phase is also a time when the traumatized person may not be able to articulate his or her experience in a fashion that could be therapeutic, especially to a relative stranger even if he or she is empathic and supportive.

There are virtually no studies of the phenomenology and time course of the immediate response to trauma. To appreciate the complex immediate aftermath of trauma, we have to infer from retrospective reports of trauma survivors, clinician observations of disaster response, and what is known about the effects of severe stress on human performance. Although there are tremendous individual differences, the traumatic stress reaction entails extreme activation of physiological and psychological resources designed to mobilize the person to respond to life threat and any uncontrollable, intense, or sustained threat to psychological integrity (such as severe dehumanization, humiliation, and degradation), a variety of negative affects (e.g., dread, anger, and horror), intense feelings of vulnerability, powerlessness, and loss of control, as well as depersonalization and derealization—being in a daze, depression, despair, and withdrawal (e.g., Herman, 1992; Horowitz, 1986; Rothbaum et al., 1992; Solomon, Laor, Weiler, & Muller, 1993; Shalev et al., 1996; Weiss, Marmar, Metzler, & Ronfeldt, 1995). In addition, the immediate impact phase is characterized by the behavioral and emotional effects of circulating epinephrine and cortisol (stress hormones), which sustain the alarm reaction (jitteriness, hypervigilance, sleep disruption, appetite suppression, etc.). These physiological and psychological states drain coping capacities, narrow or dull attention, reduce learning capacity, and affect organization of thought and experience (e.g., Christianson, 1992; Eysenck & Calvo, 1992).

It is best to be conservative with respect to estimating how long the immediate impact of trauma exposure lasts. We define the time frame for the immediate impact phase to be from the time the person is objectively safe to 2 days posttrauma. This corresponds with the 48-hour interval for an *acute stress reaction* in the 10th edition of the *International Classification of Diseases* (ICD-10; World Health Organization, 1992). Of course, there will be gray area instances in which the person is still exposed to the possibility of threat or harm to self or others—in these cases, the threat response would linger. Also, if the trauma entails loss of physical capacities (e.g., burns and injuries) or loss of significant personal resources (housing, money, food, clothing, etc.), that, if present, would promote recovery, then this time frame will expand accordingly. In addition, mental health interventions need to be secondary to efforts to secure safety and to address basic needs, which is consistent with the recommendations of the American Red Cross (1998). In addition, if the trauma entailed physical or sexual assault, safety planning and emergency stabilization should take precedence over efforts to address psychological or emotional needs (e.g., Resnick, Acierno, Holmes, Dammeyer, & Kilpatrick, 2000).

What do people need in the immediate aftermath of trauma? The answer to this question may come, for the most part, from what we would envision doing immediately after someone we love is exposed to trauma. We would ask the person what he or she needed and empower that person to decide the kind of help he or she wanted. We would provide soothing comfort, respectful and well-timed physical touch (e.g., handholding, a hug), and we would do our best to remain calm. We would accurately convey the person's experiences and we would be extremely accepting and validating. We would emphasize that that person is not alone and that we are there to help him or her. We would provide information relevant to recovery, assist with problem solving, and seek professional assistance when necessary. We would work toward reducing stigma and shame. We would not be intrusive and we would not pressure the person to disclose what happened unless he or she felt the need to. These supportive, caring, and empathic responses lie on a continuum. At the other end of the continuum are recovery environments that are impoverished, punitive, blaming, demanding, anxious, and invalidating; features that create risk for chronic PTSD (e.g., Bolton, Litz, Glenn, Orsillo, & Roemer, 2002).

The type of support that individuals need in the immediate impact phase is "psychological first aid," a term first employed by Beverley Raphael (1977; 1986), which is supportive and noninterventionist and not offered as "therapy" or "treatment." Formal mental health intervention, advice, interpretation, or other directive interventions are not to be provided during the immediate impact phase. The goal of psychological first aid is *not* to maximize therapeutic emotional processing of horrific events, as in exposure therapy (see later) but, rather, to respond to the acute need that arises in many to share their experience, at the same time respecting those who do not wish to discuss what happened (Litz et al., 2002). Added to the list of emotional support methods described previously is the goal of providing information to individuals about what they can reasonably expect in the days and weeks ahead (see U.S. Consensus Workshop on Mass Violence and Early Intervention, 2001). If feasible, clinicians should inquire briefly and respectfully about known risk factors for chronic PTSD. For example, prior trauma can be evaluated by asking the person, "Has anything like this ever happened to you before?" If the person spontaneously reports a history of severe psychological problems, if it is clear that there are inadequate social supports and ongoing stressors, and the person suffered severe exposure to particularly grotesque aspects of the event, including fatalities or salient harm, then it is prudent to offer and schedule early intervention services for a period after the immediate recovery phase has passed. If early intervention is indicated, information should also be provided about what should trigger help seeking after a few days have passed. The clinician should also find out how the person is going to take care of him- or herself in the days ahead; if necessary, the person should be prompted to find respite and to reduce demands.

One could argue that psychological first aid could be provided by significant others, and in many cases this is true. On the other hand, formal professional training in the provision of psychological first aid can be useful for several reasons. First, in some situations, people do not have available significant others, their significant others are also traumatized, or the trauma has made it difficult for them to take advantage of support systems (e.g., Riggs, Byrne, Weathers, & Litz, 1998; Solomon, Mikulincer, & Avitzur, 1988). Second, professional training is appropriate because the person providing the psychological first aid would be guaranteed to know what *not* to do (i.e., not be intrusive and demanding of self-disclosure)—some bystanders, or untrained emergency medical professionals may inadvertently be intrusive or demanding, which can be destructive. On the other hand, given that the immediate impact lasts days, sustained respectful and accommodating social support in the natural recovery environment is of obvious importance. Professionals can provide information (e.g., handouts and public service announcements) and formal education regarding recovery needs to significant others.

In an ideal world, everyone exposed to trauma would receive some kind of psychological first aid that matches the needs of the individual in the immediate impact phase. However, the scope of the traumatic events and the availability of resources affect the capacity for planning and implementing a psychological first-aid strategy. Not everyone can be offered psychological first aid and, thankfully, at least from a public health perspective, because of natural resourcefulness and resilience, not everyone needs it. Even in the context of the attack on the World Trade Center in Manhattan on 9-11-01, the majority of individuals who suffered direct trauma on that day did not receive any formal intervention, and, a year after the event, the prevalence rates for PTSD were about 10% (e.g., Galea et al., 2002). Nevertheless, there are traumatic contexts in which resources should be (and typically are) provided routinely for psychological first aid to promote recovery and service seeking (emergency room consultations with victims of violent crime and sexual assault, death notification, etc.).

It is important to underscore that there is little or no research on the effects of psychological first aid and there has been no research that has systematically explored the optimal timing interval for intervention. Although there is ample conceptual justification for psychological first aid on theoretical and human grounds, empirical research is needed to determine demonstrable and measurable impact. Improvements should be expected in perceived social support, reduced stigma, increased help seeking, and understanding and acceptance of experience. Finally, it should be noted that the immediate impact phase is a period in which basic stress management procedures and medical interventions designed to reduce arousal may be appropriate and effective (see Pitman et al., 2002).

Early preventive psychological interventions should be offered only to individuals who are at risk after the immediate impact phase has passed. Because most people are distraught initially, there is no way of knowing whether the transient reaction reflects a risk factor for chronicity. That would require a clinical assessment to determine risk at an inappropriate time for such an inquiry. In addition, the absence of visible expressions of intense emotional reaction does not necessarily signal risk. During the *acute phase* of recovery from trauma, secondary prevention interventions should be employed for those at risk for chronic posttraumatic difficulties. We define the acute phase as the interval after the immediate phase is over to 1 month posttrauma. As with the definition of the time frame for the immediate impact phase, the time frame prescribed for the acute phase is a working heuristic model rather than an absolute recommendation. Because acute stress disorder (ASD) is a major risk factor for chronic PTSD, the outer limit for the acute phase corresponds to the time frame for ASD (American Psychiatric Association, 1994). We turn now to describing early secondary prevention interventions for trauma.

EARLY INTERVENTIONS DESIGNED TO REDUCE RISK FOR POSTTRAUMATIC STRESS DISORDER

Critical Incident Stress Debriefing and Critical Incident Stress Management

CISD remains the most commonly accepted and applied method of early secondary prevention of PTSD. Throughout the world, emergency services personnel (e.g., firefighters, police, and emergency medical technicians), employee assistance programs, school counselors, the majority of governmental and nongovernmental agencies responsible for disaster and refugee mental health, and military organizations employ CISD as policy. For example, the American Red Cross policy mandates the use of CISD (American Red Cross, 1998). The American Psychological Association's task force on the mental health response to the Oklahoma City Bombing recommended extensive training in CISD and mandated the use of CISD in mass causality disasters (American Psychological Association, 1997). CISD is attractive because it is presented not as a clinical intervention but, rather, as an opportunity for individuals to share their common, normal response to extreme circumstances with CISD team members, at least one of whom is a peer highly familiar with occupational demands and concerns.

The CISD framework has been revised so that it is now considered part of a more comprehensive critical incident stress management (CISM) program (Everly & Mitchell, 2000). The CISM program is a series of interventions with high face validity designed to comprehensively address the needs of emergency services organizations and personnel. The CISM interventions are designed to psychologically prepare or prebrief individuals prior to dangerous work, meet the support needs of individuals during "critical incidents" (e.g., while Red Cross personnel are working with families who lost loved ones in a disaster), provide CISD, consult with organizations and leaders, work with the families of those directly affected by trauma, and facilitate referrals and follow-up interventions designed to address lingering stress disorders.

The cornerstone of CISM is CISD, which is a formal, group intervention with didactic and experiential components. The goal of CISD is to reduce acute stress and reduce risk for PTSD (secondary prevention; Everly & Mitchell, 2000; Mitchell & Everly, 1996). The interventions are designed (1) to educate individuals about stress reactions and ways of coping adaptively with them, (2) to instill messages about the normalcy of reactions to trauma, (3) to promote emotional processing and self-disclosure of the details of what each individual in the group experienced, and (4) to provide information about, and opportunity for, further trauma-related intervention if it is requested by the participant.

Individuals exposed to a trauma are invited, within days (often within 48 hours), to participate in a 3- to 4-hour session in which the trauma ("incident") is reviewed, akin to Marshall's original concept of debriefing. All individuals, regardless of the degree of their exposure, acute symptoms, or impairment, are invited to attend a CISD (e.g., Hokanson & Wirth, 2000). The common assumption of individuals who apply CISD is that everyone exposed to a trauma is at risk for PTSD and that everyone could benefit from an opportunity to learn about trauma and stress management and to share their experience emotionally soon after trauma. This thinking is problematic given that not everyone is equally at risk (nor does everyone need a standard intervention). Treating everyone exposed to a trauma also fails to sufficiently consider the natural resiliency of survivors and emergency care providers and their capacity to find adaptive ways of managing reactions to the stressful demands they face (e.g., Gist & Devilly, 2002; Gist & Woodall, 2000). In addition, we would argue that for some, providing a formal intervention of this kind within 48 hours is inappropriate.

In the official CISD literature, CISD is framed as a necessary and sufficient intervention to prevent PTSD in some cases and as a necessary but not sufficient intervention for severely traumatized individuals who have lingering disturbing symptoms and problems after a trauma (these individuals require follow-up care). Given the lack of prescreening, CISD is provided to people who would do well on their own anyway with the passage of time, which would suggest that their participation is unnecessary. In addition, it appears that CISD may serve to screen individuals (it is hoped) who require sustained psychological therapy to reduce the risk of chronic PTSD. For these individuals, it is entirely unclear whether the single CISD meeting has any rehabilitative benefit other than providing information about other services that may be available on down the line.

Although it makes sense, given the goals of CISD, to include peers as cofacilitators, this can create dual relationships and may make some attendees feel unsafe, which may be countertherapeutic and possibly unethical (e.g., Gist & Woodwall, 2000). Formally, the goal of including peer support personnel in a CISD team is to enhance the team's credibility and legitimacy in terms of particular work cultures. It is quite possible that this feature is important in many work contexts, although it also seems likely that it constrains the extent to which emotionally salient or inadvertently incriminating experiences are shared for some.

Another concern with the implementation of CISD is that individuals may be mandated or subtly coerced by their employers to attend a debriefing session, which could breed resentment and disengagement. For example, all 65,000 police officers in the five boroughs of New York City were mandated to attend a CISD. A related criticism of CISD is that an individual who is reluctant to disclose personal information may feel stigmatized and pressured by the group's expectations. In this context, sharing of personal experiences may have harmful rather than helpful consequences (Young & Gerrity, 1994).

One of the confusing issues in the execution of CISD is the process whereby an individual (or group of individuals) is found to be appropriate for CISD. Apparently, CISD is chiefly designed for use with emergency service workers (firefighters, rescue personnel, emergency room personnel, police officers, etc.), although CISD training materials also describe CISD as appropriate for witnesses to events and bystanders who assist in the emergency response. The literature emphasizes that "direct victims" of critical incidents, family members of those seriously injured or killed, and those seriously injured in trying to respond to an incident require more extensive early intervention treatment and should not attend a CISD. These so-called direct victims are handled in unspecified ways within the broader treatment framework of CISM. However, it is unclear whether those who practice CISD apply the intervention only to individuals secondarily exposed to trauma (Dyregrov, 1999). The American Red Cross disaster mental health manual mandates the use of CISD for all victims of trauma and loss by traumatic means (e.g., air disasters). Following the terrorist attacks on the World Trade Center, thousands of office workers and other people directly involved in the incident were provided CISD. Another issue is how direct victims of trauma are screened, operationally, in the field. Certainly, a role as the sole inclusionary criterion for CISD would be insufficient: for example, emergency workers may be exposed to severe trauma "directly" and secondarily by virtue of observing others suffer greatly.

All the foregoing points aside, by far the biggest criticism of CISD and CISM is that there is grossly insufficient evidence to support its use as a secondary prevention of PTSD. The studies that proponents of CISD/CISM use to support the efficacy of their approach are all uncontrolled (no control group, no random assignment), fail to employ well-validated measures of posttraumatic stress, fail to evaluate preintervention status and rely on posttest only data, fail to provide independent evaluations of outcome, and fail to employ treatment fidelity checks (Everly, Flannery, & Eyler, 2002). As a result, they are internally invalid and fail to reveal anything about the efficacy of CISD/CISM. Any study of an intervention provided in the immediate and acute recovery phases of traumatic adjustment that fails to evaluate preintervention baseline mental health and randomly assign subjects may appear to promote change because of the natural reduction in severity and frequency of symptoms that occurs over time.

Yet, proponents of CISD/CISM tout the empirical support their approach receives in research literature reviews, mostly published in the proprietary trade journal of their own organization (The *International Journal of Emergency Mental Health*[1]; e.g., Flannery & Everly, 2000; Everly & Mitchell, 2000; Flannery, 1999; Miller, 1999). The proponents of CISD/CISM also ignore or eschew negative findings from uncontrolled and controlled studies (see below) because of concerns that the intervention provided was not "CISD" but, rather, "psychological debriefing" of some unspecified variety. This conclusion is disingenuous. Due to the absence of treatment fidelity checks, we cannot know that CISD was employed in the uncontrolled studies used to support CISD, even if investigators claim to be using that specific approach. In Everly, Flannery, and Mitchell's (2000) review of research on CISM, the authors note the need for more empirically sound, controlled, randomized trials to test the efficacy of CISM, yet they summarize the results of uncontrolled, internally invalid studies and anecdotal evidence as proof that CISM works as an early intervention. For example, Everly et al. state that "current evidence suggests that

---

[1]From the International Critical Incident Stress Foundation (ICISF) membership information sheet: "CISM team and ICISF members responsible for implementing CISM interventions in the field have asked for a simple, concise way of keeping up with the latest advances in crisis intervention and CISM. Those who teach, train, and do research have also asked for a simple concise way of 'staying current' with the latest research and 'lessons learned' in actual CISM interventions and from the program development perspective. The *International Journal of Emergency Mental Health* can help to keep people current in the crisis intervention field."

the CISM approach appears clinically efficacious and cost effective in this era of managed health care. The current, distinguished, international body of CISM researchers suggests great promise for the development of improved CISM procedures that further minimize present suffering and prevent the development of long-term negative sequelae" (p. 37).

There have been several independent, randomized, controlled trials of psychological debriefing using the procedures of CISD with direct victims of trauma as participants (and one study using couples; Bisson, Jenkins, Alexander, & Bannister, 1997; Conlon, Fahy, & Conrory, 1999; Deahl, Srinivasan, Jones, Thomas, Neblett, & Jolly, 2000; Hobbs, Mayou, Harrison, & Warlock, 1996; Mayou, Ehlers, & Hobbs, 2000; and Rose, Brewin, Andrews, & Kirk, 1999). These studies have been discussed exhaustively in recent literature and meta-analytic reviews (Litz et al., 2002; Rose, Bisson, & Wessely, 2001; van Emmerik, Kamphuis, Hulsbosch, & Emmelkamp, 2002). Each study revealed that debriefing did not produce positive change relative to no intervention. Two widely cited studies showed debriefing to lead to small but significantly worse outcomes (Bisson et al., 1997, and Hobbs et al., 1996). Many authors have concluded from these studies that debriefing is "toxic" (e.g., Gist et al., 1997). However, in our view, it is premature to definitively conclude that CISD is harmful because of the small effect size of the negative results (Litz et al., 2002).

Contrary to the conclusions of advocates of CISD/CISM, there is no sufficiently rigorous empirical support for the use of CISD/CISM in the secondary prevention of chronic PTSD. Controlled studies reveal it to be therapeutically inert when applied to individuals. As the modal application of CISD/CISM is the group format, rigorous randomized controlled trials of group debriefing, exquisitely executed (and documented) according to the standards offered by Everly and Mitchell (2000), are needed to definitively address the controversy surrounding the approach. It would be prudent for the ICISF to fund independent, randomized, controlled trials of CISD/CISM, provided in strict accordance with the dictates of the approach. This research is needed quickly, if CISD/CISM can remain a viable approach, given the rapidly shifting tide in the early intervention field. For example, the U.S. Department of Defense, the National Institute of Mental Health, the Department of Veterans Affairs, the American Red Cross, the U.S. Department of Health and Human Services, and the Department of Justice convened a consensus conference on early interventions following mass violence in October 2001. One of the conclusions of the conference was that CISD/CISM had no rigorous empirical support, and, as a result, was not recommended (National Institute of Mental Health, 2002). In addition, the official policy of the British National Health Service is that debriefing should not be used for victims of trauma (Parry, 2001), based on the results of the Cochrane review of debriefing (Rose et al., 2001).

The Alternative to Critical Incident Stress Debriefing/
Critical Incident Stress Management:
Cognitive-Behavioral Therapy as Early Intervention

Major gains have been made in the last 15 years in the development and validation of protocols for treating adults with chronic PTSD with cognitive-behavioral therapy (CBT) as well as generating standards for evaluating the efficacy of treatments trials in PTSD research (e.g., Foa & Meadows, 1997). The majority of well-designed, randomized, controlled trials have been conducted on samples of motor vehicle accident survivors (e.g., Bryant, Harvey, Dang, Sackville, & Basten, 1998), sexual assault survivors (e.g., Foa et al., 1999; Resick, Nishith, Weaver, Astin, & Feuer, 2002), and combat veterans (Keane, Fairbank, Caddell, & Zimering, 1989). The specific techniques that have been shown to be effective within the CBT framework are exposure therapy, stress inoculation training, and cognitive restructuring (see Foa & Rothbaum, 1998). Thus far, studies have shown convincingly that CBT reduces PTSD symptom severity and related functional impairments from relatively discreet adult-onset traumas (e.g., Foa et al., 1999). Cognitive-behavioral treatment has become the prescriptive evidence-based approach to treat PTSD, recommended and endorsed by the International Society of Traumatic Stress Studies (Foa, Keane, & Friedman, 2002).

As a natural extension of empirical research on the treatment of chronic PTSD, leading clinical research groups have applied CBT as an early intervention to prevent PTSD, which represents an excellent example of how research on the treatment of chronic PTSD can be translated to the acute context. The interventions employed within CBT treatments have been shown in randomized controlled trials to prevent the development of chronic posttraumatic pathology in recent trauma victims (Bryant et al., 1998; Bryant, Sackville, Dang, Moulds, & Guthrie, 1999).

Foa, Hearst-Ikeda, and Perry (1995) were the first to examine CBT to prevent PTSD. They compared the symptom course of 10 female victims of rape or aggravated assault who received a four-session cognitive-behavioral intervention shortly after their assault with that of 10 assessment-only control victims. All participants were matched on symptom severity, type and severity of assault, demographic characteristics, and time since the assault. This individually administered intervention consisted of educating participants about common reactions to assault, relaxation training, imaginal and *in vivo* exposure, and cognitive restructuring. Two months after the assault, victims receiving CBT reported experiencing significantly fewer symptoms of PTSD than did assessment control participants. At a 5-month follow-up assessment, participants in the treatment condition reported significantly fewer symptoms of depression, although there were no differences between groups with respect to PTSD symptoms. Effect size analyses indicated that the difference in PTSD scores between the two groups at the 5-month follow-up was relatively large, but because of the small sample size, the lack of a statistically significant difference likely resulted from low statistical power. Moreover, the control group in this investigation experienced significant symptom remission that also may have contributed to the lack of a statistically significant difference in PTSD symptoms at the 5-month follow-up.

Bryant et al. (1998) also report a successful CBT program for recently traumatized individuals. This intervention specifically targeted individuals with ASD who were thus more at risk for chronic PTSD. Accordingly, their study provided a more direct test of the efficacy of brief CBT in preventing PTSD. Moreover, because control participants received supportive counseling, it was possible to evaluate the extent to which treatment promoted improvement above and beyond that resulting from nonspecific therapeutic factors (somewhat analogous to psychological first aid). Participants were survivors of motor vehicle accidents or industrial accidents who were randomly assigned to either CBT or supportive counseling. Both interventions consisted of five, 90-minute, weekly, individual therapy sessions. At posttreatment and at the 6-month follow-up, significantly fewer participants in the CBT group met diagnostic criteria for PTSD relative to the supportive counseling condition.

In a subsequent study that dismantled the components of CBT, Bryant and colleagues randomly allocated 45 civilian trauma survivors with ASD to five sessions of either (1) CBT (prolonged exposure, cognitive therapy, anxiety management), (2) prolonged exposure combined with cognitive therapy, or (3) supportive counseling (Bryant et al., 1999). This study found that, at a 6-month follow-up, PTSD was observed in approximately 20% of both active treatment groups compared to 67% of those receiving supportive counseling.

The CBT interventions share many features with psychological debriefing. For example, they both include an education component designed to inform trauma victims about common posttraumatic reactions and sequelae, both attempt to teach coping skills for managing symptoms of stress and anxiety, and both provide an opportunity for survivors to disclose and emotionally process their trauma. Given the similarity between psychological debriefing and cognitive behavioral interventions, what may account for the apparent differences in treatment efficacy? Perhaps the most prominent reason that CBT appears to be more efficacious than CISD, in particular, is that within CBT, there is an emphasis on facilitating survivors as they learn and apply adaptive coping strategies that promote recovery and lessen risk for chronic PTSD, *in vivo*, over time. In addition, there is greater emphasis on repeated, imaginal reliving of the traumatic event and graded, *in vivo* exposure of avoided trauma-reminiscent situations. In their review of the psychological debriefing literature, Bisson, McFarlane, and Rose (2000) suggest that one-session intense exposure to trauma memories that characterizes most debriefing approaches might be countertherapeutic because it may heighten arousal and distress without allowing sufficient time for extinction or resolution of intensely negative posttraumatic affect. The results of the cognitive-behavioral interventions described earlier would seem to refute the notion that early exposure per se is countertherapeutic. Rather, it is the hasty and incomplete exposure to trauma memories that typifies traditional psychological debriefing approaches that may be potentially harmful.

The CBT approaches of Foa et al. (1995) and Bryant et al. (1998; Bryant et al. 1999) also included systematic cognitive restructuring. There is evidence that acute pathological trauma responses are characterized by catastrophic cognitive styles (Smith & Bryant, 2000; Warda & Bryant, 1998). Given that there is also evidence from studies targeting chronic PTSD that cognitive restructuring is effective in reducing symptoms (Tarrier, Pilgrim, & Sommerfield, 1999), the inclusion of cognitive restructuring over repeated sessions in CBT approaches to secondary prevention of PTSD may be another reason why CBT is more effective than CISD/CISM.

Cognitive-behavioral interventions also differ from CISD/CISM efforts with respect to timing and duration of the intervention. We have argued that formal secondary prevention efforts are at risk for failure (or symptom exacerbation) if provided in the immediate impact phase after trauma exposure. The interventions developed by Foa et al. (1995) and Bryant et al. (1998) were administered an average of 10 or more days after the trauma occurred. Moreover, the interventions, though brief, consisted of four or five weekly sessions, and both encouraged extensive daily homework as an integral feature of treatment. Given the profoundly deleterious effects of trauma, single-session interventions are simply insufficient to adequately address such powerful experiences among individuals who experience chronic or severe posttraumatic pathology.

Considering the multiple differences (prolonged exposure, cognitive restructuring, delayed intervention, and multiple session treatment) between CBT and psychological debriefing, it is not possible to specify which factors— alone or in combination—are responsible for CBT promoting better posttraumatic adjustment. Future research efforts should be designed to elucidate which specific components of CBT are the necessary and sufficient factors in achieving positive change following recent traumatic exposure. It will also be necessary to replicate the findings of Foa et al. (1995) and Bryant et al. (1998; Bryant et al., 1999) with larger samples comprised of different types of trauma victims to evaluate the generality of these findings.

Indeed, considerably more research is needed to examine a number of outstanding issues in early secondary prevention of PTSD. These are (1) the optimal time frame to provide psychological first aid and early intervention, (2) how and why resilient and at-risk individuals who receive services recover from trauma over time, (3) the parameters of specific therapeutic change agents, (4) the type of postintervention behaviors that promote recovery and maintenance of change, and (5) the optimal mode and method of screening for various types of trauma (e.g., mass disaster and victims of violence presenting at emergency rooms). Although we recommend that interventions be devised to treat only those individuals who are not likely to recover over time on their own, more research is needed to determine which risk factors are optimal from empirical and public health vantage points. In addition, researchers and clinicians should be vigilant about the possibility that early identification of individuals could inadvertently produce negative iatrogenic effects (e.g., stigmatization and self-fulfilling prophecy).

In addition, research on the interaction of individual difference characteristics, response to psychological first aid, and formal secondary prevention intervention is needed. For example, some trauma survivors may feel imposed upon by peers or significant others to share their trauma experiences, preferring to avoid emotional self-disclosure, not because of a pathological response to trauma but as a result of personality characteristics. It could be that some forms of early intervention may be inappropriate, counterproductive, or destructive because they fail to acknowledge individual differences in characteristic mode of event processing. Some trauma survivors may be unduly anxious, resentful, or inhibited if they are provided group-based interventions that require self-disclosure and bearing witness to others' self-disclosure. Alternatively, some individuals in a group may be so intensely emotionally reactive to the process of sharing a narrative account of their trauma that they feel overwhelmed, which exacerbates the experience of shame and victimization. In terms of help seeking, some people may be predisposed to expect others to be a useful source of support and guidance under stressful conditions, while others prefer to work problems out on their own—also, not necessarily a sign of pathological response to trauma.

Finally, translation research is needed to test more efficient methods of delivering evidenced-based procedures in the treatment of PTSD. Although there is excellent empirical support for the use of CBT in the early intervention of trauma in adults, a practical limitation of available studies is that they are limited to individually administered therapy contexts that typically require between 8 and 12 sessions delivered in a specialty mental health care setting. From a public health perspective, the labor-intensive nature of these therapies represents a significant obstacle to provision of therapy to thousands of individuals suffering PTSD in the context of mass violence events and disasters.

Even in communities with substantial mental health infrastructure, there are rarely sufficient therapy resources to provide the form of individual, multi-session therapy described in previous outcome studies. Typically, the availability of professionals trained in comprehensive CBT procedures is limited, and many victims may not be able to access such services or may have difficulty following through with multiple visits to mental health centers. In these contexts, brief evidence-based interventions are much more cost-effective and reach a larger number of victims, which makes them attractive from a public health perspective. Accordingly, research is needed that evaluates novel, efficient modes of treatment delivery for patients with chronic PTSD that can be translated to the acute trauma context as an early intervention. For example, specially designed Internet sites or telemedicine-type methods could be employed to teach, promote, and monitor stress- and self-management skills practiced *in vivo*, over time, consistent with CBT.

REFERENCES

American Psychiatric Association. (1994). *Diagnostic and statistical manual of mental disorders* (4th ed.). Washington, DC: Author.

American Psychological Association. (1997, July). Final report. *Task Force on the Mental Health Response to the Oklahoma City Bombing.* Washington, DC: Author.

American Red Cross. (1998). *Disaster mental health services.* Washington, DC: Author.

Bisson, J. I., Jenkins, P. L., Alexander, J., & Bannister, C. (1997). Randomized controlled trial of psychological debriefing for victims of acute burn trauma. *British Journal of Psychiatry, 171,* 78–81.

Bisson, J. I., McFarlane, A. C., & Rose, S. (2000). Psychological debriefing. In E. B. Foa, T. M. Keane, & M. J. Friedman (Eds.), *Effective treatments for PTSD: Practice guidelines from the International Society for Traumatic Stress Studies* (pp. 317–319). New York: Guilford Press.

Bolton, E. E., Litz, B. T., Glenn, D. M., Orsillo, S., & Roemer, L. (2002). The impact of homecoming reception on the adaptation of peacekeepers following deployment. *Military Psychology, 14,* 241–251.

Breslau, N., Davis, G. C., Andreski, P., & Peterson, E. (1991). Traumatic events and posttraumatic stress disorder in an urban population of young adults. *Archives of General Psychiatry, 48,* 216–222.

Breslau, N., Kessler, R., Chilcoat, H., Schultz, L, Davis, G., & Andreski, P. (1998). Trauma and posttraumatic stress disorder in the community: The 1996 Detroit area survey of trauma. *Archives of General Psychiatry, 55,* 626–632.

Bryant, R. A., Harvey, A. G., Dang, S., Sackville, T., & Basten, C. (1998). Treatment of acute stress disorder: A comparison of cognitive-behavioral therapy and supportive counseling. *Journal of Consulting and Clinical Psychology, 66,* 862–866.

Bryant, R. A., Sackville, T., Dang, S. T., Moulds, M., & Guthrie, R. (1999). Treating acute stress disorder: An evaluation of cognitive behavior therapy and counseling techniques. *American Journal of Psychiatry, 156,* 1780–1786.

Christianson, S. A. (1992). Emotional stress and eyewitness memory: A critical review. *Psychological-Bulletin, 112,* 284–309.

Conlon, L., Fahy, T. J., & Conroy, R. (1999). PTSD in ambulant RTA victims: A randomized controlled trial of debriefing. *Journal of Psychosomatic Research, 46,* 37–44.

Deahl, M., Srinivasan, M., Jones, N., Thomas, J., Neblett, C., & Jolly, A. (2000). Preventing psychological trauma in soldiers: The role of operational stress training and psychological debriefing. *British Journal of Medical Psychology, 73,* 77–85.

Dollard, J., & Miller, N. E. (1950). *Personality and psychotherapy; an analysis in terms of learning, thinking, and culture.* New York: McGraw-Hill.

Dyregrov, A. (1999). Helpful and hurtful aspects of psychological debriefing groups. *International Journal of Emergency Mental Health, 3,* 175–182.

Everly, G. S. (2000). The role of pastoral crisis intervention in disasters, terrorism, violence, and other community crises. *International Journal of Emergency Mental Health, 2,* 139–142.

Everly, G. S., Flannery, R. B., & Eyler, V. A. (2002). Critical Incident Stress Management (CISM): A statistical review of the literature. *Psychiatric Quarterly, 73,* 171–182.

Everly, G. S., Flannery, R. B., & Mitchell, J. T. (2000). Critical incident stress management (CISM): A review of the literature. *Aggression and Violent Behavior, 5,* 23–40.

Everly, G. S., & Mitchell, J. T. (2000). The debriefing controversy and crisis intervention: A review of the lexical and substantive issues. *International Journal of Emergency Mental Health, 2,* 211–225.

Eysenck, M. W., & Calvo, M. G. (1992). Anxiety and performance: The processing efficiency theory. *Cognition and Emotion, 6,* 409–434.

Flannery, R. B. Jr. (1999). Psychological trauma and posttraumatic stress disorder: A review. *International Journal of Emergency Mental Health, 1,* 135–140.

Flannery, R. B., & Everly, G. S. (2000). Crisis intervention: a review. *International Journal of Emergency Mental Health, 2,* 119–125.

Foa, E. B., Dancu, C. V., Hembree, E. A., Jaycox, L. H., Meadows, E. A., & Street, G. P. (1999). A comparison of exposure therapy, stress inoculation training, and their combination for reducing posttraumatic stress disorder in female assault victims. *Journal of Consulting and Clinical Psychology, 67,* 194–200.

Foa, E. B., Hearst-Ikeda, D., & Perry, K. J. (1995). Evaluation of a brief cognitive-behavioral program for the prevention of chronic PTSD in recent assault victims. *Journal of Consulting and Clinical Psychology, 63,* 948–955.

Foa, E. B., Keane, T. M., & Friedman, M. J. (Eds.). (2002). *Effective treatments for PTSD: Practice guidelines from the International Society for Traumatic Stress Studies.* New York: Guilford Press.

Foa, E. B., & Meadows, E. A. (1997). Psychosocial treatments for posttraumatic stress disorder: A critical review. *Annual Review of Psychology, 48,* 449–480.

Foa, E. B., & Rothbaum, B. O. (1998). *Treating the trauma of rape: Cognitive-behavioral therapy for PTSD.* New York: Guilford Press.

Foy, D.W., Sipprelle, R. C., Rueger, D. B., & Carroll, E. (1984). Etiology of posttraumatic stress disorder in Vietnam veterans: Analysis of premilitary, military, and combat exposure influences. *Journal of Consulting and Clinical Psychology, 52,* 79–87.

Freedman, S. A., Brandes, D., Peri, T., & Shalev, A. (1999). Predictors of chronic post-traumatic stress disorder: A prospective study. *British Journal of Psychiatry, 174,* 353–359.

Galea, S., Ahern, J., Resnick, H., Kilpatrick, D., Bucuvalas, M., Gold, J., & Vlahov, D. (2002). Psychological sequelae of the September 11 terrorist attacks in New York City. *New England Journal of Medicine, 346,* 982–987.

Gist, R., & Devilly, G. J. (2002). Post-trauma debriefing: The road too frequently travelled. *Lancet, 360,* 741–742.

Gist, R., Lohr, J. M., Kenardy, J. A., Bergmann, L., Meldrum, L., Redburn, B. G., Paton, D., Bisson, J. I., Woodall, S. J., & Rosen, G. M. (1997). Researchers speak on CISM. *Journal of Emergency Medical Services, 22,* 27–28.

Gist, R., & Woodall, S. (2000). There are no simple solutions to complex problems. In J. M. Violanti & P. Douglas (Eds.), *Posttraumatic stress intervention: Challenges, issues, and perspectives* (pp. 81–95). Springfield, IL: Charles C Thomas.

Green, B. (1994). Psychosocial research in traumatic stress: An update. *Journal of Traumatic Stress, 7,* 341–362.

Green, B. L., Grace, M. C., Lindy, J. D., Gleser, G. C., & Leonard, A. C. (1990). Risk factors for PTSD and other diagnoses in a general sample of Vietnam veterans. *American Journal of Psychiatry, 147,* 729–733.

Green, B. L., Lindy, J. D., Grace, M. C., Gleser, G. C., Leonard, A. C., Korol, M., & Winget, C. (1990). Buffalo Creek survivors in the second decade: Stability of stress symptoms. *American Journal of Orthopsychiatry, 60,* 43–54.

Grinker, R. R., & Spiegel , J. P. (1945). *Men under stress.* Philadelphia: Blakiston.

Harvey, A. G., & Bryant, R. A. (1999). Predictors of acute stress following motor vehicle accidents. *Journal of Traumatic Stress, 12,* 519–525.

Herman, J. L. (1992). Complex PTSD: A syndrome in survivors of prolonged and repeated trauma. *Journal of Traumatic Stress, 5,* 377–391.

Hobbs, M., Mayou, R., Harrison, B., & Warlock, P. (1996). A randomized trial of psychological debriefing for victims of road traffic accidents. *British Medical Journal, 313,* 1438–1439.

Hokanson, M., & Wirth, B. (2000). The critical incident stress debriefing process for the Los Angeles County Fire Department: Automatic and effective. *International Journal of Emergency, 2,* 249–257.

Horowitz, M. J. (1986). Stress-response syndromes: A review of posttraumatic and adjustment disorders. *Hospital and Community Psychiatry, 37,* 241–249.

Kardiner, A. (1941). *The traumatic neuroses of war.* Oxford, UK: Hoeber.

Karon, B. P., & Widener, A. J. (1997). Lest we forget!: Repressed memories and World War II. *Professional Psychology: Research and Practice, 28,* 338–340.

Keane, T. M., Fairbank, J. A., Caddell, J. M., & Zimering, R. T. (1989). Implosive (flooding) therapy reduces symptoms of PTSD in Vietnam combat veterans. *Behavior Therapy, 20,* 245–260.

Keane, T. M., Scott, W. O., Chavoya, G. A., Lamparski, D. M., & Fairbank, J. A. (1985).

Social support in Vietnam veterans with posttraumatic stress disorder: A comparative analysis. *Journal of Consulting and Clinical Psychology, 53,* 95–102.

Kessler, R. C., Sonnega, A., Bromet, E., Hughes, M., & Nelson, C. B. (1995). Posttraumatic stress disorder in the National Comorbidity Survey. *Archives of General Psychiatry, 52,* 1048–1060.

King, L. A., King, D. W., Fairbank, J. A., Keane, T. M., & Adams, G. A. (1998). Resilience/recovery factors in posttraumatic stress disorder among female and male Vietnam veterans: Hardiness, postwar social support, and additional stressful life events. *Journal of Personality and Social Psychology, 74,* 420–434.

Koss, M. P. (1993). Rape. Scope, impact, interventions, and public policy responses. *American Psychologist, 48,* 1062–1069.

Kulka, R., Schlenger, W., Fairbank, J., Hough, R., Jordon, B., Marmar, C., & Weiss, D. (1988). *National Vietnam Veterans Readjustment Study (NVVRS).* Research Triangle Park, NC: Research Triangle Institute.

Litz, B. T., Gray, M. J., Bryant, R. A., & Adler, A. B. (2002). Early intervention for trauma: Current status and future directions. *Clinical Psychology: Science and Practice, 9,* 112–134.

Marshall, S. L. A. (1950). *Men against fire.* New York: William Morrow.

Martin, L., Rosen, L. N., Durand, D. B., Knudson, K., & Stretch, R. H. (2000). Psychological and physical health effects of sexual assaults and nonsexual traumas among male and female United States Army soldiers. *Behavioral Medicine, 26,* 23–33.

Mayou, R., Ehlers, A., & Hobbs, M. (2000). Psychological debriefing for road traffic accident victims: Three-year follow-up of a randomized controlled trial. *British Journal of Psychiatry, 176,* 589–593.

McCarroll, J. E., Urasano, R. J., & Fullerton, C. S. (1994). Symptoms of posttraumatic stress disorder following recovery of war dead. *American Journal of Psychiatry, 150,* 1875–1877.

Miller, L. (1999). Critical incident stress debriefing: Clinical applications and new directions. *International Journal of Emergency Mental Health, 1,* 253–265.

Mitchell, J. T. (1983). When disaster strikes: The critical incident stress debriefing process. *Journal of Emergency Medical Services, 1,* 36–39.

Mitchell, J. T., & Everly, G. S. (1996). *Critical incident stress debriefing: An operations manual for the prevention of traumatic stress among emergency services and disaster workers* (2nd ed.). Ellicott City, MD: Chevron.

National Institute of Mental Health. (2002). *Mental health and mass violence: Evidence-based early psychological intervention for victims/survivors of mass violence. A workshop to reach consensus on best practices.* Washington, DC: U.S. Government Printing Office.

Norris, F. H. (1992). Epidemiology of trauma: frequency and impact of different potentiallytraumatic events on different demographic groups. *Journal of Consulting and Clinical Psychology, 60,* 409–418.

Norris, F. H., Friedman, M. J., Watson, P. J., Byrne, C. M., Diaz, E., & Kaniasty, K. (2002). 60,000 disaster victims speak: Part I. An empirical review of the empirical literature, 1981–2001. *Psychiatry, 65,* 207–239.

North, C. S., Nixon, S. J., Shariat, S., Mallonee, S., McMillen, J. C., Spitznagel, E. L., & Smith, E. M. (1999). Psychiatric disorders among survivors of the Oklahoma City bombing. *Journal of the American Medical Association, 282,* 755–762.

Parry, G. (Chair, Development Group). (2001). *Evidence-based clinical practice guidelines for treatment choice in psychological therapies and counseling.* London, UK: Department of Health, National Health Service.

Pennebaker, J., & O'Heeron, R. (1984). Confiding in others and illness rate among spouses of suicide and accidental death victims. *Journal of Abnormal Psychology, 93,* 473–376.

Pitman, R. K., Sanders, K. M., Zusman, R. M., Healy, A. R., Cheema, F., Lasko, N. B., Cahill, L., & Orr, S. P. (2002). Pilot study of secondary prevention of posttraumatic stress disorder with propranolol. *Lancet, 360,* 766–771.

Raphael, B. (1977). The Granville train disaster: Psychological needs and their management. *Medical Journal Australia, 1,* 303–305.

Raphael, B. (1986). *When disaster strikes: How individuals cope and communities cope with catastrophe.* New York: Basic Books.

Resick, P. A., Nishith, P., Weaver, T. L., Astin, M. C., & Feuer, C. A. (2002). A comparison of cognitive-processing therapy with prolonged exposure and a waiting condition for the treatment of chronic posttraumatic stress disorder in female rape victims. *Journal of Consulting and Clinical Psychology, 70,* 867–879.

Resnick, H., Acierno, R., Holmes, M., Dammeyer, M., & Kilpatrick, D. (2000). Emergency evaluation and intervention with female victims of rape and other violence. *Journal of Clinical Psychology, 56,* 1317–1333.

Resnick, H. S., Kilpatrick, D. G., Dansky, B. S., Saunders, B. E., & Best, C. L. (1993). Prevalence of civilian trauma and posttraumatic stress disorder in a representative national sample of women. *Journal of Consulting and Clinical Psychology, 61,* 984–991.

Riggs, D., Byrne, C., Weathers, F., & Litz, B. (1998). The quality of the intimate relationships of male Vietnam veterans: Problems associated with posttraumatic stress disorder. *Journal of Traumatic Stress, 11,* 87–101.

Roberts, A. R. (1991). Delivery of services to crime victims: A national survey. *American Journal of Orthopsychiatry, 61,* 128–137.

Rose, S., Bisson, J., & Wessely, S. (2001). Psychological debriefing for preventing post traumatic stress disorder (PTSD) (Cochrane review). In *The Cochrane Library* (p. 3). Oxford, UK: Update Software.

Rose, S., Brewin, C. R., Andrews, B., & Kirk, M. (1999). A randomized controlled trial of individual psychological debriefing for victims of violent crime. *Psychological Medicine, 29,* 793–799.

Rothbaum, B., Foa, E., Riggs, D., Murdock, T., & Walsh, W. (1992). A prospective examination of post-traumatic stress disorder in rape victims. *Journal of Traumatic Stress, 5,* 455–475.

Salmon, T. S. (1919). War neuroses and their lesson. *New York Medical Journal, 108,* 993–994.

Shalev, A. Y. (1994). Debriefing following traumatic exposure. In R. J. Ursano, B. G. McCoughey, & C. S. Fullerton (Eds.), *Individual and community response to trau-*

ma and disaster: The structure of human chaos (pp. 201–219). Cambridge, UK: Cambridge University Press.

Shalev, A. Y. (2002). Acute stress reactions in adults. *Biological Psychiatry, 51,* 532–543.

Shalev, A. Y., Freedman, S., Peri, T., Brandes, D., & Sahar, T. (1997). Predicting PTSD in trauma survivors: Prospective evaluation of self-report and clinician-administered instruments. *British Journal of Psychiatry, 170,* 558–564.

Shalev, A. Y., Peri, T., Canetti, L., & Schreiber, S. (1996). Predictors of PTSD in injured trauma survivors: A prospective study. *American Journal of Psychiatry, 15,* 219–225.

Smith, K., & Bryant, R.A. (2000). The generality of cognitive bias in acute stress disorder. *Behavior Research and Therapy, 38,* 709–715.

Solomon, Z., & Benbenishty, R. (1986). The role of proximity, immediacy, and expectancy in frontline treatment of combat stress reaction among Israelis in the Lebanon War. *American Journal of Psychiatry, 143,* 613–617.

Solomon, Z., Laor, N., Weiler, D., & Muller, U. F. (1993). The psychological impact of the Gulf War: A study of acute stress in Israeli evacuees. *Archives of General Psychiatry, 50,* 320–321.

Solomon, Z., Mikulincer, M., & Avitzur, E. (1988). Coping, locus of control, social support, and combat related posttraumatic stress disorder: A prospective study. *Journal of Personality and Social Psychology, 55,* 279–285.

Tarrier N., Pilgrim H., & Sommerfield C. (1999). A randomized trial of cognitive therapy and imaginal exposure in the treatment of chronic posttraumatic stress disorder. *Journal of Consulting and Clinical Psychology, 67,* 13–18.

U.S. Consensus Workshop on Mass Violence and Early Intervention. (2001). Mental health and mass violence: Evidence-based early psychological intervention for victims/survivors of mass violence [On-line]. Available: *http://www.nimh.nih.gov/research/massviolence.pdf.*

van Emmerik, A. A. P., Kamphuis, J. H., Hulsbosch, A. M., & Emmelkamp, P. M. G. (2002). Single session debriefing after psychological trauma: A meta-analysis. *Lancet, 360,* 766–771.

Warda, G., & Bryant, R. A. (1998). Cognitive bias in acute stress disorder. *Behavior Research and Therapy, 36,* 1177–1183.

Weiss, D. S., Marmar, C. R., Metzler, T. J., & Ronfeldt, H. M. (1995). Predicting symptomatic distress in emergency services personnel. *Journal of Consulting and Clinical Psychology, 63,* 361–368.

Williams, F. D. (1990). *SLAM: The influence of S. L. A. Marshall on the United States Army.* Ft. Monroe, VA: U.S. Army, TRADOC.

World Health Organization. (1992). *International classification of diseases.* Geneva, Switzerland: Author.

Wright, K. M., Huffman, A. H., Adler, A. B., & Castro, C. A. (2002). Psychological screening program overview. *Military Medicine, 167,* 853–861.

Young, B. H., & Gerrity, E. (1994). Critical incident stress debriefing (CISD): Value and limitations in disaster response. *National Center for Post-Traumatic Stress Disorder Clinical Quarterly, 4,* 17–19.

6

Early Intervention with Infants, Toddlers, and Preschoolers

PATRICIA VAN HORN
ALICIA F. LIEBERMAN

Although there has been little systematic study of either the incidence of trauma exposure in our youngest children or effective means of treatment, social scientists are beginning to understand that traumatic life experiences can have a dramatic impact on the development of young children. This chapter explores what is known about the incidence of young children's exposure to trauma, the impact of trauma on children in their earliest developmental stages, the complexities of diagnosing trauma responses in young children, and protective factors that may moderate the impact of traumatic exposure. We focus on clinical descriptions of the phenomenology of the young child's response to trauma and examine some empirically tested treatment models to ameliorate the impact of trauma on infants and young children.

HOW MANY YOUNG CHILDREN ARE EXPOSED TO TRAUMATIC EVENTS?

As a culture, we yearn to protect our youngest children and see them as innocent and carefree. Perhaps because of our collective wish to view infancy and early childhood in this light, we have neglected to collect systematic data on the degree to which young children are exposed to interpersonal traumas, accidents, and disasters. Jenkins and Bell (1997) conducted a comprehensive review of literature on children's exposure to community violence. None of the 12 studies they reviewed inquired about the exposure of children under the age of 6.

Yet there are growing indications that many children under the age of 6 are exposed to interpersonal violence. In one study, mothers of children younger than 6 (mean age = 2.7 years) who used the pediatric service at Boston Medical Center were surveyed in the waiting room. Forty-seven percent of the mothers surveyed reported that their children had heard gunshots, and 94% of these mothers reported more than one episode. Ten percent of the children had directly witnessed a knifing or a shooting, and nearly 20% had witnessed an episode of hitting, kicking, or shoving between adults (Taylor, Zuckerman, Harik, & Groves, 1994). A study that collected data from five metropolitan areas in the United States determined that in all five areas, children under 5 were more likely than older children to be present in homes in which domestic violence occurred (Fantuzzo, Brouch, Beriama, & Atkins, 1997). Young children are also disproportionately victims of direct violence. More physical abuse and more fatal abuse occur with children in the first year of life than in any other 1-year period (Zeanah & Scheeringa, 1997). Extrapolating from data collected in 40 states that provided the age of the child in reporting to the National Center on Child Abuse and Neglect in 1995, the National Research Council (2000) found that over one-third of victims of substantiated reports to child protection agencies were 5 years old or younger, and that 77% of the child victims killed were under the age of 3.

Exposure to traumatic life events is clearly a significant problem for our youngest children. In the next section of this chapter we explore the impact of such exposure on children's development.

THE IMPACT OF EXPOSURE TO TRAUMATIC LIFE EVENTS ON YOUNG CHILDREN'S DEVELOPMENT

Pynoos, Steinberg, and Piacentini (1999) hypothesize that a child's response to a traumatic life event is multidetermined, and that a child's developmental stage at the time of the trauma is critical to understanding the child's response and predicting the child's outcome. Trauma and its effects are not uniform across ages. The impact of a violent event changes depending on the nature of the event, the child's prior experience, and the changing demands of the maturational process (Marans & Adelman, 1997; Pynoos et al., 1999).

Two of the essential developmental tasks of infancy are forming attachment relationships and accomplishing self-regulation, including regulation of emotional experience and expression (National Research Council, 2000). The abilities to enter into trusting relationships with others and to regulate and calm oneself lie at the core of emotional health. When infants and young children experience traumas, their ability to accomplish these essential tasks is compromised.

Attachment bonds are essential to the child's feeling of security and trust. Bowlby (1969/1982) suggests that babies are biologically equipped with an array of attachment behaviors designed to ensure the proximity of caregiving adults in time of threat or stress. If their attachment cues are responded to sensitively and contingently, babies will develop the belief that they are worthy of protection and that they can rely on others to protect them. Attachment bonds, then, are the foundation of the child's assumption that the world is a relatively safe place and that humans can be relied on to provide protection in times of danger. From the child's early attachment bonds, he or she forms internal working models that will influence intimate relationships throughout his or her life.

The formation of solid attachment bonds is also an essential element of the developmental task of self-regulation. Emotions are relational at their core, and a baby's first experiences of emotional regulation occur when caregivers respond to the child's feelings of distress and help restore him or her to a positive feeling state. The growing child internalizes these experiences, gradually learning to soothe him- or herself when he or she is distressed, thus regulating his or her expression of emotion (Emde, 1987, 1998).

The experience of traumatic life events, particularly interpersonal trauma, disrupts both of these essential developmental tasks, interfering with the child's attachments and his or her ability to self-regulate. As the child's own capacities are overwhelmed by trauma, his or her sense of being able to rely on attachment figures to protect her falters. The traumatic experience floods the baby or young child with terrifying sights, sounds, and feelings with which the baby cannot cope (Krystal, 1978). In that moment when the baby is not protected, the traumatic experience shatters the baby's belief that the world is a trustworthy place, and that he or she can rely on caregivers to protect him or her from harm. In addition, it destroys the developing belief that feelings and sensations can be modulated and controlled. The disruption is most profound when the victim or the perpetrator of the trauma is someone close to the child, especially a parent, because the child associates terror with the person on whom he or she relies for protection in times of fear and stress (Lieberman & Van Horn, 1998; Osofsky, 1995).

In the toddler years, the developmental challenges faced by the child change. Although toddlers continue to work toward self-regulation, they are simultaneously striving toward independence and autonomy. The toddler's ability to manage these strivings rests on receiving both active encouragement toward independence and constant reassuring support from his or her parents. As toddlers strive toward asserting autonomy and control in their world, the overwhelming unpredictability of traumatic events, especially events involving parents and caregivers, may cause toddlers to doubt their own competence and to doubt that they can rely on others for help and support (Marans & Adelman, 1997).

Preschoolers face an additional developmental challenge. Concerns about competition with the same-sex parent, power and size, and body vulnerability are of utmost importance during this stage (Marans & Adelman, 1997). Witnessing or experiencing violent traumas may make preschoolers fears for their own bodily safety, and the safety of others on whom they rely, even more profound.

Even in the earliest years of a child's life, the impact of experiencing a trauma is different depending on the developmental stage of the child. It is critical to keep these developmental demands in mind as we diagnose and intervene with young children.

THE PROBLEM OF DIAGNOSING YOUNG CHILDREN

Consideration of the impact of trauma in the early years is not new. Clinicians have long pointed to defensive disruptions in emotion regulation and attachment among children exposed to such traumas as child maltreatment. For example, Fraiberg (1982) described maltreated infants as young as 6 months of age using fighting, freezing, and avoidance to defend against overwhelming emotion. In the second year of life, Fraiberg (1982) observed an additional defensive pattern in maltreated infants: turning aggression against the self. Providing formal diagnoses for infants and young children has, however, been more difficult. The standard psychiatric disorder associated with the experience of overwhelming life events is posttraumatic stress disorder (PTSD), a nosological classification from the fourth edition of the *Diagnostic and Statistical Manual of Mental Disorders* (DSM-IV; American Psychiatric Association, 1994) that has been validated for adults and older children but which resulted in a high number of false-negative diagnoses when applied to young children (Scheeringa, Zeanah, Drell, & Larrieu, 1995). A newer nosology, traumatic stress disorder (TSD; Zero to Three, 1994), modifies the standard diagnostic criteria by requiring that the child display only one symptom in each of the three PTSD symptom clusters (reexperiencing, withdrawal, and hyperarousal), and by recognizing a fourth cluster of symptoms observed in young children: new fears and aggression. This alterative diagnostic nosology is based on observations of posttraumatic response in young children (Scheeringa et al., 1995), and on a consideration of the developmental capacities of infants, toddlers, and preschool children (Drell, Siegel, & Gaensbauer, 1993; Gaensbauer, 1995; Scheering & Gaensbauer, 2000).

The reexperiencing and avoidance symptom clusters for TSD are more behaviorally based as well as less reliant on subjective appraisal and verbal self-report than the corresponding PTSD symptoms, (Scheeringa et al., 1995). The reexperiencing phenomena are behaviorally observable (posttraumatic play, play reenactment, talking about the event outside play, nightmares, episodes with objective features of a flashback, and distress at reminders), and criteria requiring internal or external symbolic cues of the trauma are omitted. Similarly, in the avoidant cluster of symptoms, items depicting efforts to avoid thoughts and feelings, people and places associated with the trauma, and items requiring expression of lack of recall or a foreshortened future are omitted. In their place are items such as constriction in play and exploration, social withdrawal, restricted range of affect, and developmental regression. The TSD nosology also recognizes that new fears, separation anxiety, and aggressive behavior may emerge in young children after a traumatic life experience.

Children who have experienced a variety of traumas, drawn from clinical populations, have met diagnostic criteria for TSD. Lieberman and Van Horn (1998) found that 61% of a sample of children ages 3–5 who had witnessed domestic violence met criteria for the disorder. Zeanah and Scheeringa (1997) reported TSD in their sample of infants who were victims of violence. There are, however, no reliable studies of prevalence rates of PTSD in very young children (Scheeringa & Gaensbauer, 2000). The clinical picture of TSD in two young children at different developmental stages is illustrated by the examples that follow.

CASE EXAMPLE: BRIAN

When Brian was 2 years old he witnessed the drive-by shooting of his uncle. The shooting took place in front of Brian's home and Brian's parents pulled his gravely injured uncle into their living room and called for an ambulance. While they waited for the ambulance, they were screaming and crying, unable to cope with Brian's uncle's injuries or to comfort their terrified child, who sat in the corner, shaking. Six months after the shooting, Brian's mother called our clinic for help. She reported that Brian had become so aggressive that she was afraid he would hurt his baby brother. He had destroyed almost every piece of furniture in the family's living room, although he was not similarly destructive in other places. He would not go into the living room alone and refused to sleep alone. Although Brian had previously loved to play with his uncle, he refused to be near his uncle after he recovered from his injuries. On July 4th, the firecrackers in the neighborhood so frightened Brian that he spent the day cowering and crying under the kitchen table. The high levels of violence in his community intensified Brian's difficulties. There was gunfire almost every day. Almost every night, Brian woke up screaming from nightmares that he could not describe. When Brian turned 3, and it was time for him to start preschool, he refused to let his mother leave him there. Every morning after she dropped him off, he ran from the room looking for her. Even when his mother stayed in the classroom with him, he could not be calmed. The noise at recess frightened him. When children approached him to play, he hit and kicked them.

Brian was suffering from the classic cluster of symptoms of TSD. The sounds of gunfire or firecrackers and his family living room served as traumatic reminders, triggering fearfulness, nightmares, and destructive behavior. He did his best to avoid one of these reminders, the family living room, by refusing to be there by himself. He completely avoided the company of the uncle he loved. He was hyperalert to danger, and he defended himself by fighting with children who approached him to play. Noise and confusion made him jittery. He was newly aggressive with his baby brother and terrified to be separated from his mother. In addition, his symptoms were entirely behaviorally based. He did not talk about the shooting at school or with members of his family. His difficulties were exacerbated by the secondary stress of continued violence in his environment (Pynoos et al., 1999).

CASE EXAMPLE: SASHA

When Sasha was 6 months old, she was sitting in her car seat at the top of the staircase leading to her family's apartment. She and her mother had just come home, and her mother had put Sasha, sleeping in her car seat, on the floor so that she could open the door. As Sasha's mother opened the door, her father ran out, screaming. He accused Sasha's mother of trying to kill him. He grabbed her by the throat, shook her violently, and threw her down the stairs, breaking both her legs and several ribs. A downstairs neighbor called the police, who arrested Sasha's father and called an ambulance for her mother. They also called Sasha's maternal aunt who took Sasha home with her and later provided a home in which Sasha's mother could continue her convalescence after she was released from the hospital. Three months after the assault, Sasha and her mother returned to their apartment for the first time. When Sasha saw the staircase, she began to scream and twisted so violently to get away that her mother nearly dropped her. Although Sasha had seemed to do well while she and her mother were in her aunt's home, after the return to the apartment Sasha experienced night terrors. She cried and screamed whenever she saw the staircase her father had thrown her mother down. She babbled less and was less interactive with her mother and other caregivers. The staircase served as a traumatic reminder that flooded Sasha with terror each time she saw it, leading to other symptoms of numbing (diminished responsiveness) and hyperarousal (night terrors).

RESILIENCE

Although traumatic life experiences clearly have an impact on the lives of infants, toddlers, and preschoolers, not all young children exposed to such experiences develop emotional or behavioral problems or psychiatric disorders. The literature on resilience has consistently identified a small number of critical factors that protect children's development: (1) a relationship with a caring, competent adult (most often a parent); (2) a community safe haven; and (3) the child's internal resources such as an easy temperament and average or above-average intellectual capacity (Osofsky, 1999; Rutter, 1994).

Perhaps because relationships are so essential to the development of young children, the most important of these resilience factors is the presence of a caring, competent adult in the child's life. The caregiver's capacity to cope with a child's response after a trauma has been found to be the strongest predictor of child outcome, with increased levels of maternal support predicting lower levels of symptomatology and higher levels of adjustment in children (Rossman, Bingham, & Emde, 1997). Similarly, when parents are less able to provide support because they are suffering from symptoms as well, child outcomes decline. In a study of Israeli preschool children attacked by Scud missiles, Laor and colleagues (1996) found that when parents had higher levels of posttrauma symptomatology, the children experienced greater dysfunction. Similar results are reported by Rossman et al. (1997) and Scheeringa and Gaensbauer (2000). When young children suffer traumatic life experiences, the best way to ensure their return to a positive developmental trajectory is to enhance their caregivers' capacities for care and empathic responding.

INTERVENTION: WHEN AND HOW

Families of young children exposed to violence or other interpersonal trauma do not always seek help immediately. Family members may not be aware that help is available for children so young. They may hope a young child will "forget" what has happened. Indeed, at times, mental health professionals conspire with families in this hope.

CASE EXAMPLE: CHARLIE

Charlie was just over 2 years old when he witnessed an assault on his mother by two men who held up the convenience store where they were shopping. One of the assailants hit Charlie's mother on the head with a gun. She bled profusely, and for many weeks her head was bandaged. Charlie cried when he saw her bandages and stroked her head saying, "Mommy hurt. Mommy hurt." When Charlie was 3½, his mother called to ask if therapy might be helpful for him. She was worried because he still had so much trouble separating from her. He was clingy and could not sleep through the night in his own bed. He cried whenever she left his sight. Charlie's mother was concerned that it would be too hard for him to start preschool after his fourth birthday, and she wanted to get some help for him before that time arrived. She told us that she had been helped by psychotherapy but that her psychiatrist had advised her that if people did not remind Charlie of what he had seen, he would forget about it. His mother was concerned that his symptoms had persisted for so long and was beginning to believe that he had not forgotten. Indeed, he had not. When Charlie came to our clinic for treatment with his mother he played out, over a period of several weeks, not only the violence that he had seen but the guilt he had harbored for many months because he had not been able to save his mother.

Osofsky (2000) reported anecdotal evidence of the cost of treatment delay to young children served by the Violence Intervention Program for Children and Families in New Orleans. Children referred to the program 2 years or more after their exposure to a traumatic event tended to have significant learning problems, to be intensely and unpredictably aggressive, and to show significant signs of depression. All the later-referred children had memories of the violence that they had witnessed and survived, though many of them had not shared their memories with others before they came to treatment.

There is no systematic research documenting how delay in receiving treatment for their symptoms affects recovery or outcome in young children, or how timing of treatment interacts with other factors such as type of trauma, amount of exposure, or family or other support for the child. It seems clear, however, from the evidence of clinicians who have worked with young children following traumas, that children do not forget and that many of them remain symptomatic in spite of the passage of time.

When young children are symptomatic after a traumatic life event, what interventions can help? Although the research regarding interventions with young children who suffered traumas is scant, there is some empirical evidence that groupwork, cognitive-behavioral individual therapy, and child–parent psychotherapy are all effective modalities for treating young children. However, none of the studies focuses on the relative effectiveness of early intervention as opposed to treatment that is offered later. In the sections that follow, we discuss interventions, with special emphasis on the theoretical underpinnings, goals, and outcomes of child–parent psychotherapy.

GROUP TREATMENT FOR TRAUMATIZED YOUNG CHILDREN

Preschool-age children who have experienced such diverse traumas as sexual abuse and witnessing parental violence have been successfully treated using group interventions. Based on a qualitative assessment of their group treatment program, Peled and Davis (1995) developed a manual for group treatment of children of battered women that can be used with children as young as 4. Children are grouped by age, with 4-, 5-, and 6-year-olds placed together. In 10 weekly sessions, the group focuses on defining abuse, naming and exploring feelings such as sadness and anger, sharing experiences of witnessing violence, learning self-protection and assertiveness, and safety planning. Parents may attend a 10-week psychoeducational parenting group. At the end of 10 weeks, the parents and children meet together to talk about what they learned from the groups. There has been no reported study of the effectiveness of this treatment comparing it against a control group. The qualitative study (Peled & Edleson, 1992) that preceded the development of the manual reported that children's attitudes change after attending the groups, and that some of them gained self-protection and assertive conflict resolution skills. It also reported that although telling their stories relieved some children, others experienced new tensions and stresses as a result of this process. These findings, however, were based on interviews with only 30 children between the ages of 4 and 16. It is impossible to determine how effective the groups were for their youngest participants.

Sudermann, Marshall, and Loosely (2000) report on the effectiveness of a different group intervention for children of battered women. Again, the groups are designed for children between the ages of 4 and 16. Four- and 5-year-olds are grouped together, and the groups meet for 10 to 12 weeks. Topics addressed in the groups include definitions of, and language to describe, different types of violence; recognizing, understanding, and communicating feelings; talking about violence in families; anger and conflict resolution; talking about who is responsible for violence; power and control; self-esteem; and safety planning. The degree to which nonoffending parents are involved in the groups varies. Some groups are formulated as mother–child groups. Others are for children only. Still others include parallel but nonintegrated groups for mothers and children. Although the groups were evaluated using a pre–post design, only children between the ages of 7 and 15 years were included in the evaluation, making it impossible to determine how effective the groups were for 4- and 5-year-olds. The absence of a control group also makes it difficult to draw conclusions about what caused the positive changes that were reported in the evaluation.

The mother–child groups, used for children as young as 3 (Rabenstein & Lehmann, 2000), were not separately evaluated. The authors note that the mother–child group format requires that mothers be able to recognize the effects of violence on their children and offer support and assistance for their children, making the model generally not suitable for families in crisis. This may have implications for the use of a mother–child group model as a model for early intervention.

Groups have also been used as an intervention modality with young children who were sexually abused. Hyde, Bentovim, and Monck (1995) devised an intervention for sexually abused children ages 4–16 and their families. The groups met for a total of 20 weeks. The first four to six meetings were family meetings. These were followed by parallel but nonintegrated groupwork for children and parents. Although the investigators reported some positive results across time for the full sample (primarily on mother-reported outcomes), they did not report separate findings for young children.

Group models may be effective treatments for traumatized preschoolers, but as yet there is no empirical literature to support the assertion that they are effective. The particular group interventions that have been described in the literature do not appear to have been designed with the developmental needs of preschoolers in mind. Although their focus on assertive conflict resolution may be relevant to the ways in which preschooler's competitive strivings are affected by trauma exposure, they do not appear to address the developmentally salient issues of physical integrity and safety. More work is needed to create, and then rigorously test, group interventions that focus on the developmental needs of traumatized preschoolers.

INDIVIDUAL TREATMENT MODELS
FOR TRAUMATIZED YOUNG CHILDREN

More direct empirical evidence exists of the effectiveness of individual treatment with traumatized preschool children. Cohen and Mannarino (1996) evaluated a 12-session, individually administered, cognitive-behavioral protocol for treating sexually abused preschoolers, comparing it to a nondirective, supportive treatment. The cognitive-behavioral protocol contained some elements common to cognitive-behavioral therapy without a trauma focus: explanation of the distinction and relationship between thoughts, behavior, and feelings; identification of feelings; and strategies such as relaxation, thought stopping, and cognitive coping. It also contained elements of graduated exposure to upsetting aspects of the traumatic event.

Although families in both groups expressed high levels of satisfaction with the treatment they received, children in the cognitive-behavioral group showed more improvement with treatment than did children in the nondirective group on measures of home problems and sexual behavior problems and significantly more improvement on a measure of internalizing symptoms. There were no differences between the groups at the end of treatment on measures of externalizing problems or social competence. A follow-up report 1 year after treatment ended, however, revealed that the children treated with cognitive-behavioral therapy had greater improvements in both internalizing and externalizing problems, suggesting maintenance and enhancement of treatment gains for that group (Cohen & Mannarino, 1996).

Stauffer and Deblinger (1996) also evaluated a cognitive-behavioral protocol for the individual treatment of preschool children. Although they did not use a control-group design, their treatment was associated with significant pre- to postreductions in avoidance behavior and sexualized behavior, and these gains were maintained at a follow-up conducted 3 months after the end of treatment.

Both of the protocols described previously included parallel sessions for parents and were flexible enough to include one or two joint child–parent sessions at the end of the course of treatment. Stauffer and Deblinger (1996) reported decreased parenting dysfunction at the end of their treatment, according to parent self-report.

These individual modes of treatment have proven effective for preschool-age children. Work with parents is central to the healing of young children. The individual models, however, have not been used with children younger than preschool age, perhaps because of the limited developmental capacity that infants and toddlers have to talk or to play symbolically. In the next section of this chapter, we discuss child–parent psychotherapy, a modality that was developed specifically to work with traumatized infants, toddlers, and preschoolers, that recognizes the centrality of the parent–child relationship as a vehicle for the child's healing.

CHILD–PARENT PSYCHOTHERAPY[1]

Child–parent psychotherapy is a relationship-based form of intervention that focuses on the parent–child interaction and on each partner's perceptions of the other. It was developed specifically for use with children birth to 5 who have witnessed domestic violence. (Lieberman & Van Horn, 2002). More recently we have begun to investigate the utility of child–parent psychotherapy to help young children who have experienced other kinds of interpersonal traumas, including sexual abuse, physical abuse, and witnessing violence in the community. The chief theoretical principle that underlies child–parent psychotherapy is the premise that emotional and behavioral problems in infancy and early childhood need to be addressed in the context of the child's primary attachment relationships (Fraiberg, 1980; Lieberman, Silverman, & Pawl, 2000). Because the young child's sense of self evolves in the context of relationships with primary caregivers, enhancing the emotional quality of those relationships is the most effective vehicle for promoting the child's healthy development. Especially when the young child's trust in the reliability of his or her caregivers has been shattered by trauma, working to repair misperceptions in the parent–child relationship is critical if the child is to be restored to the expectation that other people are trustworthy sources of help. When both the parent and the child have been traumatized, as in cases of domestic violence, both are likely to have perceptions of self and other distorted by trauma. If these distortions are not corrected, they can act as self-fulfilling prophesies, distorting the child's development (Lieberman, 1999).

CASE EXAMPLE: JAMAL

Jamal, 15 months old, and his family came to treatment because his mother had suffered domestic violence during all of her 5-year-long relationship with Jamal's father. She had recently left him and had sought help for herself and her children. During a session early in the treatment, Jamal

---

[1]The treatment model described here was developed with the support of the National Institute of Mental Health and the support of private foundations including the Irving Harris Foundation, the Miriam and Peter Haas Fund, the Francis North Foundation, and the Pinewood Foundation.

was toddling around the living room where his mother, his 3-year-old brother, and the therapist were talking. He approached a tower of blocks that his brother had built and, reaching out to touch it, knocked it over. His brother screamed at him and Jamal turned to his mother with his arms outstretched, entreating her to pick him up. Instead she also screamed at him, "Don't hit me! I've told you and told you not to hit me!" In that moment Jamal's mother's view of her toddler was distorted by her own traumatic experiences, and she saw him not as a little boy in need of her help but as a potential dangerous threat. Jamal's mother's loud voice frightened him, and he backed away, lost his balance and fell, banging his head on the floor. As he lay on the floor crying, his mother turned to the therapist and said, "You're the psychologist. You fix him."

The therapist asked permission to pick Jamal up, which his mother granted. She held Jamal and sat on the floor near his mother and spoke to him quietly. She said, "Your mommy didn't mean to scare you. But when you put your hands out to your mommy it scared her, because sometimes when people have put their hands out to her, they've hit her, and it's hurt. Now, whenever she sees that, she gets frightened, and sometimes when grownups are frightened, they act angry. I think that's all that happened with your mommy."

This intervention worked for both the parent and the child. It calmed them so that they were able to attend and hear. More than that, the words spoken to the baby, but intended for the mother, explained her misattribution to her son in a nonjudgmental way that the mother could understand but that did not make her defensive. It linked her current fear to her past experience of violence.

To intervene in these trauma-based misattributions, child–parent psychotherapy uses developmental guidance, behavior-based strategies, play, and verbal interpretation as agents of change. It focuses on using the simplest interventions first. For example, when working with a traumatized infant, developmental guidance is often the most helpful intervention.

CASE EXAMPLE: SASHA

In the case of Sasha, the 9-month-old infant responding with avoidance and night terrors to the sight of her family's front staircase, the therapist explained the basis of Sasha's fears to her mother. She helped Sasha's mother plan strategies that would calm her baby. Although Sasha could not talk, her receptive language was good. The therapist explained to Sasha's mother that the baby could understand far more than she could say. They experimented with things that the mother might tell Sasha as they approached the staircase together as they came and went from home. Sasha's mother learned to say things such as, "You were so scared the day that daddy pushed me down the stairs. I was hurt but now I'm fine. I'm here to take care of you. I won't fall down the stairs again. It won't happen again." She talked in a similarly soothing way during Sasha's night terrors. Gradually, Sasha's fears diminished and she became once again more joyful in her interactions.

Child–parent psychotherapy has a number of goals that are related to trauma treatment. First and foremost, it encourages a valuing of safety in the environment and in the parent–child relationship. Until these basic needs are met, the parent and child are not free to focus on the work of healing from trauma.

Specific trauma-related goals of child–parent psychotherapy are:

1. *Fostering an increased capacity to respond realistically to threat.* Promoting safety is based on the ability to evaluate whether a situation may involve danger. Traumatized children and adults are often impaired in their ability to appraise and respond to cues of danger. They may either minimize or exaggerate danger, and sometimes do both, overreacting to minor stimuli and overlooking serious threats. In children, this tendency is manifested in an alternation of recklessness and accident proneness. The treatment focuses on developing more accurate perceptions of danger and appropriate responses to it.

2. *Maintaining regular levels of affective arousal.* Traumatic events impair the ability to regulate emotion. This impairment creates a "biopsychosocial trap" because neurophysiological disruptions in the regulation of arousal affect other self-regulatory healing mechanisms. For example, children appear to be especially prone to sleep disturbances after trauma, including somnambulism, vocalization, motor restlessness, and night terrors (Pynoos, 1996). Sleeplessness can make children more prone to overreact and respond to mild aversive events with anger and aggression. These changes in physiological reactivity are a behavioral analogue of traumatic expectations (Pynoos, Steinberg, & Goenjian, 1996). Intervening to help with emotion regulation is especially critical during the early years of life because children are actively working on attaining this capacity during this developmental phase.

3. *Reestablishing trust in bodily sensations.* The body is the primary stage where affects are experienced and where the memory of the trauma lives on. As a result, the body itself may become something to be feared and avoided, defensively shutting down sensations and closing off the possibility of intimacy and pleasure with another. For young children, for whom touching and being touched are essential building blocks for a healthy relationship to them-

selves and others, the recovery of trust in one's body and the body of the caregiver is an essential component of developmental progress. The intervention must give the message that one can safely touch and be touched, and that the pleasure of safe touching is something to be cherished. This message can be given by encouraging expressions of affection between the parent and the child, by accepting naturally, but without excessive enthusiasm, the expressions of physical affection of the child to the therapist, and by not recoiling from casual physical contact in the context of play or other activities.

4. *Restoration of reciprocity in intimate relationships.* If the loss of a secure base is the earliest and most damaging consequence of psychological trauma, its reconstruction is essential to recovery. As the case of Jamal illustrates, battered women can be impaired in their ability to foster an emotionally reciprocal relationship with their children because of emotional numbing and hyperarousal, which may lead them to ignore or overreact to their children's behavior, or attribute dangerous motives to their children's behavior. Children exposed to violence, for their part, may engage in internalizing and externalizing behavioral problems that are likely to exacerbate the mother's maladaptive responses. The intervention must involve a search for solutions to failures of reciprocity that are both developmentally appropriate and within the scope of the psychological resources of the parent and the child.

5. *Normalization of the traumatic response.* Traumatized adults often worry that they are "crazy"; children harbor fantasies that they are "bad" and "unlovable" when their behaviors evoke negative responses from others. For adults as well as for children, treatment focuses on establishing a frame of meaning and validating the legitimacy and universality of the traumatic responses.

6. *Encouraging a differentiation between reliving and remembering.* Being flooded by intrusive recollections is one of the frequent sequelae of trauma. In children, it is manifested in repeated reenactment of the traumatic scenes either through action or through play. Treatment involves helping adults or children realize the connection between what they are doing and feeling in the moment and the traumatic experience, stressing the difference between the past and present circumstances, and increasing their awareness of the current, safer surroundings.

7. *Placing the traumatic experience in perspective.* Treatment focuses on helping the adult or the child to gain control over the uncontrolled emotions evoked by the memory of the trauma. Children and adults are encouraged to achieve a balance where the memory of the trauma is not eradicated but there is a marked decrease in being preoccupied by it. Instead, the person is encouraged to take pleasure in rewarding life events and personal characteristics and to make space to appreciate the positive and enriching aspects of life.

We are currently engaged in a clinical trial comparing child–parent psychotherapy to "community standard" treatment. In the pilot investigation that preceded that clinical trial, child–parent psychotherapy was associated with improvement in both children's and mother's functioning. Children's internalizing and externalizing behaviors improved significantly by their mother's report. Children's scores on a measure of cognitive functioning improved significantly. Mother's symptoms of PTSD sharply declined. Assessors observed improvements in the quality of the parent–child relationship. We are encouraged that this model, based specifically on the developmental needs of young children exposed to traumas, shows such promising results.

FUTURE DIRECTIONS FOR RESEARCH

Although there are some promising trends in intervention with very young children who have suffered traumatic life experiences, much is left to do. Specifically, we suggest the following research agenda:

1. Basic research is needed to establish the incidence and prevalence of exposure to various types of trauma during early childhood and to establish the incidence and prevalence of development of traumatic stress disorder following exposure.
2. Treatment modalities that are designed with the developmental needs of very young children in mind must be created and assessed using rigorous control-group designs.
3. Mental health professionals and others must be trained to recognize symptoms of trauma exposure in early childhood and to intervene effectively, and the effectiveness of the training must be empirically established.
4. Treatment modalities should be assessed using samples that are large enough to determine whether young children benefit more from treatment that is delivered immediately after a trauma than they do from later-delivered intervention.

REFERENCES

American Psychiatric Association. (1994). *Diagnostic and statistical manual of mental disorders* (4th ed.). Washington, DC: Author.
Bowlby, J. (1982). *Attachment and loss* (Vol. 1). New York: Basic Books. (Original work published 1969)

Cohen, J. A., & Mannarino, A. P. (1996). A treatment outcome study for sexually abused preschool children: Initial findings. *Journal of the American Academy of Child and Adolescent Psychiatry, 35,* 42–50.

Drell, M. J., Siegel, C. H., & Gaensbauer, T. J. (1993). Posttraumatic stress disorder. In C. H. Zeanah (Ed.), *Handbook of infant mental health* (pp. 291–304). New York: Guilford Press.

Emde, R. N. (1987). The infant's relationship experience: Developmental and affective aspects. In A. J. Sameroff & R. N. Emde (Eds.), *Relationship disturbances in early childhood* (pp. 33–51). New York: Basic Books.

Emde, R. N. (1998). Early emotional development: New modes of thinking for research and intervention. In J. G. Warhol (Ed.), *New perspectives in early emotional development* (pp. 29–45). New Brunswick, NJ: Johnson & Johnson Pediatric Institute.

Fantuzzo, J. W., Brouch, R., Beriama, A., & Atkins, M. (1997). Domestic violence and children: Prevalence and risk in five major U.S. cities. *Journal of the American Academy of Child and Adolescent Psychiatry, 36,* 116–122.

Fraiberg, S. (Ed.). (1980). *Clinical studies in infant mental health.* New York: Basic Books.

Fraiberg, S. (1982). Pathological defenses in infancy. *Psychoanalytic Quarterly, 51,* 612–635.

Gaensbauer, T. (1995). Trauma in the preverbal period: Symptoms, memories, and developmental impact. *Psychoanalytic Study of the Child, 50,* 122–149.

Hyde, C., Bentovim, A., & Monck, E. (1995). Some clinical and methodological implications of a treatment outcome study of sexually abused children. *Child Abuse and Neglect, 19,* 1387–1399.

Jenkins, E. J., & Bell, C. C. (1997). Exposure and response to community violence among children and adolescents. In J. Osofsky (Ed.), *Children in a violent society* (pp. 9–31). New York: Guilford Press.

Krystal, H. (1978). Trauma and affects. *Psycholanalytic Study of the Child, 33,* 81–116.

Laor, N., Wolmer, L., Mayes, L. C., Golomb, A., Silverberg, D. S., Wiezman, R., & Cohen, D. I. (1996). Israeli preschoolers under Scud Missile attack: A developmental perspective on risk modifying factors. *Archives of General Psychiatry, 53,* 416–423.

Lieberman, A. F. (1999). Negative maternal attributions: Effects on toddlers' sense of self. *Psychoanalytic Inquiry, 19,* 737–756.

Lieberman, A. F., Silverman, R., & Pawl, J. H. (2000) Infant–parent psychotherapy: Core concepts and current approaches. In C. H. Zeanah (Ed.), *Handbook of infant mental health* (2nd ed., pp. 472–484). New York: Guilford Press.

Lieberman, A. F., & Van Horn, P. (1998). Attachment, trauma, and domestic violence: Implications for child custody. *Child and Adolescent Clinics of North America, 7*(2), 423–443.

Lieberman, A. F., & Van Horn, P. (2002). *Manual of child–parent psychotherapy for infant, toddler and preschooler witnesses of domestic violence.* Unpublished manuscript.

Marans, S., & Adelman, A. (1997). Experiencing violence in a developmental context.

In J. Osofsky (Ed.), *Children in a violent society* (pp. 202–222). New York: Guilford Press.

National Research Council and Institute of Medicine. (2000). *From neurons to neighborhoods: The science of early childhood development.* Washington, DC: National Academy Press.

Osofsky, J. D. (1995). The effects of exposure to violence on young children. *American Psychologist, 50,* 782–788.

Osofsky, J. D. (1999). The impact of violence on children. *Domestic Violence and Children: The Future of Children, 9*(3), 33–49.

Osofsky, J. D. (2000). Treating traumatized children: The costs of delay. In J. D. Osofsky & E. Fenichel (Eds.), *Protecting young children in violent environments: Building staff and community strengths* (pp. 20–24). Washington, DC: Zero to Three, National Center for Infants, Toddlers, and Families.

Peled, E., & Davis, D. (1995). *Groupwork with children of battered women.* Thousand Oaks, CA: Sage.

Peled, E., & Edleson, J. (1992). Multiple perspectives on groupwork with children of battered women. *Violence and Victims, 7,* 327–346.

Pynoos, R. S., Steinberg, A. M., & Goenjian, A. (1996). Traumatic stress in childhood and adolescence: Recent developments and current controversies. In B. A. van der Kolk, A. C. McFarlane, & L. Weisaeth (Eds.), *Traumatic stress: The effects of overwhelming experience on mind, body, and society* (pp. 331–358). New York: Guilford Press.

Pynoos, R. S., Steinberg, A. M., & Piacentini, J. C. (1999). A developmental psychopathology model of childhood traumatic stress and intersection with anxiety disorders. *Biological Psychiatry, 46,* 1542–1554.

Rabenstein, S., & Lehmann, P. (2000). Mothers and children together: A family group approach to treatment. In R. A. Geffner, P. G. Jaffee, & M. Sudermann (Eds.), *Children exposed to domestic violence: Current issues in research, intervention, prevention, and policy development* (pp. 185–206). New York: Haworth Press.

Rossman, B. B. R., Bingham, R. D., & Emde, R. N. (1997). Symptomatology and adaptive functioning for children exposed to normative stressors, dog attack, and parental violence. *Journal of the American Academy of Child and Adolescent Psychiatry, 36,* 1089–1097.

Rutter, M. (1994). Resilience: Some conceptual considerations. *Contemporary Pediatrics, 11,* 36–48.

Scheeringa, M. S., & Gaensbauer, T. J. (2000). Posttraumatic stress disorder. In C. H. Zeanah, Jr. (Ed.), *Handbook of infant mental health* (2nd ed., pp. 369–381). New York: Guilford Press.

Scheeringa, M. S., Zeanah, C. H., Drell, M. J., & Larrieu, J. A. (1995) Two approaches to the diagnosis of posttraumatic stress disorder in infancy and early childhood. *Journal of the American Academy of Child and Adolescent Psychiatry, 34,* 191–200.

Stauffer, L. B., & Deblinger, E. (1996). Cognitive behavioral groups for nonoffending mothers and their young sexually abused children: A preliminary treatment outcome study. *Child Maltreatment, 1,* 65–76.

Sudermann, M., Marshall, L., & Loosely, S. (2000). Evaluation of the London (Ontario) community group treatment programme for children who have witnessed woman abuse. In R. A. Geffner, P. G. Jaffee, & M. Sudermann (Eds.), *Children exposed to domestic violence: Current issues in research, intervention, prevention, and policy development* (pp. 127–146). New York: Haworth Press.

Taylor, L., Zuckerman, B., Harik, V., & Groves, B. (1994). Witnessing violence by young children and their mothers. *Journal of Developmental and Behavioral Pediatrics, 15,* 120–123.

Zeanah, C. H., & Scheeringa, M. S. (1997). The experience and effects of violence in infancy. In J. D. Osofsky (Ed.), *Children in a violent society* (pp. 97–123). New York: Guilford Press.

Zero to Three, National Center for Clinical Infant Programs. (1994). *Diagnostic classification: 0-3. Diagnostic classification of mental health and developmental disorders of infancy and early childhood.* Washington, DC: Author.

7

Early Mental Health Interventions for Trauma and Traumatic Loss in Children and Adolescents

JUDITH A. COHEN

Although there is growing information about effective mental health treatments for children and adolescents with posttraumatic stress disorder (PTSD) and other trauma-related conditions, no empirical studies have evaluated psychological debriefing (PD) or other "early" mental health interventions for these populations (i.e., those that are completed within the first 3 months after exposure to a traumatic event.) There are several reasons for this paucity of research, which are important to address in planning, providing, and evaluating interventions for such children.

Children rarely ask for or present themselves for mental health treatment; they are almost always dependent on adults to recognize that a mental health problem exists, to recognize that the problem may be related to exposure to traumatic events, and to seek or accept professional help for them. The younger the child, the more complete this dependency is likely to be. In cases of interpersonal trauma such as child abuse, bullying, or witnessing violence, adults' ability to access appropriate care for the traumatized child may be impeded by the child's failure to disclose his or her traumatic exposure. The sexually abused child may have compelling reasons not to disclose the abuse: The abuser may have threatened the child or the child's loved ones, or the child may fear not being believed when accusing an older child or adult. If the perpetrator is a family member, the child may have ambivalent feelings about getting the family member into trouble and may fear causing emotional, legal, or financial trouble for the family. Children exposed to domestic violence may fear for their own physical safety and that of the abused parent and may believe that disclosure to an outside party may exacerbate the abusive parent's violent behavior. Similarly, children who have been the direct victim of or witness to community or school violence may fear retribution from the perpetrator if they tell someone; they may also fear not being believed. Thus, in some cases, the parent or other concerned adult will not know that the child has been traumatized in the immediate aftermath of exposure, and therefore the child will not receive early mental health interventions.

Another problem that arises is that once parents know about the child's traumatic exposure, they may hesitate to seek help due to fear of legal involvement, fear of having Child Protective Services (CPS) remove the child from their home, or fear of retribution from the perpetrator. Parents may also fail to seek treatment for the child because they do not recognize the seriousness of the child's symptoms. PTSD and other internalizing disorders are often difficult to detect unless the child verbally expresses symptoms, or until the illness becomes so severe that secondary difficulties such as suicidality, substance use, school failure, or delinquency develop. In other cases, children's somatic symptoms may be mistakenly diagnosed as physical disorders (such as migraine or irritable bowel disease), leading to extensive medical tests and interventions rather than early psychological assessment and treatment.

Because of the importance of avoiding professional role conflicts, many therapists will not begin treating a child who has alleged abuse until an independent evaluator has confirmed that child abuse occurred, or until CPS or police have completed their investigations (Mannarino & Cohen, 2001). Thus, even after the child has disclosed abuse and the parent has decided to seek help, there may be further systemic delays in receiving therapeutic interventions.

In the case of disasters, where whole communities experience traumatic exposure, other barriers typically prevent children from receiving early mental health screening and interventions (Chemtob, Nakashima, & Hamada, 2002). School boards, school personnel, and parents are understandably protective of their students. In addition, these adults have also been exposed to the disaster and may be dealing with their own trauma symptoms. Unless a previous relationship existed between the school and mental health providers with expertise in child trauma, it is unlikely that screening or treatment for symptomatic children will occur within weeks of the disaster. Although the psychological screening of schoolchildren that occurred 7 weeks after the Oklahoma City bombing (Pfefferbaum et al., 1999) was exceptional, the more typical course is illustrated by the New York City experience following the terrorist attacks on the World Trade Center, where representative samples of children were screened 6 months after the event. Universal student screening has not yet been implemented.

Another difficulty in providing and testing early mental health interventions for traumatized children is that they are not a homogeneous group with regard to disorder: These children develop a wide variety of psychiatric difficulties and thus may require a variety of different interventions. Although most of the known, effective treatments for these children have addressed their PTSD symptoms, few studies have evaluated the efficacy of these interventions for other anxiety disorders, depression, substance abuse, or externalizing disorders, all of which are common in traumatized children. Thus, the complexity of children's responses to trauma complicates efforts to design universally appropriate interventions.

Finally, conducting treatment outcome research with children is more complex than with adults because of added protection for children (who are identified as a vulnerable population), and because both parental consent and child assent for research participation are required. These requirements impede the implementation of such studies in the school setting, which is the most feasible site in which to conduct PD or other early interventions.

Thus, there are many more barriers to children and adolescents receiving early mental health interventions, and to researchers empirically evaluating the efficacy of such treatments, than there are for adults, who can simply seek and accept treatment for themselves. For this reason, the term "early mental health interventions" in this chapter has been revised to refer to treatments provided within the first 12 months after the most recent traumatic exposure.

EPIDEMIOLOGY

Research indicates that substantial numbers of children and adolescents experience traumatic life events. One national survey found that one-third of students in eighth and tenth grade in the United States had been threatened with bodily harm, 16% had been physically assaulted in their neighborhoods, and one-third had been threatened, whereas 13% reported being attacked in school during the past year (American School Health Association, 1989). Inner-city youth appear to be at even greater risk of exposure to interpersonal violence: One study documented that 42% reported seeing someone shot and

22% reported seeing someone killed (Schubiner, Scott, & Tzelepis, 1993). Another study found that, although exposure to sexual abuse or violence in the home was greater for girls than boys, with 12–17% of girls reporting sexual abuse and 34–56% of girls reporting being hit, slapped, or punched at home, male adolescents reported higher rates than females for all other forms of victimization (Singer, Anglin, Song, & Lunghofer, 1995). This study also documented that whereas youths attending school in cities experienced higher rates of exposure to severe violence, males attending suburban schools also experienced substantial rates of lesser forms of violence.

An epidemiological population study conducted in North Carolina indicated that one-quarter of children and adolescents had experienced at least one "high magnitude" (PTSD-type) traumatic event by age 16, with 6% experiencing such an event within the past 3 months. In this study one-third had experienced a "low magnitude" traumatic event (such as death of a grandparent) within the past 3 months (Costello, Erkanli, Fairbank, & Angold, 2002). This study also found that family relationship problems, parental psychopathology, and familial adversity such as poverty increased the likelihood of children's exposure to traumatic life events. Thus, trauma exposure is a fairly common occurrence in children's lives.

Not all children will develop PTSD or other significant psychopathology following traumatic experiences. Rates of PTSD in children who have been exposed to traumatic events have varied from study to study (American Academy of Child and Adolescent Psychiatry, 1998); this may reflect differences in responses to specific types of traumatic events as well as the difficulty in accurately assessing PTSD in children (American Academy of Child and Adolescent Psychiatry, 1998). Large-scale community-based studies have documented that the level of trauma exposure, having psychiatric difficulties prior to the traumatic event, female gender, and disruption of social support networks most strongly predict psychiatric symptomatology in children exposed to traumatic events (reviewed in Pine & Cohen, 2002). This may have important implications for screening children in need of early mental health interventions, as discussed next.

MEASUREMENT ISSUES

To screen children for trauma symptoms or to assess the efficacy of providing early mental health interventions for traumatized children, it is critical to consider what will be measured and how to optimally measure it. In adult studies of early trauma interventions, PTSD symptoms have typically been the focus of attention. Measuring this disorder in children is particularly difficult, as almost half of the diagnostic criteria depend on the child's ability to accurately report his or her internal emotional state (Scheeringa, Zeanah, Drell, & Larrieu, 1995). In very young children, the use of additional criteria appears to improve diagnostic reliability and validity (Scheeringa, Peebles, Cook, & Zeanah, 2001). However, using this approach, or other structured interviews, which are the standard for research diagnosis (American Academy of Child and Adolescent Psychiatry, 1998), is too time-consuming in typical clinical or community settings, where early mental health interventions are most likely to be provided.

Several brief self-report instruments to assess childhood PTSD are available. The UCLA PTSD Index for the fourth edition of the *Diagnostic and Statistical Manual of Mental Disorders* (DSM-IV; American Psychiatric Association, 1994) includes child, adolescent, and parent versions and is the most widely used self-report instrument for childhood PTSD (Pynoos, Rodriguez, Steinberg, Stuber, & Frederick, 1998). The psychometric properties of this revision of the original Reaction Index have not been published. The Child PTSD Symptom Scale (CPSS) is a self-report scale for DSM-IV PTSD, and also includes a scale to assess adaptive functioning (Foa, Johnson, Feeny, & Treadwell, 2001). This instrument has high test–retest reliability, internal consistency, and convergent validity with the UCLA PTSD Index for DSM-IV, with the CPSS showing evidence of better discriminant validity. The Child PTSD Checklist (Amaya-Jackson et al., 2000) also has high content validity, test–retest reliability, internal consistency, and divergent validity and is particularly "child-friendly" in its wording. Several other instruments are also available to measure childhood PTSD and other specific trauma-related difficulties (reviewed in American Academy of Child and Adolescent Psychiatry, 1998). Use of at least one psychometrically strong, self-report PTSD instrument is probably critical to assessing the efficacy of early mental health interventions for traumatized children.

In addition to PTSD, other psychiatric conditions are common among children who have experienced traumatic life events. Many children who do not meet full PTSD diagnostic criteria are, nevertheless, significantly functionally impaired (Carrion, Weems, Ray, & Reiss, 2002). These children should also be provided with early mental health interventions to address their functional difficulties and also to prevent their PTSD symptoms from worsening to the point where they meet full criteria for this disorder. Children exposed to trauma may have depressive or other anxiety symptoms, either comorbid with PTSD or without prominent traumatic stress symptoms. Obviously these children also deserve early interventions, although the exact nature of such treatment should vary according to the child's diagnosis and known effective treatments for that disorder. Appropriate instruments with established psychometric properties should be used to document the course of improvement of these disorders as treatment progresses. The complexity of children's responses to trauma suggests that comprehensive assessment of symptomatic children be conducted prior to providing early mental health interventions, in order to optimally address the individual needs of each child and family. Though providing such evaluations in school or community settings in the days or weeks after trauma exposure presents numerous challenges, conducting early screening in these settings may allow for the timely identification of more symptomatic children, who should then be referred for more comprehensive evaluation.

Although there is a growing consensus regarding the definition of childhood traumatic grief (CTG; Cohen, Mannarino, Greenberg, Padlo, & Shipley, 2002), the measurement of this condition is in its infancy. Only one instrument, the UCLA-BYU Expanded Grief Inventory (EGI; Layne, Savjak, Saltzman, & Pynoos, 2001), purports to measure CTG. The Traumatic Intrusion and Avoidance subscale of the EGI measures symptoms of CTG; other scales of the EGI include normal grief reactions and existentially complicated grief reactions. The psychometric properties of the EGI are currently being established.

EARLY PSYCHOSOCIAL INTERVENTIONS FOR TRAUMA IN CHILDREN

A number of treatment outcome studies for traumatized children have been published (reviewed in Cohen, Berliner, & March, 2000). Unfortunately, many of these studies do not specify the length of time between the most recent traumatic experience and the start of treatment; others only note percentages of children with acute PTSD (i.e., within the first 3 months following trauma exposure) versus chronic PTSD (longer than 3 months posttrauma). Thus, in many of these studies it is not possible to determine whether or what proportion of participants received "early" mental health interventions (i.e., within the first year).

Two randomized controlled psychosocial treatment studies examined sexually abused children treated within 1 to 6 months of the most recent abuse episode. One of these studies documented the superiority of trauma-focused cognitive-behavioral therapy (TF-CBT) in decreasing PTSD, sexual behavior problems, internalizing and externalizing symptoms when compared to non-directive play therapy for 3- to 7-year-old children and nondirective supportive therapy for their nonoffending parents (Cohen & Mannarino, 1996a). This study also documented that greater parental emotional distress about the child's abuse strongly predicted higher levels of child symptomatology at posttreatment (Cohen & Mannarino, 1996b). The second study documented that TF-CBT was superior to nondirective supportive therapy in reducing depression and improving social competence in sexually abused 8–14-year-olds (Cohen & Mannarino, 1998), and that parental support strongly predicted treatment outcome (Cohen & Mannarino, 2000). At 1-year follow-up, those who completed treatment and received TF-CBT had significantly greater improvement in PTSD and dissociation. An intent to treat analysis indicated significant group × time effects favoring TF-CBT for depression, anxiety, and sexual problems (Cohen, Mannarino & Knudsen, 2003). A third study included a preponderance (66%) of children who received treatment within 6 months of the most recent abuse episode (Deblinger, Lippmann, & Steer, 1996). This study similarly indicated that TF-CBT was superior to community treatment as usual in reducing PTSD symptoms. The design of this study, in which individual TF-CBT was provided either to the abused child only, to the nonoffending parent only, or to both the child and parent, also allowed the authors to evaluate the importance of including a parental treatment component. They found that providing treatment directly to the child (in either the child-only or child-and-parent treatment condition) resulted in more improvement in PTSD symptoms, but providing treatment directly to the parent (in either the parent-only or child-and-parent treatment condition) resulted in greater improvement in child-reported depression as well as externalizing behavior problems.

The only published study using PD in children (Stallard & Law, 1993) did not provide the intervention until 5 months after the index event (a school minibus crash). It also suffered from significant methodological shortcomings: The study included only five children, had no random assignment to an alternative treatment condition, and did not include a posttreatment measure of PTSD. The remaining published treatment studies of traumatized children have not provided early interventions. For example, a study treating single-episode trauma included subjects whose mean duration of PTSD symptoms was 1½ years for child and 2½ years for adolescent participants (March, Amaya-Jackson, Murray, & Schulte, 1998). In disaster treatment studies, interventions were provided 1½ years (Goenjian et al., 1997) to 2–3 years (Chemtob, Nakashima, Hamada, & Carlson, 2002) after exposure to the disaster. Several other studies of sexually abused children (Celano, Hazard, Webb, & McCall, 1996; Trowell et al., 2002) also included a predominance of children with chronic PTSD. The majority of these studies documented the efficacy of some form of TF-CBT in decreasing PTSD symptoms. One (Trowell et al., 2002) supported the efficacy of individual psychodynamic therapy.

Based on current research, TF-CBT currently has the strongest evidence of efficacy for traumatized children with PTSD symptoms (Cohen et al., 2000).

However, many questions remain about the utility of TF-CBT or other interventions in the acute aftermath of trauma exposure. TF-CBT, as it has been tested thus far, includes several distinct components, including stress inoculation training, creating a trauma narrative (also called "gradual exposure" because it encourages the child to directly discuss more details about the traumatic experience over time), cognitive processing, psychoeducation, and, often, a parental treatment component. We have little information regarding which of these elements is most critical to improving PTSD or other symptomatology. We also do not know the optimal dosage of such interventions; the treatment studies that have demonstrated the efficacy of TF-CBT have typically provided 10–18 treatment sessions, whereas acute interventions such as PD are typically provided in much smaller dosages (one to three sessions). It is not clear whether current forms of TF-CBT would be effective if provided in such dosages. A multi-site study is currently underway to study these issues.

As has been discussed elsewhere in this volume, PD and other acute interventions have the potential for worsening outcomes in trauma-exposed adults. We have no information regarding whether these same risks are present for children. There are developmental reasons to suggest that providing treatment that focuses on the trauma in the immediate aftermath of a traumatic event may not be helpful to some children. This may be particularly true for brief interventions such as PD, which may sensitize the child to trauma reminders without providing an adequate opportunity to process or resolve the trauma experience.

Children's perceptions and understanding of events are influenced by the reactions of adults and children around them. This "social referencing" may diminish as children mature. An intervention such as PD, where adults call attention to the traumatic nature of the event, may inadvertently heighten children's perception of that experience as being horrifying or frightening. This may lead to a worsening of symptoms in some children. Because early interventions such as PD are typically provided in a group setting, it is also possible that exposure to the frightening, trauma-related stories shared by other children, or observing other children's fearful reactions, may increase children's physiological arousal and/or alter their cognitive understanding in the direction of perceiving the event as more threatening than initially thought. If this occurs, PTSD symptoms could be expected to worsen.

From a psychobiological perspective, it is clear that interpersonal trauma such as child abuse can result in serious and long-lasting psychobiological abnormalities, and that the severity of these changes may be related to the age at which traumatic exposure began and how long PTSD symptoms have been present (DeBellis et al., 1999). This would suggest that it is crucial to provide effective treatments to symptomatic children as early as possible following trauma exposure. However, we do not yet know whether there is a "critical period" during which some traumatized children's biological stress systems spontaneously normalize, and, if this exists, whether it might be detrimental to provide early treatment to such children, particularly one (e.g., PD or TF-CBT) that focuses ongoing attention on the traumatic event. More research with regard to the timing of psychobiological changes associated with childhood PTSD may be helpful in answering these questions. Thus, there are reasons to be concerned about the impact of providing early trauma-focused interventions to children, particularly to those who are not displaying significant signs of distress. More research is needed to determine whether such interventions are beneficial for some children in the acute aftermath of trauma exposure, and, if so, how to identify those children who may benefit versus those whose symptoms may be exacerbated by such interventions.

EARLY PHARMACOLOGICAL INTERVENTIONS FOR TRAUMA IN CHILDREN

Given the numerous barriers to accessing early mental health interventions for children, it is not surprising that most early pharmacological studies have been conducted with children who came to treatment for serious trauma-related *physical,* rather than psychological, injuries. Specifically, two studies have evaluated pharmacological treatment in severely burned children. The only published pharmacological randomized clinical trial for traumatized children compared imipramine (a tricyclic antidepressant) to chloral hydrate (a sedative) in treating severely burned children with acute stress disorder (ASD; Robert, Blackeney, Villarreal, Rosenberg, & Meyer, 1999). This study documented that the children who received imipramine developed PTSD at a significantly lower rate than those who received chloral hydrate. A naturalistic study found a significant relationship between dosage of morphine given to acutely burned children and 6-month reduction in PTSD symptoms (Saxe et al., 2001). It is not known whether children who did not experience the physiological insults associated with severe burns would respond similarly to these medications or whether the potential benefits of providing such treatments would justify the risks associated with these particular medications.

An open study using propranolol in an A–B–A design (medication–no medication–medication) treated abused children with acute PTSD and found that PTSD symptoms were significantly less in the medication condition (Famularo, Kinscherff, & Fenton, 1988). Another study included six children with acute PTSD but did not analyze their results separately from those of the 18 children with chronic or delayed PTSD. This study (Seedat et al., 2002) found that citalopram (a serotonergic antidepressant) decreased PTSD symptoms in children and adolescents to a comparable degree as it did in adults. Neither of these studies included randomization, blinding procedures, or placebo control conditions. Several other pharmacological studies for chronic childhood PTSD have been published but suffer from similar methodological weaknesses (Pine & Cohen, 2002). However, the success of various pharmacological agents in these trials suggests that further evaluation in double-blind, placebo-controlled trials is warranted. It is risky to assume that effective early pharmacological treatments for adults will have similar effects with comparable side-effect profiles in children. Therefore, extrapolating findings from adult pharmacological studies to children is unwarranted (Cohen, 2001). Thus, it will be important to conduct well-designed studies of acute pharmacological interventions for traumatized children.

EARLY TREATMENTS FOR CHILDHOOD TRAUMATIC GRIEF

As noted earlier, the definition and measurement of CTG are currently evolving. The available empirical data suggest that this condition is somewhat different from adult complicated bereavement (Cohen et al., 2002). Our current concept is that following the traumatic death of a loved one, children may develop PTSD symptoms that interfere with their ability to navigate the typical grieving process. In traumatic grief, the child has difficulty reminiscing about the deceased person, because any thoughts or reminders of that person (even happy, loving memories) segue into reminders of the traumatic manner of the death and are accompanied by psychological distress and physiological arousal. This leads to avoidance of reminiscing about the lost loved one or processing the meaning of the death. Because these tasks are integral to normal grieving, these symptoms prevent the child from successfully grieving the loss (Pynoos, 1992).

As with other traumatized children, there are barriers to accessing early mental health interventions for children with traumatic grief. If the loved one died under circumstances associated with social stigma (e.g., through suicide or drug overdose), this potential stigmatization may impede the family's willingness to seek treatment. Bereaved adults may be less able to perceive the child's trauma symptoms, particularly when these are predominantly avoidant in nature. Such adults may be using avoidant coping responses themselves and thus may be reticent to seek treatment related to the death of the loved one. Coping with the practical impact of the trauma/loss, such as loss of housing (e.g., if the death occurred in a fire which destroyed the family's home), income (if the deceased was the primary wage earner for the family), or health insurance (which may preclude receiving mental health interventions), and the need to attend to matters such as burial and accessing life insurance and other financial resources may take precedence over seeking mental health intervention in the acute aftermath of fatal traumas. Thus, it is not surprising that no studies have yet evaluated the impact of early interventions for such children.

The only published treatment study for CTG evaluated the impact of trauma- and loss-focused treatment modules for Bosnian adolescents exposed to war. This study (Layne, Pynoos, et al., 2001) provided group treatment 2 to 4 years after the end of the war in Bosnia and Hercegovina. The treatment model included trauma and grief-focused CBT components provided in distinct modules in school settings by trained school personnel. The five treatment modules were traumatic experiences, trauma and loss reminders, postwar adversities, bereavement and the interplay of trauma and grief, and developmental impact. Due to logistical problems, some children received all five treatment modules, whereas others received only the trauma-focused interventions. Both groups experienced significant improvements in PTSD and depressive symptoms, but the group that received both trauma and bereavement interventions experienced more improvement in traumatic grief symptoms than those that only received the trauma-focused interventions. Although there was no control condition or randomization, these findings provide promising support for the efficacy of combined trauma- and grief-focused CBT interventions for CTG in adolescents.

Another open trial of individual trauma and grief-focused CBT for CTG is currently being conducted for children and their surviving parents who lost loved ones due to a variety of traumas such as suicide, accidents, substance abuse, or community violence (Cohen, Mannarino, Stubenbort, Padlo, & Shipley, 2001). The majority of these children are receiving acute interventions, often within the first 1–2 months after the traumatic loss. In response to the tragic events of 9-11-01, the Silver Shield Foundation has funded a randomized clinical trial for children who lost their firefighter parents in the terrorist attacks on the World Trade Center in New York. This study is comparing trauma- and grief-focused CBT to child-centered therapy for these children and their surviving parents (Brown & Goodman, 2002). These studies will, ideally, enhance our understanding of effective early interventions for CTG.

THE VALUE OF EARLY SCREENING

The treatment studies described in this chapter have focused on symptomatic children and adolescents. There is no evidence that providing treatment to trauma-exposed children with no or minimal symptoms is beneficial. In fact, there are developmental reasons to be concerned that trauma-focused interventions may worsen symptoms in such children, as discussed earlier. This suggests the value of focusing early interventions on those children with significant acute stress symptoms, or those at highest risk of developing PTSD. There is evidence that early screening can successfully identify such children soon after trauma exposure. For example, Yule and Udwin (1991) demonstrated that administering a screening battery 10 days after the sinking of a cruise ship accurately identified children who reported higher levels of PTSD, depression, and anxiety symptoms 5 months later. These children were also more likely to be participating in counseling 5 months after the sinking. Brent, Moritz, Bridge, Perper, and Canobbio (1996) also found that early screening of suicide survivors accurately identified youth who had PTSD or depression 3 years later. Chemtob, Nakashima, and Hamada (2002) demonstrated the feasibility of conducting communitywide, school-based screening of disaster-exposed public school children to identify those most in need of treatment. Thus, even in the absence of research supporting the efficacy of early mental health treatment, early identification and follow-up of highly symptomatic children are likely warranted. This would indicate that when community-level traumas occur, public health resources should be devoted to conducting early, universal screening for highly symptomatic and/or high-risk children. As discussed earlier, there are numerous obstacles to conducting such screening in the acute aftermath of these disasters. Developing ongoing relationships between public health/mental health professionals and school systems will likely be necessary to overcome these barriers in the future (Chemtob, Nakashima, & Hamada, 2002).

SUMMARY

At the present time, few studies have evaluated the efficacy of early mental health interventions for children exposed to traumatic life events. There is growing evidence that TF-CBT is effective in decreasing a variety of symptoms and improving adaptive functioning in children exposed to a variety of traumatic life events (child abuse, disaster, single episode traumas, war), and that early TF-CBT interventions are effective for sexually abused children. In addition, there is preliminary evidence that early pharmacological interventions may be effective in decreasing acute stress symptoms in burned children or abused children, although these findings have yet to be replicated in randomized trials. Furthermore, there is support for the idea that early universal screening of trauma-exposed children is helpful in identifying those who are highly symptomatic and/or at high risk of developing PTSD. Additional research is needed to better understand what types and dosages of early mental health interventions may be valuable to which children, and when such interventions should be provided.

ACKNOWLEDGMENTS

Preparation of this chapter was supported in part by grants K2MH01938 (NIMH) and SM 54319 (SAMHSA). I gratefully acknowledge the assistance of Anthony P. Mannarino, PhD, Matthew Friedman, MD, PhD, and Ann Marie Kotlik in the preparation of this chapter.

REFERENCES

Amaya-Jackson, L., Newman, E., Lipzchitz, D., Davis-Rosenbalm, K., Billingslea, E., & Ymanis, N. (2000). The Child and Adolescent PTSD Checklist in three clinical research populations. In V. Carrion (Chair), *New methods and practice in assessing pediatric posttraumatic stress disorder.* Symposium presented at the annual meeting of the American Academy of Child and Adolescent Psychiatry, New York.
American Academy of Child and Adolescent Psychiatry. (1998). Practice parameters for the assessment and treatment of children and adolescents with PTSD. *Journal of the American Academy of Child and Adolescent Psychiatry, 37*(Suppl. 10), 4–26.
American Psychiatric Association. (1994). *Diagnostic and statistical manual of mental disorders* (4th ed.). Washington, DC: Author.
American School Health Association. (1989). *The National Adolescent Student Health Survey: A report on the health of America's youth.* Oakland, CA: Third Party Publishing.
Brent, D. A., Moritz, G., Bridge, J., Perper, J., & Canobbio, R. (1996). Long-term impact of exposure to suicide: A three year controlled follow-up. *Journal of the American Academy of Child and Adolescent Psychiatry, 35*, 646–653.
Brown, E. B., & Goodman, R. (2002). *Treating children with traumatic grief following 9/ 11.* Grant funded by the Silver Shield Foundation, New York.
Carrion, V. G., Weems, C. F., Ray, R., & Reiss, A. L. (2002). Toward an empirical definition of pediatric PTSD: The phenomenology of PTSD symptoms in youth. *Journal of the American Academy of Child and Adolescent Psychiatry, 41*, 166–173.
Celano, M., Hazzard, A., Webb, C., & McCall, C. (1996). Treatment of traumagenic beliefs among sexually abused girls and their mothers: An evaluation study. *Journal of Abnormal Psychology, 24*, 1–17.
Chemtob, C. M., Nakashima, J. P., & Hamada, R. S. (2002). Psychosocial intervention for postdisaster trauma symptoms in elementary school children. *Archives of Pediatric and Adolescent Medicine, 146*, 211–216.
Chemtob, C. M., Nakashima, J., Hamada, R., & Carlson, J. (2002). Brief treatment for elementary school children with disaster-related posttraumatic stress disorder: A field study. *Journal of Clinical Psychology, 58*, 99–112.

Cohen, J. A. (2001). Pharmacologic treatment of traumatized children. *Trauma, Violence and Abuse: A Review Journal, 2,* 155–171.

Cohen, J. A., Berliner, L., & March, J. S. (2000). Treatment of children and adolescents. In E. B. Foa, T. M. Keane, & M. J. Friedman (Eds.), *Effective treatments for PTSD: Practice guidelines from the International Society for Traumatic Stress Studies* (pp. 106–138). New York: Guilford Press.

Cohen, J. A., & Mannarino, A. P. (1996a). A treatment outcome study for sexually abused preschool children: Initial findings. *Journal of the American Academy of Child and Adolescent Psychiatry, 35,* 42–50.

Cohen, J. A., & Mannarino, A. P. (1996b). Factors that mediate treatment outcome of sexually abused preschool children. *Journal of the American Academy of Child and Adolescent Psychiatry, 35,* 1402–1410.

Cohen, J. A., & Mannarino, A. P. (1998). Interventions for sexually abused children: Initial treatment findings. *Child Maltreatment, 3,* 17–26.

Cohen, J. A., & Mannarino, A. P. (2000). Predictors of treatment outcome in sexually abused children. *Child Abuse and Neglect, 24,* 983–994.

Cohen, J. A., Mannarino, A. P., Greenberg, T., Padlo, S., & Shipley, C. (2002). Childhood traumatic grief: Concepts and controversies. *Trauma, Violence and Abuse: A Review Journal, 3,* 307–327.

Cohen, J. A., Mannarino, A. P., & Knudsen, K. (2003, May). *Treating sexually abused children: One-year follow-up of a randomized controlled trial.* Paper presented at the 156th annual meeting of the American Psychiatric Association, San Francisco.

Cohen, J. A., Mannarino, A. P., Stubenbort, K., Padlo, S., & Shipley, C. (2001). *Treating traumatic bereavement in children.* Grant no. SM 54319 funded by the SAMHSA Center for Mental Health Services, Child Abuse and Traumatic Loss Treatment Development Center.

Costello, E. J., Erkanli, A., Fairbank, J. A., & Angold, A. (2002). The prevalence of potentially traumatic events in childhood and adolescence. *Journal of Traumatic Stress, 15,* 99–112.

DeBellis, M. D., Keshavan, M. S., Clark, D. B., Casey, B. J., Giedd, J. N., Boring, A. M., Frustaci, K., & Ryan, N. D. (1999). Developmental traumatology. Part II: Brain development. *Biological Psychiatry, 45,* 1271–1284.

Deblinger, E., Lippman, J., & Steer, R. (1996). Sexually abused children suffering posttraumatic stress symptoms: Initial treatment outcome findings. *Child Maltreatment, 1,* 310–321.

Famularo, R., Kinscherff, R., & Fenton, T. (1988). Propranolol treatment for childhood PTSD, acute type. *American Diseases of Children, 142,* 1244–1247.

Foa, E. B., Johnson, K. M., Feeny, N. C., & Treadwell, K. R. H. (2001). The Child PTSD Symptom Scale: A preliminary examination of its psychometric properties. *Journal of Clinical Child Psychology, 30,* 376–384.

Goenjian, A. K., Karayan, I., Pynoos, R. S., Minassian, D., Najarian, L. M., Steinber, A. M., & Fairbanks, L. A. (1997). Outcome of psychotherapy among early adolescents after trauma. *American Journal of Psychiatry, 154,* 536–542.

Layne, C. M., Pynoos, R. S., Saltzman, W. R., Arslanagic, B. G., Black, M., Savjak, N.,

Popovic, T., Durakovic, E., Music, M., Campara, N., Djapo, N., & Houston, R. (2001). Trauma/grief focused group psychotherapy: School-based postwar intervention with traumatized Bosnian youth. *Group Dynamics: Theory, Research and Practice, 5,* 277–290.

Layne, C. M., Savjak, N., Saltzman, W. R., & Pynoos, R. S. (2001). *UCLA/BYU Expanded Grief Inventory.* Unpublished instrument. Brigham Young University, Provo, UT.

Mannarino, A. P., & Cohen, J. A. (2001). Treating sexually abused children and their families: Identifying and avoiding professional role conflicts. *Trauma, Violence and Abuse: A Review Journal, 2,* 331–342.

March, J. S., Amaya-Jackson, L., Murray, M. C., & Schulte, A. (1998). Cognitive-behavioral psychotherapy for children and adolescents with PTSD after a single-episode stressor. *Journal of the American Academy of Child and Adolescent Psychiatry, 37,* 585–593.

Pfefferbaum, B., Nixon, S. J., Tucker, P. M., Tivis, R. D., Moore, V. L., Gurwitch, R. H., Pynoos, R. S., & Geis, H. R. (1999). Posttraumatic stress responses in bereaved children after the Oklahoma City bombing. *Journal of the American Academy of Child and Adolescent Psychiatry, 38,* 1372–1379.

Pine, D. S., & Cohen, J. A. (2002). Trauma in children and adolescents: Risk and treatment of psychiatric sequelae. *Biological Psychiatry, 51,* 519–531.

Pynoos, R. S. (1992). Grief and trauma in children and adolescents. *Bereavement Care, 11,* 2–10.

Pynoos, R. S., Rodriguez, P., Steinberg, A., Stuber, M., & Frederick, C. J. (1998). *UCLA PTSD Index for DSM-IV.* Unpublished instrument, University of California-Los Angeles.

Robert, R., Blackeney, P. E., Villarreal, C., Rosenberg, L., & Meyer, W. J. (1999). Imipramine treatment in pediatric burn patients with symptoms of adult stress disorder. *Journal of the American Academy of Child and Adolescent Psychiatry, 38,* 873–882.

Saxe, G., Stoddard, F., Courtney, D., Cunningham, K., Chawla, N., Sheridan, R., King, D., & King, L. (2001). Relationship between acute morphine and the course of PTSD in children with burns. *Journal of the American Academy of Child and Adolescent Psychiatry, 40,* 915–921.

Scheeringa, M. S., Peebles, C. D., Cook, C. A., & Zeanah, C. H. (2001). Toward establishing procedural criterion and discriminant validity for PTSD in early childhood. *Journal of the American Academy of Child and Adolescent Psychiatry, 40,* 52–60.

Scheeringa, M. S., Zeanah, C. H., Drell, M. J., & Larrieu, J. A. (1995). Two approaches to diagnosing PTSD in infancy and early childhood. *Journal of the American Academy of Child and Adolescent Psychiatry, 34,* 191–200.

Schubiner, H., Scott, R., & Tzelepis, A. (1993). Exposure to violence among inner-city youth. *Journal of Adolescence Health, 14,* 214–219.

Seedat, S., Stein, D. J., Ziervogel, C., Middleton, T., Kaminer, D., Emsley, R. A., & Rossouw, W. (2002). Comparison of response to a selective serotonin reuptake inhibitor in children, adolescents, and adults with PTSD. *Journal of Child and Adolescent Psychopharmacology, 12,* 37–46.

Singer, M. I., Anglin, T. M., Song, L. Y., & Lunghofer, L. (1995). Adolescents' exposure to violence and associated symptoms of psychological trauma. *Journal of the American Medical Association, 273,* 477–482.

Stallard, P., & Law, F. (1993). Screening and psychological debriefing of adolescent survivors of life threatening events. *British Journal of Psychiatry, 163,* 660–665.

Trowell, J., Kelvin, I., Weeramanthi, T., Sadowski, H., Berelowitz, M., Glasser, D., & Leitch, I. (2002). Psychotherapy for sexually abused girls: Psychopathological outcome findings and patterns of change. *British Journal of Psychiatry, 160,* 234–247.

Yule, W., & Udwin, D. (1991). Screening child survivors for PTSD: Experiences from the "Jupiter" sinking. *British Journal of Psychology, 30,* 131–138.

8

Early Mental Health Interventions for Traumatic Loss in Adults

BEVERLEY RAPHAEL
SALLY WOODING

Recent tragedies have highlighted the shock, horror, and profound aftermath of terrorist attacks such as those in New York on September 11th, 2001, and the Bali bombing on October 12th, 2002. There have, of course, been many other terrorist activities that have impacted on communities acutely and over a prolonged time. The numbers of deaths, their sudden and violent occurrence, the threat to life, the injuries, and destruction to buildings, homes, and communities all contribute major stressors. These are public events, seen and experienced directly by many. The purpose of terrorism is to have a maximal impact on populations. Terrorists and their acts are seen repeatedly on television and through the media; so the impact is extended beyond those who experienced the attack directly. Terrorism, and its effects, is one theme through which such experiences can be studied for their impact on the health and well-being of societies.

Many other "traumatic" experiences occur. For instance Breslau, Davis, Andreski, and Peterson (1991) found that more than one-third of population groups studied had experienced at least one traumatic event. In the National Comorbidity Study, Kessler, Sonnega, Bromet, Hughes, and Nelson (1995) found that more than 60% of men and 50% of women had experienced at least one traumatic event in their lifetime. Traumatic events such as violent assaults, major accidents, homicides, fires, rape, and other horrific events can cause other stressors to emerge (e.g., loss of resources), which can affect individuals and their families. Of special concern is the impact these events may have on mental health. The aforementioned events have all been the source of studies in the conceptual framework of posttraumatic stress disorder (PTSD) with variable rates of PTSD reported over time for those directly exposed (Davidson & Foa, 1991; Kessler et al., 1995; North et al., 1999). Similarly, studies of major disasters have been undertaken, again with a primary focus on PTSD (Shore, Tatum, & Volmer, 1986; McFarlane, 1986, 1988a, 1988b; Ursano, McCaughey, & Fullerton, 1994). Despite the focus on the development of PTSD after trauma, it is clear that the majority of people exposed to these events, while distressed and suffering at the time and in the immediate aftermath, do not develop PTSD but recover fully.

Most often, traumatic events are indexed in terms of the number of deaths that have resulted, just as battles are judged by the "body count" of casualties. However, some of the most complex and profound psychological and social morbidity can result from the bereavements that have occurred. In contrast to natural deaths, "good" deaths, timely deaths, or peaceful deaths at the end of a fulfilled life, bereaved individuals in traumatic circumstances have to contend with unexpected and tragic loss. These deaths, be they through violent and horrific personal disasters or major catastrophes, such as terrorism, are likely to be traumatic and to lead to traumatic bereavement. The limited research and clinical data available highlight the complexity of dealing with such events and resolving these losses and the substantial risk to well-being and mental health that may result.

In the case of terrorism, it is likely that deaths will lead to particularly complex and problematic bereavements. These deaths are sudden, unexpected, untimely, and violent. There may be prolonged uncertainty about the fate of loved ones. In addition to the circumstances surrounding the death of the loved one, the bereaved are likely to be experiencing other major stressors as well, particularly if they have been involved in and survived the terrorist episode themselves. There are multiple and public losses. Balancing these factors, individuals bereaved by terrorist attacks are likely to experience enormous public support for recognition of the loss and grief, and public ritual and recognition of the needs of the bereaved. Recent epidemiological studies of the mental heath impact of 9-11 report almost exclusively on the traumatic stress phenomena related to direct exposure to life threat (Schuster et al., 2001; Schlenger et al., 2002; Silver, Holman, McIntosh, Poulin, & Gil-Rivas, 2002). However, one study conducted by Galea et al. (2002) reported on the impact of the loss as well as the impact of traumatic stress effects. Their results indicated that "experiences involving exposure to the attacks predicted current PTSD and that loss as a result of the attack predicted current depression" (p. 346).

It is important to note that bereavement is a part of everyday life and that most deaths do not occur as a consequence of terror or horrific incidents. Grief, as the emotional reaction to such loss, is a normal human emotional response attesting to the value and significance of human attachments and the pain of losing them. Grief is not a disease (Engel, 1961).

Understanding the phenomenology of the normal reaction to loss is an important step to a better understanding of abnormal patterns that may be indicative of the need for interventions to prevent or treat the occurrence of bereavement-related morbidity. Research in the field of normal and pathological grief responses is evolving, but it is still limited in many respects. As with traumatic stress reactions, there are methodological and ethical difficulties in conducting research with acutely distressed populations. Sampling may also be a problem. Instruments to accurately measure the reactive phenomenology are frequently measures of disorders. For instance with traumatic stress reactions, symptom measures for PTSD are used; and for bereavement, until recently, symptom measures for depression have often been used by default. In the future, specific checklists and instruments will be of value to quantify reactive processes and monitor these over time.

Tailored assessment is important both to improving understanding and as a basis for appropriate intervention. This is more so as bereavement was initially classified as part of the stress response syndrome in Horowitz's original model, and the phenomenology of traumatic grief was considered exclusively in this context (e.g., Horowitz, 1976). It was also seen as a reactive depression (Clayton, 1990; Parkes, 1970; Parkes & Weiss, 1983). Bereavement and depression are distinct entities, although depression may be one adverse outcome after loss. In addition, as discussed later, there is now general agreement that the phenomena of bereavement and posttraumatic stress syndromes are separate reactions to different stressors, although they may occur concurrently (Pynoos, Frederick, et al., 1987; Pynoos, Nader, Frederick, Gonda, & Stuber, 1987; Raphael & Martinek, 1997; Rynearson, 2002).

An understanding of the overlapping and distinct features of PTSD, depression, and traumatic grief is critical to assessing and providing an appropriately tailored response or intervention for people bereaved in such circumstances. It is also vital that research on the longitudinal course and outcome of loss delineates the risk and protective factors that contribute to whether or not pathology occurs as a consequence of, or in association with, these life events (see King, Vogt, & King, Chapter 3, this volume). Research on risk and resilience factors will greatly inform decisions about intervention.

In terms of evidence-based interventions for prevention and treatment of traumatic bereavement, a number of approaches have been discussed (Raphael, Minkov, & Dobson, 2001; Stroebe, Hannson, Stroebe, &, Schut, 2001). Support for these varies. The critical components of any effective intervention for bereavement-related distress and other problems are human compassion and concern as well as genuine warmth and empathy, within the therapeutic relationship, for those who have lost faith in the security of their personal world (Raphael, Middleton, Martinek, & Misso, 1993). This is likely to be particularly important for those who have lost a primary attachment figure. Meta-analysis has indicated modest treatment effects for bereavement interventions (Neimeyer, 2000). Despite the difficulty in comparing studies, there is a clear trend that benefits are most likely when interventions are targeted to those at higher risk of adverse outcomes. Questions then include the following: Should early intervention be provided? What should the aims and goals of an intervention be? What sort of intervention should be done and what is its rationale? What are the intended outcomes?

PHENOMENOLOGY OF BEREAVEMENT

Bereavement processes have been studied in a number of ways: retrospective surveys of reactions reported by bereaved people, clinical studies, questionnaires to populations of bereaved people, "prospective" studies with families of the terminally ill, studies that follow "total" or representative samples of all those bereaved after a series of deaths, and epidemiological research correlating poorer health and social outcomes with bereavement status. These different research methods have led to a great deal of information about bereavement; however it is often difficult (and methodologically questionable) to compare or pool studies in order to define what is "normal" and what is "pathological."

Recent research has focused on the systematic study of the reactive process using standardized measures (and the development of assessment measures). This research is informed by theories on the nature of bereavement reactions, most frequently of John Bowlby's attachment theory (Middelton, Moylan, Raphael, Burnett, & Martinek, 1993; Raphael, 1983). Measures used include, but are not limited to, the Texas Revised Inventory of Grief (TRIG; Faschingbauer, Zisook, & DeVaul, 1987), the Grief Experience Inventory (Sanders, 1980), measures of separation distress and mourning (Jacobs, 1993; Jacobs, Kasl, Ostfeld, Berkman, & Charpentier, 1986; Jacobs et al., 1986) and measures of Core Bereavement Phenomena (Core Bereavement Items, CBI; Burnett, Middleton, Raphael, & Martinek, 1997).

The findings from the use of such measures are fairly consistent. There are initial periods of shock and numbness, especially if bereavement is unexpected, but also in terms of the reality of the death, and the news of the loss and the way it is communicated. High levels of distress appear, and, initially, this represents separation distress and anxiety. There is intense longing for loved ones, "searching behaviors," yearning and pining for them, though intellectually it is known that the loved one will not return. The bereaved may experience difficulties concentrating as well as cognitive distortions such as misperceiving the face of the deceased and "hallucinating" their image, touch, or voice. Angry protest is also a frequent part of this with feelings of "why me" and "why my loved one" and an ongoing sense of abandonment. These feelings may lead to psychological mourning processes where the reality and finality of the death are progressively accepted and there is a preoccupation with and focus on memories of the loved one. These memories, along with the possessions of the deceased, are "sorted through." There is sadness at what has been lost with the relationship as vivid memories of it are reviewed, and for what can no longer be and the loss of what was hoped for the future. Feelings of guilt and anger may also surface during this time. Functioning may be difficult initially but gradually returns.

In normal bereavements, the intense distress lessens progressively through the first month to 6 weeks, and gradually thereafter but is likely to return with reminders over the first year and even subsequently. Bereavement is not "packaged" so that it is all fixed or "resolved" by a certain period of time. Thoughts, memories, and sadness may return over many years, as may a sense of unfinished business with the deceased. Nevertheless functioning and interpersonal relations continue, as does adapting to "getting on with life" without the deceased. Middleton, Raphael, Burnett, and Martinek (1998) have demonstrated this pattern in adults following the death of a partner/spouse, child, or parent, showing similar phenomena for each type of loss, although with varying intensity (loss of child being most intense and parent least for the adult). No clear-cut "stages" of grief have been validated by any researcher, but rather what has been discerned is a variable progression over time.

The emotional reactions associated with grief may also be extremely intense. Many bereaved people describe them as unlike anything else they have felt, and some have feared they were "going mad." Initially, sleep disturbances are common as are frequent and realistic dreams of the deceased, which can cause the bereaved to awake believing that the deceased person is still alive or has returned. As the grieving process continues, the bereaved individual may dream of illness and farewell.

Abnormal bereavement phenomena have been ambiguously defined. In a survey of experts in the field, Middleton, Burnett, Raphael, and Martinek

(1996) found that there was not a great deal of consensus and few agreed-on operational definitions of commonly used terms such as "abnormal grief," "chronic grief," "delayed grief," "absent grief," "distorted grief," and so forth. Middleton et al.'s survey reported that the most agreement centered on "chronic grief," which was seen as intense and prolonged patterns of the heightened distress of the acute phase. Recent studies have attempted to define pathological grief, which they identify as being characterized by intense and prolonged separation distress (Prigerson & Jacobs, 2001). Prigerson and Jacobs (2001) initially called this traumatic grief but acknowledge that it does not necessarily reflect the traumatic grief that follows a shocking and horrific death and trauma and grief as is discussed later. Prigerson and colleagues have now adopted the broader and more valid term, "complicated grief" (see Gray, Prigerson, & Litz, Chapter 4, this volume). Horowitz et al. (1997) have focused a similar form of grief, which they define as "complicated grief disorder." Similar qualities are used by both research groups to describe these terms, and both groups have developed potential diagnostic criteria.

Middleton et al. (1996) as well as other research using the same assessment of phenomenology (e.g., Byrne & Raphael, 1994, 1997; after bereavement in the elderly) have shown that about 9% of those in a well-sampled population are likely to demonstrate chronic grief on the CBI (Middleton et al., 1996). That is, high levels of continuing intense distress (as in acute grief) at 6 months and 13 months after the bereavement.

PATHOLOGIES AND OUTCOMES OF BEREAVEMENT

Whether or not a bereavement can be described as "pathological" has been discussed by Bowlby (1969, 1973, 1980), Lindemann (1944), and Parkes and Weiss (1983), as well as those researching complicated, chronic, and abnormal grief (Horowitz et al., 1997; Raphael & Minkov, 1999; Prigerson & Jacobs, 2001). Other aspects of pathological outcome in relation to bereavement should also be taken into account when the need for intervention is being assessed. These include the development of other disorders in association with bereavement such as anxiety disorders, depressive disorders, substance disorders, the precipitation of psychoses, and so forth (Jacobs, 1993; Stroebe et al., 2001). Of particular interest is the development of depressive disorders and PTSD, as is discussed in the following paragraphs.

Physical health problems, such as heightened mortality for older bereaved men (including but not only due to suicide or health-related behavior change, Byrne & Raphael, 1997, 1999), heightened utilization of health services such as primary care, and increased risk of cardiovascular problems, cancer, and other adverse health outcomes such as disrupted sleep and lowered immune functioning (Hall & Irwin, 2001; Prigerson et al., 1997), have also been reported in bereaved individuals.

However, it must be emphasized that these outcomes are by no means inevitable. Though the majority of bereaved people may experience distress and anguish over their loss, they recover and adapt well in their ongoing lives. They remember their loved ones with nostalgia and sadness, but they regain their positive involvement in life. There is clearly a need for much more collaborative, broadly based, and sophisticated research to extend knowledge about potentially influential variables and to determine, at a population level, the patterns and the positive and negative outcomes over time. It must also be noted that positive outcomes also occur with internalizations and strengths and personal growth may follow (e.g., Vaillant, 1988).

PHENOMENOLOGY OF POSTTRAUMATIC STRESS REACTIONS

Threat to life and exposure to shocking and horrific events, to the gruesome and mutilating deaths of others, are the types of stressors that lead to reactive processes of posttraumatic stress reactions. Although some of these reactions were initially understood in terms of war syndromes that resulted from combat (e.g., shell shock and traumatic neurosis), the phenomena were most clearly postulated in Horowitz's (1976) classic work, *Stress Response Syndromes*. He identified the shock and numbness that might be initial reactions, but more specifically the ongoing phenomena of reexperiencing and avoidance which were systematically measured using the Impact of Event Scale (IES; Horowitz, Wilner, & Alvarez, 1979), which his group developed.

Studies of these phenomena and other reactions to such shocking events were also advanced by the work of Weisaeth (1989), who studied a total population of workers immediately after a paint factory explosion and fire and followed them over time. He demonstrated clearly the dose–response effect of degree of exposure (closeness to center) and level of reactive processes (anxiety and cognitive phenomena) as well as a relationship between these variables and the development of posttraumatic syndromes. These phenomena have also been extensively studied with Vietnam veterans, rape victims, assault victims, and accident victims as well as victims of war, conflict, and disasters. Numerous measures (some providing dimensional, categorical, or both approaches to PTSD) have been used including checklists reflecting the symptoms of disorder as defined in DSM manuals, structured interviews such as the Clinician-Administered PTSD Scale (CAPS; Blake et al., 1995), versions of the Minnesota Multiphasic Personality Inventory (Keane, Malloy, & Fairbanks, 1984), and a revised version of the IES (Weiss & Marmar, 1997).

As with bereavement, there has been research such as that reported by

Davidson et al. which shows that prolonged and heightened initial distress may continue into posttraumatic stress syndromes such as PTSD (Davidson & Foa, 1993). As is the case with bereavement, heightened distress beyond the first month posttrauma increases the likelihood that disorders will develop. If symptoms persist beyond 3–4 months, a chronic disorder such as PTSD is more apt to appear (Raphael & Minkov, 1999).

Acute stress reaction phenomena of great intensity in association with dissociative phenomena, in the early days following trauma, have been identified as a syndrome (acute stress disorder; ASD), predicting the development of PTSD (Harvey & Bryant, 1998), although this diagnostic syndrome is somewhat contentious (Harvey & Bryant, 2002). McFarlane (1988a) described the delayed onset of this reactive process and/or disorder. Normally, with the passage of time, reactive processes progressively diminish. The event and the fear it evoked are no longer a central preoccupation, and function returns. This is not the case with pathology, where preoccupation continues as a major theme, dominating the person's life (see discussion in Raphael, 1997).

PATHOLOGIES AND OUTCOMES OF TRAUMATIC STRESS

While the major syndrome studied in almost every piece of research dealing with disasters and major incidents is PTSD, more recent work has highlighted other pathologies. For instance, comorbid or independent major depression, panic disorder and other anxiety disorders, substance use disorder, personality changes as a result of profound and ongoing stressor exposure, and the impact on physical health and health care utilization (Ullman & Siegel, 1996; Taft, Stern, King, & King, 1999; Wagner, Wolfe, Rotnitsky, Proctor, & Erickson, 2000) have all been studied. In addition, social functioning has also been found to be significantly impaired (i.e., social isolation, interpersonal relationships, and capacity to work). Neuroendocrine and central nervous system changes have also been reviewed (Yehuda, 1999). However, it should again be acknowledged that positive outcomes and personal growth may occur, even following the most stressful experiences (Davidson, 2002; Hull, Alexander, & Klein, 2002; Tedeschi & Calhoun, 1996).

SOCIAL CONSTRUCTIONS AND PHENOMENA OF LOSS AND TRAUMATIC STRESS

Social meanings, social recognition, and social and cultural rituals, as well as social support and response, may influence how the phenomena of loss and traumatic stress are perceived and dealt with. These variables may also affect certain outcomes posttrauma or loss. All these variables must be taken into account when considering a health or mental health intervention. For instance, there may be strong cultural prescriptions about how death is viewed, religious requirements about the disposal of the body of the deceased, or social requirements and practices around grief and mourning and the roles and rights of the bereaved. Failure to meet these prescriptions may complicate and interfere with the psychological processes of grief and mourning. Legal requirements, such as autopsy, legal inquiries, and trials, may also affect how trauma and loss are processed (e.g., after a homicide). Medical requirements may also affect adaptive processes (e.g., as in the case of death from highly infectious diseases). Also, some bereavements may be more stigmatized (e.g., AIDS deaths and suicide in some societies). In addition, some sections of society may be expected to behave in certain ways (e.g., for men to contain grief, or to be "strong" despite the experience of severe life threat and traumatic stress).

Rituals for traumatic stress frequently performed in some cultures or subcultures have included informal and formal debriefing, the telling of war stories, and healing and cleansing rituals. Rituals recognizing heroes who have survived traumatically stressful experiences may support adaptation for the traumatized, as may memorialization. However, other traditions/rituals may be exclusory, failing to acknowledge those who may have had greater exposure or need. For both preventive and treatment interventions for loss, trauma, and traumatic loss, these features need to be taken into account.

Another important component that has been repeatedly seen to be influential in such circumstances of adversity is social support—provided by confidants, family members, and communities to members who are profoundly affected (Maddison & Walker, 1967; Murphy, 1998). Assessing social support and its role may be essential before intervention is decided on. For instance, bereaved individuals who perceive social support to be inadequate or unhelpful are at heightened risk of adverse outcomes and more likely to benefit from intervention (Raphael, 1977b). It should be noted, however, that intervention should not replace the normal, helpful social networks which bereaved and traumatized individuals will use, over time, to deal with their experiences.

CONCURRENT TRAUMATIC STRESS AND LOSS

It is essential to understand the overlapping and complex phenomena that occur when traumatic stress and loss are concurrent so that these complex interactions and reactive processes may be evaluated to provide appropriate, well-timed interventions in the right form, as needed.

Traumatic loss occurs when there is sudden, violent, and shocking death or deaths. Many circumstances could contribute to the occurrence of traumatic loss, some of which include terrorism, mass violence, homicide, instances in which the deceased's body is not found in circumstances of violence and uncertainty or in which the body is so severely damaged or disintegrated that identification is possible only by forensic means. In addition, traumatic loss is more likely when there was a risk or threat to life, when the death is associated with gruesome, mutilating injury to the body, or is the consequence of human malevolence purposely or coincidentally perpetrated against the deceased, and thus also the bereaved, as with homicide. Other deaths that may involve shock or horror include the death of a child in an accident or from abuse, sudden infant death, multiple deaths of family members, or death with other serious concurrent losses. Death by suicide may also be particularly shocking or horrifying, especially if the bereaved was the one to find the deceased hanging or shot. Deaths in disasters, particularly "man-made" disasters, and deaths resulting from mass shootings or terrorist attack are also all potentially traumatic losses of this kind. Bearing in mind that many terrorist attacks and disasters have higher levels of deaths than physical casualties, there is the potential for significant levels of morbidity as a consequence, which will have an impact on the well-being and functioning of a great many individuals and communities (Lundin, 1984; Raphael & Martinek, 1997; Singh & Raphael, 1981).

The risk of postincident morbidity increases in cases of traumatic loss due to several factors, including complex, multiple stressors (i.e., survivor guilt and survivor "responsibility"—the feeling that the survivor contributed to the death, by what he or she did or did not do; Hull et al., 2002), a lack of or breakdown of social support due to the impact of the event, as well as the lack of effective interventions available to treat large numbers of at-risk individuals. Other risk factors for adverse outcomes of bereavement include the untimely nature of the deaths (e.g., the death of a child), heightened ambivalence or dependence in the relationship the bereaved had with the deceased, personality factors and coping styles (e.g., neuroticism), or deprivations and issues from earlier life (e.g., the death of a parent in childhood). A number of studies have highlighted such risks (e.g., Lundin, 1984; Parkes & Weiss, 1983; Raphael, 1977b ; Raphael & Maddison, 1976). Given these risk factors, interventions are likely to be necessary to prevent adverse effects, or to treat them once they have arisen. Early intervention is an important part of the intervention spectrum offering the chance for benefit before morbidity and associated impairments become established or the person becomes fixed in identity and the role of victim.

In assessing reactions to trauma and traumatic loss, Table 8.1 is a useful guide to determine the need and type of intervention and to judge their outcomes. Although traumatic stress and loss are described separately, it is nevertheless fully acknowledged and recognized that they commonly co-occur. As can be seen in Table 8.1, there are often co-occurring and interacting patterns of symptomatology.

TABLE 8.1. Phenomena of Bereavement and Posttraumatic Reactions

Posttraumatic phenomena	Bereavement phenomena
Cognitive phenomena	
• Intrusions of *scene of trauma* (e.g., death) Not associated with yearning or longing Associated with distress, anxiety at image	• Image of *lost person* constantly comes to mind (unbidden or bidden) Associated with yearning or longing Distress that person is not there
• Preoccupation with the *traumatic event* and circumstances of it	• Preoccupation with the *lost person* and loved images of him or her
• *Memories* usually of the *traumatic* scene	• *Memories of person* associated with affect relevant to memory (often positive)
• Reexperiencing of threatening aspects of the event	• Reexperiencing of *person's presence,* as though he or she were still there (e.g., hallucinations of sound, tough, sight)
Affective phenomena	
Anxiety	
• Anxiety as the principal affect *General* and generated by threat Fearful of *threat/danger* Precipitated by *reminders, intrusions*	• Anxiety, when present, is *separation* anxiety Specific and generated by separation from lost person Generated by imagined futures without lost person Precipitated by his or her *failure to return*
Yearning/longing	
• These are not prominent features Not person oriented; if occurs, is for things to have been as they were before—for the return of innocence of death and the sense of personal invulnerability	• Yearning for lost person Intense, painful, profound Triggered by reminders of him or her Yearning for him or her to return, to be there
Sadness	
• Sadness not commonly described	• Sadness frequent and profound
• Nostalgia for event not described	• Feelings of nostalgia common and persistent
Avoidance phenomena	
• *Avoids* reminders of event, including places	• May search for and *seek out* places of familiarity, *treasured objects* (e.g., linking objects, photos and images) • May try to *avoid reminders of the absence* of the lost person

(continued)

TABLE 8.1. *(continued)*

Posttraumatic phenomena	Bereavement phenomena
Avoidance phenomena (continued)	
• Attempts to lessen affect; numbing, lessened feelings generally	• May try to *mitigate* pangs of grief but only temporarily, including distracting, but also seeks to express grief as normal
• May have great difficulty talking of event during avoidance times, although at others may be powerfully driven to talk of experience (but not person)	• May be very driven to talk of lost relationship and lost person
• Withdrawal from others (protective of self)	• May seek others for support, or to talk of deceased
• *Oriented to threat* and danger	• *Oriented to lost person*
• General *scanning and alertness to danger,* fearfulness	• General *scanning* of *environment for lost one or cues* of them
• Exaggerated *startle* response (i.e., response to minimal threat)	• Generates *searching* behavior
• Overresponse to cues of trauma	• Overresponse to cues of lost person

A spectrum of interventions has been defined as part of a public health or population health approach to lessening morbidity and the burden and health impact of disorders. In this instance it can be used to conceptualize the interventions that may be needed to prevent or treat the consequences of traumatic loss (Mrazek & Haggerty, 1994). Figure 8.1 summarizes these interventions.

EARLY INTERVENTION

Although there are a number of potential entry points for early intervention with bereaved people and for those traumatized, any interventions must also fit with the need and readiness of those affected (see Litz, Gray, Bryant, & Adler, 2002).

Universal and Population-Wide Interventions

Universal and population-wide interventions may be proposed for those who are likely to become traumatized and bereaved. Education dealing with normal reactions to trauma and bereavement and what can be expected and effective social supports to utilize after the incident are important parts of this type of intervention. In addition, strengthening natural networks of support and education about self-help and what to do for others may all be of assistance in general ways, although there is no study demonstrating the effectiveness of such interventions and their outcomes. When considering the types of interventions applicable on a large scale, several areas need to be taken into account:

1. The social, health, and legal processes that often surround traumatic losses need to be developed, with special sensitivity to the needs of the bereaved. Intervention in these areas may serve to mitigate the stresses and stressor effects surrounding the circumstances of the deaths. Special provisions can be made to assist bereaved people in traumatic circumstances such as mass violence by a clear source of information about loved ones, whose whereabouts may be uncertain or who may be deceased. A place to go to receive support and accurate, regularly updated information can lessen stresses such as searching for the whereabouts of loved ones in hospitals, disaster sites, or morgues. The bereaved are acknowledged and supported by such a process. Information lines and police or other emergency programs can assist with this process.

2. Support and comfort for the bereaved need to be put into place around the identification process. This includes the provision of a skilled bereavement support worker who can provide information, check issues of iden-

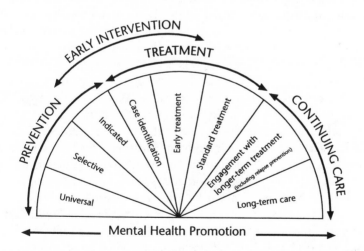

FIGURE 8.1. The spectrum of interventions for mental health problems and mental disorders. Adapted from Mrazek and Haggerty (1994). Copyright 1994 by the National Academy of Sciences, courtesy of the National Academies Press, Washington, DC. Reprinted in Commonwealth Department of Health and Aged Care (2000), p. 28.

tification, and deal with the bereaved's fears and anxieties in an honest and straightforward way while offering reassurance and support. For example, questions about what to tell children or whether or not the deceased suffered before death are often at the forefront of people's minds at such times. In addition, the support worker must be familiar with, and inform the bereaved of, legal issues surrounding autopsy and release of the remains for burial. Practical matters such as funeral and burial arrangements must also be addressed, with special attention to any social, personal, cultural, or religious practices that may apply.

Two other types of support may also be provided during this time, the first of which is "psychological first aid" (Raphael, 1977a, 1986; New South Wales Health Department, 2000; National Institute of Mental Health, 2001). This term was first coined by Raphael in 1977 and indicates the provision of comfort and support, as well as ensuring survival, if this is required (Raphael, 1977a). It also includes the provision of sources of information. While providing psychological first aid, the bereavement worker may also assess need for future follow-up or intervention based on risk status or need.

It should be noted that psychological debriefing, in any form, is *not* included among the list of interventions or support that should be offered at this time; even if the bereaved person has been exposed to traumatic stressors. There is *no* evidence that debriefing can prevent PTSD or other adverse reactions to major stressors/traumas. In addition, there is every indication that it is specifically contraindicated for those recently and traumatically bereaved. A study by Polak, Egan, Vanderbergh, and Williams (1973) which provided psychological interventions to bereaved individuals and required provisions in the first 48 hours or so failed to show benefit.

3. Community processes that acknowledge the needs of the bereaved and the tragic nature of the death may provide support for the bereaved. When there have been larger-scale incidents with many deaths, the responses of community leaders and the media in demonstrating "grief leadership" may be helpful to those who have lost loved ones. This support is likely to continue and may be a source of comfort to the bereaved throughout funeral and memorial processes. This type of support attests to the value of the persons lost, pays tribute to the deceased, and acknowledges the bereaved's grief.

Examples of some of the processes discussed previously were implemented in response to the terrorist attacks of 9-11-01, in the United States and the 2002 terrorist bombing in Bali, including the provision of places of information for loved ones, the creation of places for people to leave candles or other tokens of remembrance, memorial ceremonies and publications honoring the lives of those who died, the recognition of babies born after 9-11 who were fathered by victims of the attack, which showed support for the victim's widows and families, as well as the leadership of Mayor Giuliani in the days and weeks following the attacks in New York City. The ongoing provision of counseling will be described later.

The terrorist bombings of 2002, which occurred on the Indonesian island of Bali, injured and killed many Australian citizens who were vacationing, living, or visiting the island at the time of the attack. The Bali bombing was a traumatically stressful experience both for those who were there and for those who had a loved one who might have been injured or killed. After the attack, places to gather and disseminate information were rapidly established and formal disaster victim identification processes were supported by skilled bereavement workers. These workers were also available to help loved ones in Australia to understand what needed to happen and to answer any questions these loved ones might have. To reduce any additional stress on the bereaved, the workers also assisted in the return of the deceased who were Australian back to the country, and with the coronial and legal requirements that needed to be handled. Though every effort was made to reduce the stress of the bereaved, the requirement of forensic identification in Bali and the wait for the return of loved ones caused anguish for many families, as did one brief misidentification.

Journeying to Bali for those seeking family members was facilitated. All returning families were met by outreach support workers who assisted them with the reentry, coronial, and legal processes until the bodies of loved ones were released for burial. Support and respect were emphasized during the formal return of bodies in order to maintain the dignity of and compassion for both the deceased and the bereaved.

Additional support was provided when the Prime Minister of Australia visited Bali and offered both compassion and government support to the victims and their families. The losses suffered by the Indonesian people were also recognized in Australia. Healing and cleansing ceremonies at the site in Bali respected local cultural traditions and were widely and positively reported. The media and community both provided strong support for the bereaved and recognition of the deceased. In these ways, the response to the Bali terrorist bombing demonstrated the three broad strategies of universal application: strengthening social, health, and legal processes; supportive outreach for the bereaved; and grief leadership and community recognition for the suffering.

4. Population-level interventions need to also take into account individual circumstances of traumatic loss, such as homicide deaths and other violent deaths. For those bereaved through "individual circumstances," there is less likely to be overwhelming public support, particularly in cases of murder when the killer's identity is uncertain. Addressing social, health, and legal processes may be helpful and appropriate and thus may mitigate the stressor im-

pacts. Supportive general outreach is often provided in forms such as victims' groups (e.g., Homicide Victim Support Groups). The community may also be a source of support, though, in cases in which the death is stigmatized, support may not be forthcoming. As Rynearson (2002) has highlighted in his program to assist those bereaved by violent death, in some cases assistance may be needed over an extended period. Only over the course of months or years can those affected deal with the social requirements (e.g., due to the trial of the perpetrator) as well as the traumatic stress and grief.

Early Intervention for Those at Heightened Risk

An essential first step in the early intervention process is outreach to those bereaved, particularly when a traumatic loss has occurred and traumatic bereavement is likely. This outreach may or may not be welcomed, but it is most useful to the bereaved when it is part of the practical response to need and indicates compassion and concern for those suffering. Outreach allows needs to be assessed and engages the individual for further follow-up and early intervention when necessary.

Before discussing early interventions, it is important to acknowledge that in the initial weeks following trauma, the bereaved may be focused on survival. The primary task of those providing assistance is to help with recovery without intruding or forcing interventions upon individuals who are neither ready nor able to effectively use them. Although physical survival needs are usually obvious (e.g., after a life-threatening injury or when food, shelter, and safety from any ongoing threat are needed), psychological survival needs may be less obvious. A bereaved individual may appear to be coping extremely well, carrying on with tasks, and not openly grieving when there has been overwhelming trauma and loss. The bereaved may appear preoccupied with practical tasks or with the needs of others. Though, for some, this may be a well-tried and effective coping strategy, for others such a response is their only defense against the overwhelming need and fear of decompensation. This situation is exemplified by the case of a man who lost his wife and four children in a disaster while he was away from his home rescuing others. Media interviewers projected him as "unaffected" and "brave," whereas, in fact, as he revealed much later when he felt it was possible to touch on his loss, that he just kept going because he knew he "had to survive."

In these circumstances, victims may initially feel overwhelmed with helplessness, reawakened early loss, trauma, or deprivation. As with children, only later do they feel ready to express their grief, sadness, and yearning over the loss of their loved one. In cases such as these, it is inappropriate to assume, as some cultures of bereavement counseling have suggested, that the bereaved should be made to talk about their loss or their loved one. This course of action is likely to be ineffective and possibly damaging to the processes of adjustment and adaptation over time.

KEY ELEMENTS OF INTERVENTION

Workers who have attempted to provide early intervention with traumatically bereaved individuals include Lindemann (1944), who first described his work with victims and those who were bereaved following the Coconut Grove nightclub fire. He described his work as facilitating the normal grief process by supporting the person as he or she shifted from pathological patterns of grief. In a study involving victims of another nightclub fire, Lindy, Green, Grace, and Tichener (1983) concluded that it was necessary to deal with the effects of traumatic stress before grieving could take place. Though their study did not include an early intervention, they found that outreach and intervention in the psychotherapeutic modality was not readily used. When this type of intervention was performed, they found that it was only likely to be sustained with some benefit when those conducting the intervention were skilled, experienced psychotherapists.

In a community study of recently bereaved widows, participants were assessed for traumatic stress effects related to circumstances of death on adaptation (Raphael & Maddison, 1976). In another study, bereavement interventions began soon after a major rail disaster (Raphael, 1979–1980). Results showed that the interventions were only of value if they were perceived as helpful, but that other factors, such as not having a body or being able to say good-bye, were likely to override positive results and contribute to negative outcomes (Singh & Raphael, 1981).

Early Interventions for Trauma

Bryant and colleagues have shown the benefits of cognitive-behavioral therapy interventions (CBT) for those who are at high risk for traumatic stress effects through high levels of initial reactive processes that would meet criteria for ASD (Bryant, Harvey, Dang, & Sackville, 1998; Bryant, Sackville, Dang, Moulds, & Guthrie, 1999). This work involved review of the incident and exposure through discussion combined with cognitive therapy and, in one treatment group, anxiety management. Treatment was aimed at gradually decreasing arousal and was sensitive to clinical response. In controlled trials, these interventions have been demonstrated to be effective for individuals who were traumatized by motor vehicle and industrial accidents (Bryant, Harvey, Dang,

& Sackville, 1998; Bryant et al., 1999). Other interventions in the cognitive-behavioral modality have been shown to be of value following rape, violent crime, and other traumas (see Foa & Rothbaum, 1998; Foa et al., 1999).

As summarized by Solomon (1999), such specific interventions are best provided after the first 10 days or so, as this allows the normal processes of gradual recovery to commence ensuring that intervention does not interfere with adaptation and is provided only to those who need it. Some have recently suggested using pharmacological interventions aimed at altering physiological response to trauma; however, the effectiveness of this type of intervention is untested on the wider scale (Davidson, 2002; Pitman et al., 2002; Robert, Blakeney, Villarreal, Rosenberg, & Meyer, 1999). In addition, it may be difficult to persuade bereaved individuals to accept this type of intervention, as they often fear medications will stop their grieving process.

Early Interventions for Bereavement

Early interventions for the bereaved have been most frequently tested with high-risk widows. For instance, Vachon, Lyall, Rogers, Freedman-Letofsky, and Freeman (1980) showed that women at risk because of heightened and ongoing initial distress who completed a widow-to-widow outreach program led by trained volunteers showed more improvement when compared to a control group. In addition, Raphael (1977b) demonstrated the benefits of an intervention aimed at facilitating grief and mourning in widows who were at high risk. Risk level was determined by independently rated criteria which included a preexisting, complex relationship with the deceased (high levels of ambivalence or dependence), traumatic circumstances of the death, and perceptions of an unsupportive social network. Furthermore, interventions in the weeks and months after a loss have been found to be effective in several other populations, including parents who are at high risk following a stillbirth, neonatal death, or sudden infant death syndrome (Murray, 1998); parents whose children suffered a violent death (Murphy et al., 1998); the elderly (Casserta & Lund, 1993; Gerber, Wiener, Battin, & Arkin, 1975); those who have lost a loved one to suicide (Dunne, 1992; Valente & Saunders, 1993); and those who have lost someone in a homicide (Rynearson, 1996).

Not all interventions have been provided during the early posttrauma phase; however, studies of these interventions may nevertheless be useful in determining the effective components of intervention. For example, the work of Schut, Stroebe, de Keijser, and van den Bout (1997) has examined problem- and emotion-focused counseling for prolonged, high levels of distress experienced by widows and widowers 11 months after the death. The men benefited most from the emotion-focused counseling, while the women showed the most improvement with problem-focused counseling. These results have yet to be confirmed in the acute distress period where coping is less stable. In other work, Schut, Stroebe, van den Bout, and Terheggen (2001) review and highlight the methodological problems and mixed findings of many intervention studies.

One particular study of interest that focused on early intervention was conducted by Murphy et al. (1998). This study was aimed at preventive/early intervention with parents who had recently lost a child by homicide, suicide, or accident—generally violent circumstances of traumatic loss. Mothers with high levels of distress and grief at baseline who completed the intervention improved significantly more than controls. However, the intervention did not appear to improve posttraumatic stress symptoms. Research on early intervention with high-risk parents after the deaths of children (Lake, Johnson, Murphy, & Knuppel, 1987; Videka-Sherman & Lieberman, 1985) did not show benefits, while Forrest, Standish and Baum (1982) conducted a study which showed better outcomes at initial evaluation, but these results were not sustained. The work of Sireling, Cohen, and Marks (1988) has illustrated the benefits of guided mourning for prolonged avoidant grief, while other studies suggest that behavioral interventions may be of value (e.g., Mawson, Marks, Ramm, & Stern, 1981; Ramsay, 1977). Kavanagh (1990) has reported on cognitive-behavioral interventions and their effectiveness for bereavement.

From these various studies, several principles can be gleaned to inform early intervention for those who are bereaved by a traumatic loss. First, interventions should be focused on those at heightened risk. Interventions may not be helpful and may lead to negative outcomes for those who do not need them. Those interventions that assist with "grief work," the facilitation of "normal grieving" (Lindemann, 1944; Parkes, 1981; Raphael, 1977b), and deal with the "tasks" of grieving (Worden, 1991) are all seen as potentially beneficial; however, only a few studies (e.g., Parkes 1981; Raphael 1977b) are randomized controlled trials. Behavioral strategies have also been used effectively, although they have not yet been tested as early interventions for the bereaved.

There are also interventions that have been used for bereavement pathology, particularly when traumatic bereavements are part of the target group (see Jacobs & Prigerson, 2000). The work of Kleber and Brom (Brom, Kleber, & Defares, 1989; Kleber & Brom, 1992) has shown benefits for psychodynamic, behavioral, and hypnotherapy psychotherapeutic interventions. Other studies have dealt with grief and posttraumatic stress disorder in chronically affected populations, while Horowitz, Marmar, Weiss, De Witt, and Rosenbaum (1984) have also shown benefits of brief psychotherapy for bereavement pathologies. As noted earlier, Schut et al.'s (1997) work has provided studies that have also demonstrated benefits. Rynearsons's (1996, 2002) work with homicide-bereaved families also supports the value of intervention, although this intervention is usually provided after some months. These studies, taken together, help inform future directions, particularly the need for early intervention studies with high-risk traumatized and bereaved populations.

Early Intervention for Those Bereaved by Traumatic Loss

Those bereaved by traumatic loss are likely to be at heightened risk by the very nature of the circumstances surrounding this type of death. Risk may also increase with heightened levels of posttraumatic reactivity, which may be assessed clinically or using self-report measures such as the IES (Horowitz et al., 1979; Weiss & Marmar, 1997), the ASD measure (Bryant, Harvey, Dang, & Sackville, 1998), or other posttraumatic stress phenomenology assessments. Heightened distress due to grief phenomena may be assessed clinically or using measures such as the CBI (Burnett et al., 1997; Middleton et al., 1996), the Texas Revised Inventory of Grief (TRIG; Fashingbauer et al., 1987), or other such measures. Heightened general psychological symptomatology and distress, as measured by the General Health Questionnaire (GHQ; Goldberg & Hillier, 1979), has also been shown to be predictive of bereavement-related distress, and, possibly, traumatic stress (Parker, 1977). Assessment of perceptions of social support is also important, as these variables are relevant to bereavement and trauma adaptation. Other risk variables, such as past or recent trauma or loss, as well as other current or past adversities, may be taken into account as part of the therapeutic engagement with the bereaved.

Therapeutic assessment, which takes into account the potential for the assessment to be conducted in ways that may facilitate "normal" grieving processes, has been used with bereavement (Raphael & Martinek, 1997). This involves exploring four key domains: (1) the circumstances of the death and issues surrounding it; (2) a history of the relationship with the deceased; (3) the bereaved person's life context, such as social support; and (4) progress and changes over time since the death. These explorations are therapeutic, potentially preventive (in that they explore risk and protective factors), and should not harm. An in-depth exploration of each of these four domains as they may be applied for intervention in traumatic loss follows:

Exploration of the Circumstances of the Death

Exploration of the circumstances surrounding a death allows for understanding of the realities of the loss and grief and how they are perceived by the bereaved. It also allows the therapist to assess the traumatic stress phenomena the individual might be experiencing. This exploration includes both details of what happened and how the person died as well as the bereaved's perceptions of the events and progressive exposure and desensitization to the horrors surrounding the circumstances of the death stressor to be dealt with. Separation of images, cognitive processes, and affects related to the deceased and lost relationship can be addressed progressively as the bereaved is ready. Gradual review of painful memories and feelings combined with cognitive processing are cognitive-behavioral techniques that can be applied to the traumatic stressor components to assist the bereaved in progressively dealing with these effects. These techniques are similar to CBT strategies shown to be useful in the treatment of acute and chronic PTSD (Bryant & Friedman, 2001; Bryant, Harvey, Dang, Sackville, & Basten, 1998; Bryant et al., 1999; Foa & Rothbaum, 1997; Foa et al., 1999).

A History and Review of the Relationship with the Deceased

Collecting a history of the bereaved's relationship with the deceased facilitates the psychological mourning process. This allows the ambivalence and dependence of the relationship to be explored as well as allowing for the identification and expression of affects related to yearning and longing for the deceased. Over time, the bereaved will shift their focus from the horrific and traumatic details of the death to memories of the person when he or she was alive. Feelings of yearning and longing, affection, and sadness are often experienced as the bereaved slowly comes to terms with the finality of the separation and loss. During this time, any feelings of anger, regret, and guilt that surface can be explored to assist the bereaved to deal with these aspects of grief. This progressive "history" and review is a core part of working through grief, with all its sadness. As identified by Gray, Prigerson, and Litz (Chapter 4, this volume) working through a "history" also creates an opening though which pathologies related to unexpressed yearning or intense and ongoing separation distress may be explored.

Other Aspects of the Person's Life That Inform His or Her Response

Exploration of these issues helps to identify the other processes that need to be understood and that may need to be addressed in an intervention. These may include perceptions of support and enhancing support, practical needs, any additional stressors, past traumas, and losses that resurface and may need to be dealt with at that time and subsequently, as well as evolving disorders that may require specific treatments.

Assessing Changes and Progress over Time

This provides a picture of the trajectory of the reactive processes over time and whether pathological outcomes are evolving or resolution in a more positive direction is taking place. It is important to note, however, that both bereavement and trauma reactive processes may ebb and flow with time and thus clinical judgment is necessary to determine the nature and timing of therapeutic strategies to promote recovery, resolution, and maintenance of changes. Clinical judgment in each case is especially necessary considering that there is no agreed operationalization of "resolution and recovery" in the field.

Timing and Duration of Early Intervention for Traumatic Loss

There are two interpretations of early intervention in this context: (1) intervention that occurs soon after a traumatic event or (2) an intervention that occurs early in the course of any evolving problems due to the traumatic loss. As discussed earlier, interventions that occur soon after a traumatic event, but not immediately following it, are the ideal. In this context, an intervention should not be conducted in the immediate period unless integrated with, but not limited to, initial supportive outreach. Early interventions are more feasible at this stage if they also incorporate practical issues and the needs of the bereaved, alongside a sophisticated and sensitive therapeutic approach. Acceptance of early intervention by the bereaved may be more likely in the context of an outreach. Open discussion of the ways in which the intervention may help the bereaved cope with symptoms may also assist (e.g., decreasing arousal and helping functioning). If avoidance of the traumatic stress aspects of the death is prominent, it may need to be dealt with in a more sensitive and subtle manner. Another therapeutic challenge may arise on the opposite end of the spectrum, if, on the other hand, there is intense rumination and retelling of the story and the bereaved seems to be locked into the role of traumatized victim. This type of narrative is reflective of ongoing traumatization, not resolution.

Early intervention may not be appropriate for all bereaved individuals. Some will only be ready at a later time, perhaps after some months when the tasks of survival are securely achieved and they feel they have the emotional strength to face what has happened (i.e., time for the "luxury" of grief). In cases such as these, "early" interventions may still be provided at this early phase of actively dealing with the traumatic loss. Clearly further research is necessary to clarify such issues, which are discussed here only in terms of clinical experience.

It is also likely that treatment sessions will be longer than the traditional therapeutic hour and many take up to 90 minutes or more, though beyond 2 hours the bereaved may have exhausted opportunities for further constructive work. Early intervention should be focused not on "fixing" the bereavement and the effects of trauma but rather on goals of facilitating a positive trajectory to adaptation, while recognizing that the processes of grieving will occur progressively over a significant time period.

If necessary, more in-depth psychotherapeutic work should be negotiated when these first-level goals have been achieved. It may take considerable psychotherapeutic skill to negotiate these complexities, so it is useful to discuss with the bereaved what is offered and why and what it is hoped they will achieve. This discussion should not only be part of the informed consent process but part of their active participation in the process as well. Six to eight sessions may be necessary, or perhaps 12, but beyond this point, the direction of future interventions and care should be thoroughly examined.

Group processes have also been used to help the traumatically bereaved. The advantages of a group format include the opportunity for the provision of mutual support, sharing of strategies for adaptation, advocacy, information sharing, and the chance to work through traumatic experiences and grief in a collaborative way (Dembert & Simmer, 2000; Raphael & Wooding, in press; Rynearson, 2002; Weisaeth, 2000). However, most group interventions tend to be a source of mutual support and advocacy and practical strategies for role redefinition and identity, more than intensive psychotherapeutic work. For distressed and traumatized people, a sensitive and compassionate individual or family process is often required for therapeutic interventions in the early stages.

Families that have been traumatized and bereaved should be allowed to work through the trauma and loss together, whenever possible. Family members may be caring for others who need help. They may be feeling overwhelmed by the break in the family nexus or intensely fearful. Each member may also be processing the experience in different ways on different timelines. Individual- and family-centered work should aim to carefully address the impact of trauma, including the possible development of isolation and avoidance, as well as the need for closeness, comforting, and sharing of memories. Work conducted by Kissane has provided a valuable model of family grief, identifying families at risk, and effective intervention, although this work has tended to focus on terminal care and circumstances of prolonged illness/death and bereavement (Kissane, 1998; Kissane & Bloch, 1994).

Additional Stressor Impact: Human Malevolence

A particular problem occurs when the death, loss, and traumatic experience are a consequence of deliberate human malevolence (e.g., homicide, terrorist attacks, and violent assaults; Raphael & Wooding, 2002). Psychological adaptation under these conditions may be significantly hampered; however, there is a paucity of research in this area (National Institute of Mental Health, 2001).

When an individual is bereaved because of an act of human malevolence, he or she may feel preoccupied with why this happened (i.e., the search for meaning), the perpetrator, thoughts of revenge, or the search for justice. This may be a defense against facing the trauma and accepting and dealing with the reality of the loss. The search for "justice" may represent a wish to regain a sense of personal invulnerability that has been lost or for things to be the way they were before the deceased was gone forever. While psychotherapeutic work may assist in dealing with these issues, further research is necessary to determine both the dynamics of dealing with such human malevolence and how the bereaved can "resolve" these issues. On a broader scale, matters such as the social processes of human rights courts, tribunals, and the truth and reconciliation commission require consideration (Raphael & Wooding, 2002; Silove 1999).

Therapist Roles

It is highly stressful for those who work with the traumatically bereaved. Workers may identify with the bereaved, wish to "make things right," fear for their own loved ones, feel a sense of helplessness in the face of such horror, or fear their own fantasies and destructiveness. The bereaved may project intense fear and dependence, which may at times challenge professional boundaries. In addition, workers may develop "burnout" or compassion fatigue, be vicariously traumatized by the stories of the bereaved and the images they generate, or become enmeshed and overinvolved or cold and distant. Appropriate clinical skills and training, structure and limitations on tours of duty and client load, professional clinical supervision, case review, and ongoing training and education will all mitigate such risk.

For service systems responding to mass incidents, it may prove extremely difficult to gather enough properly trained workers to handle the immediate and overwhelming need.

RESEARCH AND EVALUATION

There are numerous ethical difficulties in researching acutely distressed populations. Practical concerns include contact and engagement of participants for an intervention, not to mention research. Nonetheless, there is the need for more systematic research and appropriate studies of these evolving phenomenologies of reaction, the emergence of positive outcomes and personal growth, and the development of pathology, as well as the factors influencing these processes and their trajectories. Future research needs to be population based and use sound methodologies, allowing risks to be quantified and the potential benefits of different interventions in mitigating adverse outcomes and promoting positive adaptation to be carefully measured.

Current methodologies can be complex and difficult to put into place at trying times; thus there is a need to find new methods of researching these sensitive issues and the interplay of trauma and loss phenomenologically and physiologically. Qualitative and quantitative methods can contribute. In addition, testing and evaluation of both preventive and therapeutic interventions are essential next steps. Furthermore, collaborative strategies across regional and international boundaries could potentially increase the power and significance of future studies.

With current concerns about terrorism and the background of heightened anxiety and uncertainty, and the likelihood that traumatic loss will be a prominent feature of any terrorist attack, systems need to be prepared to research not only the effects of traumatic stress but also the traumatic losses involved.

REFERENCES

Blake, D. D., Weathers, F. W., Nagy, L. M., Kaloupek, D. G., Gusman, F. D., Charney, D. S., & Keane, T. M. (1995). The development of a Clinician-Administered PTSD scale. *Journal of Traumatic Stress, 8,* 75–90.

Bowlby, J. (1969). *Attachment: Vol. 1. Attachment and loss.* London: Hogarth Press.

Bowlby, J. (1973). *Attachment and loss: Vol. 2. Separation: Anxiety and anger.* London: Hogarth Press.

Bowlby, J. (1980). *Attachment and loss: Vol. 3. Loss, sadness, and depression.* London: Hogarth Press.

Breslau, N., Davis, G. C., Andreski, P., & Peterson, E. (1991). Traumatic events and post-traumatic stress disorder in an urban population of young adults. *Archives of General Psychiatry, 48,* 216–222.

Brom, D., Kleber, R. J., & Defares, P. B. (1989). Brief psychotherapy for posttraumatic stress disorders. *Journal of Consulting and Clinical Psychology, 57,* 607–612.

Bryant, R. A., & Friedman, M. (2001). Medication and non-medication treatments of posttraumatic stress disorder. *Current Opinion in Psychiatry, 14,* 119–123.

Bryant, R. A., Harvey, A. G., Dang, S. T., & Sackville, T. (1998). Assessing acute stress disorder: Psychometric properties of a structured clinical interview. *Psychological Assessment, 10,* 215–220.

Bryant, R. A., Harvey, A. G., Dang, S. T., Sackville, T., & Basten, C. (1998). Treatment of acute stress disorder: A comparison of cognitive-behavioral therapy and supportive counselling. *Journal of Consulting and Clinical Psychology, 66,* 862–866.

Bryant, R. A., Sackville, T., Dang, S. T., Moulds, M., & Guthrie, R. (1999). Treating acute stress disorder: An evaluation of cognitive-behavior therapy and supportive counseling techniques. *American Journal of Psychiatry, 156,* 1780–1786.

Burnett, P., Middleton, W., Raphael, B., & Martinek, N. (1997). Measuring core bereavement phenomena. *Psychological Medicine, 27,* 49–57.

Byrne, G. J., & Raphael, B. (1994). A longitudinal study of bereavement phenomena in recently widowed elderly men. *Psychological Medicine, 24,* 411–421.

Byrne, G. J., & Raphael, B. (1997). The psychological symptoms of conjugal bereavement in elderly men over the first 13 months. *International Journal of Geriatric Psychiatry, 12,* 241–251.

Byrne, G. J., & Raphael, B. (1999). Depressive symptoms and depressive episodes in recently widowed older men. *International Psychogeriatrics, 11,* 67–74.

Caserta, M. S., & Lund, D. A. (1993). Intrapersonal resources and the effectiveness of self-help groups for bereaved older adults. *Gerontologist, 33,* 619–629.

Clayton, P. J. (1990). Bereavement and depression. *Journal of Clinical Psychiatry, 51,* 34–40.

Commonwealth Department of Health and Aged Care. (2000). *Promotion, prevention and early intervention for mental health—A monograph.* Canberra, Australia: Mental Health and Special Programs Branch, Commonwealth Department of Health and Aged Care.

Davidson, J. R. T. (2002). Surviving disaster: What comes after the trauma? *British Journal of Psychiatry, 181,* 366–368.

Davidson, J. R. T., & Foa, E. B. (1991). Diagnostic issues in posttraumatic stress disorder: Considerations for the DSM-IV. *Journal of Abnormal Psychology, 100,* 346–355.

Davidson, J. R. T., & Foa, E. B. (Eds.). (1993). *Posttraumatic stress disorder: DSM-IV and beyond.* Washington, DC: American Psychiatric Press.

Dembert, M. L., & Simmer, E. D. (2000). When trauma affects a community: Group interventions and support after a disaster. In R. H. Klein & V. L. Schermer (Eds.), *Group psychotherapy for psychological trauma* (pp. 239–264). New York: Guilford Press.

Dunne, E. J. (1992). Psychoeducational intervention strategies for survivors of suicide. *Crisis, 13,* 35–40.

Engel, G. L. (1961). Is grief a disease?: A challenge for medical research. *Psychosomatic Medicine, 23,* 18–22.

Faschingbauer, T. R., Zisook, S., & DeVaul, R. (1987). The Texas revised inventory of grief. In S. Zisook (Ed.), *Biopsychosocial aspects of bereavement* (pp. 111–124). Washington, DC: American Psychiatric Press.

Foa, E. B., Dancu, C. V., Hembree, E. A., Jaycox, L. H., Meadows, E. A., & Street, G. P. (1999). A comparison of exposure therapy, stress inoculation training, and their combinations for reducing posttraumatic stress disorder in female assault victims. *Journal of Consulting and Clinical Psychology, 67,* 194–200.

Foa, E. B., & Rothbaum, B. O. (1998). *Treating the trauma of rape: Cognitive-behavioral therapy for PTSD.* New York: Guilford Press.

Forrest, G. C., Standish, E., & Baum, J. D. (1982). Support after perinatal death: A study of support and counselling after perinatal bereavement. *British Medical Journal, 285,* 1475–1479.

Galea, S., Ahern, J., Resnick, H., Kilpatrick, D., Bucuvalas, M., Gold, J., & Vlahov, D. (2002). Psychological sequelae of the September 11 terrorist attacks in New York City. *New England Journal of Medicine, 346,* 982–987.

Gerber, I., Wiener, A., Battin, D., & Arkin, A. M. (1975). Brief therapy to the aged bereaved. In B. Schoenberg & I. Gerber (Eds.), *Bereavement: Its psychosocial aspects* (pp. 310–333). New York: Columbia University Press.

Goldberg, D., & Hillier, V. F. (1979). A scaled version of the General Health Questionnaire. *Psychological Medicine, 9,* 139–145.

Hall, M., & Irwin, M. (2001). Physiological indices of functioning in bereavement. In. M. S. Stroebe, R. O. Hannson, W. Stroebe, & H. Schut (Eds.), *Handbook of bereavement research: Consequences, coping, and care* (pp. 473–492). Washington, DC: American Psychological Association.

Harvey, A. G., & Bryant, R. A. (1998). The relationship between acute stress disorder and posttraumatic stress disorder: A prospective evaluation of motor vehicle accident survivors. *Journal of Consulting and Clinical Psychology, 66,* 507–512.

Harvey, A. G., & Bryant, R. A. (2002). Acute stress disorder: A synthesis and critique. *Psychological Bulletin, 128,* 886–902.

Horowitz, M. J. (1976). *Stress response syndromes.* New York: Jason Aronson.

Horowitz, M. J., Marmar, C., Weiss, D. S., DeWitt, K. N., & Rosenbaum, R. (1984). Brief psychotherapy of bereavement reactions: The relationship of process to outcome. *Archives of General Psychiatry, 41,* 438–448.

Horowitz, M. J., Siegel, B., Holen, A., Bonanno, G. A., Milbrath, C., & Stinson, C. H. (1997). Diagnostic criteria for complicated grief disorder. *American Journal of Psychiatry, 154,* 904–910.

Horowitz, M. J., Wilner, N., & Alvarez, W. (1979). Impact of Event Scale: A measure of subjective distress. *Psychosomatic Medicine, 41,* 209–218.

Hull, A. M., Alexander, D. A., & Klein, S. (2002). Survivors of the Piper Alpha oil platform disaster: Long-term follow-up study. *British Journal of Psychiatry, 181,* 433–438.

Jacobs, S. (1993). *Pathologic grief: Maladaptation to loss.* Washington, DC: American Psychiatric Press.

Jacobs, S., Kasl, S., Ostfeld, A., Berkman, L., & Charpentier, P. (1986). The measurement of grief: Age and sex variation. *British Journal of Medical Psychology, 59,* 305–310.

Jacobs, S. C., Kasl, S. V., Ostfeld, A. M., Berkman, L., Kosten, T. R., & Charpentier, P. (1986). The measurement of grief: Bereaved versus non-bereaved. *Hospice, 2,* 21–36.

Jacobs, S., & Prigerson, H. (2000). Psychotherapy of traumatic grief: A review of evidence for psychotherapeutic treatments. *Death Studies, 24,* 479–496.

Kavanagh, D. J. (1990). Towards a cognitive-behavioural intervention for adult grief reactions. *British Journal of Psychiatry, 157,* 373–383.

Keane, T. M., Malloy, P. F., & Fairbanks, J. A. (1984). Empirical development of an MMPI subscale for the assessment of combat-related posttraumatic stress disorder. *Journal of Consulting and Clinical Psychology, 52,* 888–891.

Kessler, R. C., Sonnega, A., Bromet, E., Hughes, M., & Nelson, C. B. (1995). Posttraumatic stress disorder in the National Comorbidity Survey. *Archives of General Psychiatry, 52,* 1048–1060.

Kissane, D. W. (1998). A controlled trial of family intervention to promote healthy family functioning in at-risk palliative care families. *Australian and New Zealand Journal of Psychiatry, 32*(Suppl. 8), A16.

Kissane, D. W., & Bloch, S. (1994). Family grief. *British Journal of Psychiatry, 164,* 728–740.

Kleber, R. J., & Brom, D. (1992). *Coping with trauma: Theory, prevention, and treatment.* Amsterdam, PA: Swets & Zeitlinger.

Lake, M. F., Johnson, T. M., Murphy, J., & Knuppel, R. A. (1987). Evaluation of a perinatal grief support team. *American Journal of Obstetrics and Gynaecology, 157,* 1203–1206.

Lindemann, E. (1944). Symptomatology and management of acute grief. *American Journal of Psychiatry, 101,* 141–148.

Lindy, J. D., Green, B. L., Grace, M., & Tichener, J. (1983). Psychotherapy with survivors of the Beverly Hills Supper Club fire. *American Journal of Psychotherapy, 37,* 593–610.

Litz, B.T., Gray, M.J., Bryant, R.A., & Adler, A.B. (2002). Early intervention for trauma: Current status and future directions. *Clinical Psychology: Science and Practice, 9*(2), 112–134.

Lundin, T. (1984). Morbidity following sudden and unexpected bereavement. *British Journal of Psychiatry, 144,* 84–88.

Maddison, D. C., & Walker, W. L. (1967). Factors affecting the outcome of conjugal bereavement. *British Journal of Psychiatry, 113,* 1057–1067.

Mawson, D., Marks, I. M., Ramm, L., & Stern, R. S. (1981). Guided mourning for morbid grief: A controlled study. *British Journal of Psychiatry, 138,* 185–193.

McFarlane, A. C. (1986). Chronic post-traumatic morbidity of the natural disaster: Implications for disaster planners and emergency services. *Medical Journal of Australia, 145,* 561–631.

McFarlane, A. C. (1988a). The longitudinal course of posttraumatic morbidity: The range of outcomes and their predictors. *Journal of Nervous and Mental Disease, 176,* 30–39.

McFarlane, A.C. (1988b). The phenomenology of post-traumatic stress disorders following a natural disaster. *Journal of Nervous and Mental Disease, 176,* 22–29.

Middleton, W., Burnett, P., Raphael, B., & Martinek, N. (1996). The bereavement response: A cluster analysis. *British Journal of Psychiatry, 169,* 167–171.

Middleton, W., Moylan, A., Raphael, B., Burnett, P., & Martinek, N. (1993). An international perspective on bereavement related concepts. *Australian & New Zealand Journal of Psychiatry, 27,* 457–463.

Middleton, W., Raphael, B., Burnett, P., & Martinek, N. (1998). A longitudinal study comparing bereavement phenomena in recently bereaved spouses, adults, children and parents. *Australian & New Zealand Journal of Psychiatry, 32,* 235–241.

Mrazek, P. J., & Haggerty, R. J. (Eds.). (1994). *Reducing risks for mental disorders: Frontiers for preventive intervention research.* Washington, DC: National Academy Press.

Murphy, S. A. (1988). Mediating effects of intrapersonal and social support on mental health 1 and 3 years after a natural disaster. *Journal of Traumatic Stress, 1,* 155–172.

Murphy, S. A., Johnson, C., Cain, K. C., Das Gupta, A., Dimond, M., & Lohan, J. (1998). Broad-spectrum group treatment for parents bereaved by the violent deaths of their 12- to 28-year-old children: A randomized controlled trial. *Death Studies, 22,* 209–236.

Murray, J. (1998). Caring families affected by infant death: Evaluating an intervention. In J. Murray (Ed.), *Grief matters* (p. 4). Melbourne, Australia: Centre for Grief Education.

National Institute of Mental Health. (2001). *Mental health and mass violence: Evidence-based early psychological intervention for victims/survivors of mass violence. A workshop to reach consensus on best practices* (NIH Publication No. 02-5138). Washington, DC: U.S. Government Printing Office.

Neimeyer, R. A. (2000). Searching for the meaning of meaning: Grief therapy and the process of reconstruction. *Death Studies, 24,* 541–558.

New South Wales Health Department. (2000). *Disaster mental health response handbook.* Sydney, Australia: New South Wales Health and the Centre for Mental Health.

North, C. S., Nixon, S. J., Shariat, S., Mallonee, S., McMillen, J. C., Spitznagel, E. L., & Smith, E. M. (1999). Psychiatric disorders among survivors of the Oklahoma City bombing. *Journal of the American Medical Association, 282,* 755–762.

Parker, G. (1977). Cyclone Tracy and Darwin evacuees: On the restoration of the species. *British Journal of Psychiatry, 130,* 548–555.

Parkes, C. M. (1970). The first year of bereavement: A longitudinal study of the reaction of London widows to the death of their husbands. *Psychiatry, 33,* 444–467.

Parkes, C. M. (1981). Evaluation of a bereavement service. *Journal of Preventive Psychiatry, 1,* 179–188.

Parkes, C. M., & Weiss, R. S. (1983). *Recovery from bereavement.* New York: Basic Books.

Pitman, R. K., Sanders, K. M., Zusman, R. M., Healy, A. R., Cheema, F., Lasko, N. B., Cahill, L., & Orr. S. P. (2002). Pilot study of secondary prevention of posttraumatic stress disorder with propranolol. *Biological Psychiatry, 51,* 189–192.

Polak, P. R., Egan, D. J., Vanderbergh, R. H., & Williams, W. W. (1973). Crisis intervention in acute bereavement: A controlled study of primary prevention. *Community Mental Health Journal, 12,* 128–136.

Prigerson, H. G., Bierhals, A. J., Kasl, S. V., Reynolds, C. F., Shear, M. K., Day, N., Beery, L. C., Newsom, J. T., & Jacobs, S. (1997). Traumatic grief as a risk factor for mental and physical morbidity. *American Journal of Psychiatry, 154,* 616–623.

Prigerson, H. G., & Jacobs, S. C. (2001). Traumatic grief as a distinct disorder: A rationale, consensus criteria, and a preliminary empirical test. In M. S. Stroebe, R. O. Hansson, W. Stroebe, & H. Schut (Eds.), *Handbook of bereavement research: Consequences, coping, and care* (pp. 613–646). Washington, DC: American Psychological Association.

Pynoos, R. S., Frederick, C., Nader, K., Arroyo, W., Steinberg, A., Eth, S., Nunez, F., & Fairbanks, L. (1987). Life threat and posttraumatic stress in school-age children. *Archives of General Psychiatry, 44,* 1057–1063.

Pynoos, R. S., Nader, K., Frederick, C., Gonda, L., & Stuber, M. (1987). Grief reactions in school age children following a sniper attack at school. *Israeli Journal of Psychiatry and Related Sciences, 24,* 53–63.

Ramsay, R. W. (1977). Behavioural approaches to bereavement. *Behaviour Research and Therapy, 15,* 131–135.

Raphael, B. (1977a). The Granville train disaster: Psychological needs and their management. *Medical Journal of Australia, 1,* 303–305.

Raphael, B. (1977b). Prevention intervention with the recently bereaved. *Archives of General Psychiatry, 34,* 1450–1454.

Raphael, B. (1979–1980). A primary prevention action programme: Psychiatric involvement following a major rail disaster. *Omega, 10,* 211–225.

Raphael, B. (1983). *Anatomy of bereavement.* New York: Basic Books.

Raphael, B. (1986). *When disaster strikes: How individuals and communities cope with catastrophe.* New York: Basic Books.

Raphael, B. (1997). The interaction of trauma and grief. In D. Black, M. Newman, J. Harris-Hendricks, & G. Mezey (Eds.), *Psychological trauma: A developmental approach* (pp. 31–43). London: Gaskell/Royal College of Psychiatrists.

Raphael, B., & Maddison, D. C. (1976). The care of bereaved adults. In O. W. Hill (Ed.), *Modern trends in psychosomatic medicine* (pp. 491–506). London: Butterworth.

Raphael, B., & Martinek, N. (1997). Assessing traumatic bereavement and posttraumatic stress disorder. In J. P. Wilson & T. M. Keane (Eds.), *Assessing psychological trauma and PTSD* (pp. 373–395). New York: Guilford Press.

Raphael, B., Middleton, W., Martinek, N., & Misso, V. (1993). Counseling and therapy of the bereaved. In M. S. Stroebe, W. Stroebe, & R. D. Hansson (Eds.), *Handbook of bereavement: Theory, research, and intervention* (pp. 427–453). New York: Cambridge University Press.

Raphael, B., & Minkov, C. (1999). Abnormal grief. *Current Opinion in Psychiatry, 12,* 99–102.

Raphael, B., Minkov, C., & Dobson, M. (2001). Psychotherapeutic and pharmacological intervention for bereaved persons. In M. S. Stroebe, R. O. Hansson, W. Stroebe, & H. Schut (Eds.), *Handbook of bereavement research: Consequences, coping, and care* (pp. 587–612). Washington, DC: American Psychological Association.

Raphael, B., & Wooding, S. (2002, September 11). *Violence and prevention.* Paper presented at the second world conference: The Promotion of Mental Health and Prevention of Mental and Behavioural Disorders, London.

Raphael, B., & Wooding, S. (in press). Group intervention for the prevention and treatment of acute initial stress reactions in civilians. In L. A. Schein, H. I. Spitz, G. M. Burlingame, & P. R. Muskin (Eds.), *Group approaches for the psychological effects of terrorist disasters.* New York: Haworth Press.

Robert, R., Blakeney, P. E., Villarreal, C., Rosenberg, L., & Meyer, W. J. (1999). Imipramine treatment in pediatric burn patients with symptoms of acute stress disorder: A pilot study. *Journal of the American Academy of Child and Adolescent Psychiatry, 38,* 873–882.

Rynearson, E. K. (1996). Psychotherapy of bereavement after homicide: Be offensive. *Psychotherapy in Practice, 2,* 47–57.

Rynearson, E. K. (2002). *Retelling violent death.* Philadelphia: Brunner-Routledge.

Sanders, C. M. (1980). A comparison of adult bereavement in the death of a spouse, child and parent. *Omega, 10,* 303–322.

Schlenger, W. E., Caddell, J. M., Ebert, L., Jordan, B. K., Rourke, K. M., Wilson, D., Thalji, L., Dennis, J. M., Fairbank, J. A., & Kulka, R. L. (2002). Psychological reactions to terrorist attacks: Findings from the National Study of Americans' Reactions to September 11. *Journal of the American Medical Association, 288,* 581–588.

Schuster, M. A., Stein, B. D., Jaycox, L. H., Collins, R. L., Marshall, G., Elliott, M. N., Zhou, A. J., Kanouse, D. E., Morrison, J. L., & Berry, S. H. (2001). A national survey of stress reactions after the September 11, 2001, terrorist attacks. *New England Journal of Medicine, 345,* 1507–1512.

Schut, H. A., Stroebe, M. S., de Keijser, J., & van den Bout, J. (1997). Intervention for the bereaved: Gender differences in the efficacy of two counselling programmes. *British Journal of Clinical Psychology, 36,* 63–72.

Schut, H., Stroebe, M. S., van den Bout, J., & Terheggen, M. (2001). The efficacy of bereavement interventions: Determining who benefits. In M. S. Stroebe, R. O. Hansson, W. Stroebe, & H. Schut (Eds.), *Handbook of bereavement research: Consequences, coping, and care* (pp. 705–737). Washington, DC: American Psychological Association.

Shore, J. H., Tatum, E. L., & Vollmer, W. M. (1986). Psychiatric reactions to disaster: The Mount St. Helens experience. *American Journal of Psychiatry, 143,* 590–595.

Silove, D. (1999). The psychosocial effects of torture, mass human rights violations, and refugee trauma: Toward an integrated conceptual framework. *Journal of Nervous and Mental Disease, 187,* 200–207.

Silver, R. C., Holman, E. A., McIntosh, D. N., Poulin, M., & Gil-Rivas, V. (2002). Nationwide longitudinal study of psychological responses to September 11. *Journal of the American Medical Association, 288,* 1235–1244.

Singh, B., & Raphael, B. (1981). Post disaster morbidity of the bereaved: A possible role for preventive psychiatry. *Journal Nervous and Mental Disease, 169,* 203–212.

Sireling, L., Cohen, D., & Marks, I. (1988). Guided mourning for morbid grief: A controlled replication. *Behavior Therapy, 19,* 121–132.

Solomon, Z. (1999). Interventions for acute trauma response. *Current Opinion in Psychiatry, 12,* 175–180.

Stroebe, M. S., Hannson, R. O., Stroebe, W., & Schut, H. (Eds.). (2001). *Handbook of bereavement research: Consequences, coping, and care.* Washington, DC: American Psychological Association.

Taft, C. T., Stern, A. S., King, L. A., & King, D. W. (1999). Modeling physical health and functional health status: The role of combat exposure, posttraumatic stress disorder, and personal resource attributes. *Journal of Traumatic Stress, 12,* 3–23.

Tedeschi, R. G., & Calhoun, L. G. (1996). The posttraumatic growth inventory: Measuring the positive legacy of trauma. *Journal of Traumatic Stress, 9,* 455–471.

Ullman, S. E., & Siegel, J. M. (1996). Traumatic events and physical health in a community sample. *Journal of Traumatic Stress, 9,* 703–720.

Ursano, R. J., McCaughey, B. G., & Fullerton, C. S. (Eds). (1994). *Individual and community responses to trauma and disaster: The structure of human chaos.* Cambridge, UK: Cambridge University Press.

Vachon, M. L., Lyall, W. A., Rogers, J., Freedman-Letofsky, K., & Freeman, S. J. (1980). A controlled study of self-help intervention for widows. *American Journal of Psychiatry, 137,* 1380–1384.

Vaillant, G. E. (1988). Attachment, loss and rediscovery. *Hillside Journal of Clinical Psychiatry, 10,* 148–164.

Valente, S. M., & Saunders, J. M. (1993). Adolescent grief after suicide. *Crisis, 14,* 16–22.

Videka-Sherman, L. & Lieberman, M. (1985). The effects of self-help and psychotherapy intervention on child loss: The limits of recovery. *American Journal of Orthopsychiatry, 55,* 70–82.

Wagner, A. W., Wolfe, J., Rotnitsky, A., Proctor, S. P., & Erickson, D. J. (2000). An investigation of the impact of posttraumatic stress disorder on physical health. *Journal of Traumatic Stress, 13,* 41–55.

Weisaeth, L. (1989). The stressors and the post-traumatic stress syndrome after an industrial disaster. *Acta Psychiatrica Scandinavica, Supplementum, 355,* 25–37.

Weisaeth, L. (2000). Briefing and debriefing: Group psychological interventions in acute stressor situations. In B. Raphael & J. Wilson (Eds.), *Psychological debriefing: Theory, practice and evidence* (pp. 43–57). Cambridge, UK: Cambridge University Press.

Weiss, D. S., & Marmar, C. R. (1997). The impact of event scale—revised. In J. P. Wilson & T. M. Keane (Eds.), *Assessing psychological trauma and PTSD* (pp. 399–411). New York: Guilford Press.

Worden, J. W. (1991). *Grief counselling and grief therapy: A handbook for the mental health practitioner.* New York: Springer.

Yehuda, R. (1999). Linking the neuroendocrinology of post-traumatic stress disorder with recent neuroanatomic findings. *Seminars in Clinical Neuropsychiatry, 4,* 256–265.

9

Methodological and Ethical Issues in Early Intervention Research

MATT J. GRAY
BRETT T. LITZ
AMY R. OLSON

Despite widespread recognition among researchers and clinicians that trauma can result in profound psychological and emotional distress for a small but substantial proportion of victims, and despite the intuitive appeal of providing mental health services soon after traumatic exposure in order to prevent chronic psychopathology, we continue to be faced with the uncomfortable fact that, at present, a compelling evidentiary base in support of such services is lacking. Although some promising early interventions for trauma have recently been developed (e.g., Foa, Hearst-Ikeda, & Perry, 1995; Bryant, Harvey, Dang, Sackville, & Basten, 1998), their clinical utility with varied trauma populations and their applicability to diverse posttraumatic contexts (e.g., incidents of mass violence) remain to be empirically investigated in controlled clinical trials. Arguably, psychological debriefing (PD) generally, and critical incident stress debriefing (CISD) specifically are presently the "standard of treatment" in the immediate aftermath of trauma as evidenced by their ubiquitous application. CISD is used throughout the world following disasters, incidents of mass violence, transportation accidents, and so forth. This is due, in part, to the fact that the American Red Cross mandates the use of CISD as formal policy (American Red Cross, 1998). Unfortunately, although these forms of intervention are widely disseminated and implemented as a result of their intuitive appeal, coupled with the supportive conclusions of several uncontrolled investigations attesting to their efficacy, recent comprehensive reviews of controlled investigations of debriefing-based interventions have concluded that in terms of reducing the prevalence or incidence of posttraumatic stress disorder and other problems implicated by trauma, these "treatments" are seemingly inert (Litz, Gray, Bryant, & Adler, 2002; Rose, Bisson, & Wesseley, 2001).

There is an understandable humanitarian desire to help those who are suddenly confronted with unimaginable pain and distress in the wake of a horrific traumatic event. Unfortunately, well-intentioned but ineffective interventions have been developed, widely disseminated, and implemented, as our efforts to help have greatly outpaced our knowledge of what is needed and what is actually effective. To prevent the emergence and persistence of unhelpful interventions, it is not only necessary to develop truly beneficial interventions but to subject these interventions to rigorous empirical scrutiny. Failure to do so may paradoxically increase the likelihood that victims' posttraumatic distress will persist as they may be less likely to seek out alternative interventions, and clinicians may be less likely to pursue alternate treatment avenues, believing that the "standard of care" is more effective than it actually is.

Accordingly, the primary goal of this chapter is to delineate standards of evidence for deeming an early posttraumatic intervention to be effective. These standards are not meant to restrict pilot work and initial treatment-development research, but they should be met or approximated prior to widespread adoption of an intervention by major federal agencies and disaster relief organizations. Improvements in experimental design and greater attention to methodology of early trauma intervention studies will no doubt result in the development of optimal interventions for at-risk victims and will enhance the quality of services proffered in the early posttraumatic environment. In this chapter, we also outline practical and ethical issues that necessarily threaten the internal validity of early intervention studies. We argue for the necessity of randomized clinical trials (RCTs)—even in the early intervention context, and we describe methodological considerations and imperatives for this line of inquiry.

PRACTICAL AND ETHICAL BARRIERS
TO CONDUCTING SOUND EARLY INTERVENTION RESEARCH

The most defensible statement that may be made about the efficacy of early intervention for trauma is that, at present, there exists no empirically validated form of treatment that can be recommended as a standard therapeutic response to meet the needs of victims of diverse traumas. Although trauma-specific interventions have yielded promising results in preliminary empirical investigations, it is unclear whether these results would hold in larger samples or in other posttraumatic contexts. The limitations of the existing evidentiary base may not be attributed to lack of innovation or effort. Rather, there are significant complications and barriers to conducting rigorous investigations in a typically chaotic posttraumatic environment. Such barriers certainly present a formidable challenge to early intervention researchers, but we contend that such challenges are not necessarily insurmountable. Indeed, the very future of early intervention rests on researchers' collective capacity to overcome the challenges inherent in this type of research.

Certainly, one of the most common practical barriers to conducting methodologically sound early intervention research pertains to access to, and continued contact with, trauma victims. Given the inordinate distress that most trauma victims experience acutely, they are often unwilling or unable to discuss their experiences or emotional state. In the context of large-scale technological or natural disasters or mass violence, many survivors may flee the area and seek refuge with relatives or friends. Thus, available samples may not always be representative.

One of the more prevalent difficulties experienced by those who do report chronic distress is posttraumatic stress disorder (PTSD). Because a hallmark feature of PTSD is marked avoidance of reminders of the traumatic event (including discussions of the trauma; American Psychiatric Association, 1994), those who are most distressed may avoid contact with mental health clinicians and researchers. Participating in a longitudinal study of PTSD symptom course necessarily involves continued revisiting of a painful memory—a process that the most distressed survivors may seek to avoid. The difficulty of accessing victims of a large-scale trauma and studying that sample longitudinally is perhaps best evidenced by a comprehensive review of postdisaster research studies published between 1981 and 2001, in which Norris and colleagues (Norris, Friedman, Watson, et al., 2002; Norris, Friedman, & Watson, 2002) found that two-thirds of these studies involved a single postdisaster assessment. The practical barriers to conducting longitudinal investigations of victims' response to intervention are compounded in instances of large-scale disasters such as the terrorist attacks of 9-11-01. Not only does the sheer number of victims make it difficult to access and track a large representative sample of the afflicted population, but the fact that many are forced to flee their homes and neighborhoods makes follow-up contact inordinately difficult.

There are also a number of ethical issues in the context of the immediate posttraumatic treatment environment which have yet to be satisfactorily addressed. The lack of consensus among trauma researchers on these issues is one of the primary factors contributing to the present state of early intervention research. One such issue is whether trauma victims are capable of providing fully informed consent in the immediate aftermath of trauma. Informed consent is an obvious mandatory prerequisite to participating in a clinical trial of an early intervention for trauma. The fact that this remains an open empirical question has disturbing implications for investigations of treatments delivered early after exposure to a traumatic event (e.g., debriefing-based interventions).

Although we are unaware of any empirical investigations documenting difficulties with the informed consent process immediately after a traumatic event, it seems reasonable to suppose that victims may be too overwhelmed, distraught, or impressionable in the early stages following traumatic exposure to fully process or comprehend information provided about the risks and benefits of the investigation or the requirements of their participation. Indeed, a diagnosis of acute stress disorder cannot be given within the first 2 days of traumatic exposure (American Psychiatric Association, 1994) in recognition of the fact that most individuals experience pronounced emotional distress and shock during the period immediately following the traumatic event— even those who will not experience more enduring difficulties.

Because trauma typically involves legitimate life threat and/or actual or threatened serious injury, the stress reaction involves the mobilization of physiological and psychological resources to respond to such threat. Accordingly, in addition to understandable deleterious psychological consequences (e.g., dread, horror, and intense helplessness), higher circulating levels of epinephrine and cortisol can act in concert with emotional distress to impair coping, attention, and information-processing capacities (e.g., Christianson, 1992; Eysenck & Calvo, 1992). For these reasons, we have argued in this volume (Litz & Gray, Chapter 5) and elsewhere (Litz et al., 2002) that it is difficult to defend initiating formal complex or demanding psychological interventions during the *immediate impact phase*—the initial 48 hours after the trauma. Though restrictions within the 48-hour period may seem rather arbitrary, and tremendous individual variability will mean that exceptions to this rule will abound, it does afford a degree of protection from well-intentioned, but perhaps ill-timed, treatment efforts. A period of quiescence will allow the initial shock of trauma to wane and will increase the likelihood that victims are able to fully process the information presented. Presumably, this reasoning would hold true for the informed consent process as well. Subsequent empirical inquiry may ultimately alter this time frame, but, at present, it would seem prudent to refrain from providing formal emotionally and cognitively complex and demanding treatment or obtaining informed consent for such procedures within the first few days following traumatic exposure.

Additional ethical considerations relevant to early intervention research include concerns about the random assignment of participants to treatment conditions when one condition is expected to promote better posttraumatic adjustment and whether it is ethical to randomly assign recent trauma victims to no-treatment or to nonspecific factors/placebo control conditions.

It is helpful to consider both of these issues with reference to the concept of "clinical equipoise" (Freedman, 1987). Ethical clinical research requires a state of equipoise or genuine uncertainty concerning the relative merits of interventions being evaluated. Specifically, if one intervention is known to be superior to another, equipoise has been violated and it is unethical, in the context of an RCT, to assign participants to the inferior treatment. Similarly, if, during the course of an investigation, it becomes abundantly clear that the merits of one arm of a clinical trial (i.e., one of the treatments) far outweigh those of the other arm(s), it is incumbent upon investigators to terminate the investigation and recommend the more effective treatment to all study participants (Freedman, 1987). One of the most famous instances of the premature termination of an investigation due to the clear superiority of one arm of a clinical trial was the investigation by the Steering Committee of the Physicians' Health Study Research Group (1988) which established that regular aspirin intake significantly reduces the risk of heart attack. Despite the minuscule effect size, the aspirin component of the larger-scale investigation was terminated due to the clinical significance of the findings, and all study participants were informed of the benefits of taking aspirin every other day. This investigation used a sample of several thousand participants; thus investigators were able to discern highly significant findings in the middle of the investigation. Typically, the superiority of one intervention relative to others will not be evident until the conclusion of the study.

Some investigators have misconstrued the concept of clinical equipoise and have applied it, not at the level of the scientific community but at the level of the individual experimenter. This means that if an investigator believes—even in the absence of compelling data—that one intervention is likely to be superior, then equipoise is disturbed and the trial cannot ethically continue (Enkin, 2000). Freedman (1987) refers to this as "theoretical equipoise" as opposed to clinical equipoise and notes that it is "conceptually odd and ethically irrelevant" (p. 143) because it is subject to the idiosyncrasies of the investigator and mandates that a trial be discontinued whenever the investigator perceives a slight superiority of one treatment over another—regardless of whether such a difference actually exists. Any bias or hunch would be grounds for discontinuing an investigation. Thus, the very reason for a clinical trial—substantive disagreement among a community of clinicians and scholars—takes a back seat to the subjective intuition of a single individual. Only a controlled clinical trial is capable of resolving legitimate disagreement of the clinical community. Intuition and hunches can only serve to perpetuate confusion and, in the absence of compelling data, can never resolve pressing clinical dilemmas. A controlled clinical trial should be conducted even if the experimenter believes in the superiority of one of the interventions relative to the alternatives, provided that other learned colleagues are in disagreement (Weijer, Shapiro, & Glass, 2000). Freedman (1987) points out that "persons are licensed . . . after they demonstrate the acquisition of professionally validated knowledge, not after they reveal a superior capacity for guessing" (p. 144).

Disagreement among the professional community most certainly exists regarding the appropriate early intervention (if any) for trauma victims. Given that the standard of treatment (i.e., variants of PD) has been shown to be inert in a number of controlled clinical trials (Litz et al., 2002; Mayou, Ehlers, & Hobbs, 2000; Rose, Brewin, Andrews, & Kirk, 1999; Rose et al., 2001) a state of clinical equipoise unequivocally exists. A failure to conduct controlled RCTs with promising, innovative treatments is arguably more unethical than conducting such investigations. It is clear that a small but significant proportion of trauma survivors develop chronic psychopathology (e.g., Breslau et al., 1998; Kessler, Sonnega, Bromet, & Nelson, 1995). At present, however, intervention options seem to consist of employing traditional but ineffective treatments (i.e., debriefing) or waiting for chronic pathology to develop before implementing valid treatments. This approach is unacceptable. Brief, multisession, early interventions have been developed and appear to hold great promise but await evaluation in the context of RCTs before they can be routinely recommended. Researchers bear the ethical responsibility of developing and implementing valid treatments. However, one could argue that ineffective early interventions have been allowed to take root precisely because the field has relied on the subjective intuition of well-intentioned clinicians rather than insisting on empirically rigorous trials.

Regarding the use of nonspecific factors/placebo control conditions in early intervention research, it is difficult to appreciate ethical objections which may be tendered given that the present standard treatment is, if anything, inert—and some have contended that it may be detrimental (Bisson, Jenkins, Alexander, & Bannister, 1997). The principle of clinical equipoise implies that placebos are unacceptable in any situation in which validated effective treatment exists (Young, Annable, & Stat, 2002). Early intervention for trauma clearly does not meet this criterion. There appears to be increasing convergence among the research community on this point, as the Declaration of Helsinki, the World Medical Association Council, the Canadian Institutes of Health Research, the Natural Sciences and Engineering Research Council of Canada, the Social Sciences and Humanities Research Council, and the U.S. Food and Drug Administration all condone the use of placebos in instances in which no standard treatment exists that has been shown to be more effective than no treatment (Young et al., 2002). In sum, given the status of the present evidentiary base for early trauma interventions, it is not only permissible to use RCTs to test promising new interventions for trauma victims and to employ placebo/nonspecific factors control conditions, but it is arguably unethical to fail to do so as this will likely perpetuate our present state of futility in attempting to alleviate the suffering of the recently traumatized.

EVALUATION AND ASSESSMENT: IDENTIFYING THOSE LIKELY TO BENEFIT FROM EARLY INTERVENTION

As noted elsewhere in this volume, early intervention for all trauma victims is ill advised, given that the vast majority will return to baseline levels of functioning in the absence of treatment. Efforts to provide universal early intervention will necessarily involve a considerable waste of resources (this is especially true in the context of mass violence or large-scale disaster), thereby decreasing the likelihood that the most needy individuals will receive necessary services. From a methodological standpoint, attempting to intervene with any and all trauma victims without regard to differences in risk for developing sustained distress increases the likelihood of falsely identifying cases of pathology when they do not exist (Type II error). Specifically, if all trauma victims are randomly assigned to various treatment conditions of a clinical trial, all conditions will invariably be associated with large decrements in average symptom levels over time because the vast majority of trauma survivors experience pronounced, but relatively transient, distress following traumatic exposure. Thus, because inert conditions will be characterized by tremendous spontaneous symptom remission, it will be difficult to document the incremental validity of truly effective treatments because 90% of participants in both active and inert conditions will return to baseline levels of function. In contrast, if clinical trials target individuals who exhibit some degree of risk for developing chronic posttraumatic difficulties, it will be easier to document the efficacy of truly helpful treatments because symptom reduction will be unique to those conditions and ineffective treatments will be exposed. For far too long, inert treatments have been touted as necessary interventions because evidence for their efficacy has capitalized on inevitable symptom remission. However, the true measure of early intervention effectiveness is documented symptom improvement among those who are likely to experience persistent distress in the absence of treatment.

ATTENTION TO RISK AND RESILIENCY FACTORS

King, Vogt, and King (Chapter 3, this volume) extensively review risk factors and risk mechanisms that are known to predict sustained posttraumatic distress. Researchers and clinicians alike should attend to these factors carefully in making decisions about appropriate candidates for early intervention. This will allow the ethical, practical, and methodological problems noted previously to be avoided. Investigations designed with attention to, and consideration of, risk factors will also shed light on the complex interplay between and among risk mechanisms in producing or increasing pathology. As noted by Norris, Friedman, and Watson (2002), with respect to pre-, peri-, and posttraumatic risk factors, "despite some synergism, we now must think of them as additive and propose that an individual's risk will increase along with the number of risk factors present and decrease along with the number of protective factors present" (p. 247). Such is the present understanding of how risk mechanisms may operate; only investigations designed to explicitly test alternative mediational models of risk and resiliency will allow for more sophisticated prediction of chronic posttraumatic distress. Readers are encouraged to refer to King et al. (Chapter 3, this volume) for a thoughtful delineation of methodological and statistical considerations specific to evaluating risk and resiliency factors in traumatic stress research. As these researchers note, risk factors are often identified in specific contexts or with specific trauma populations and may depend on the admixture of variables studied. Researchers and clinicians alike should exercise caution when using specific risk and resiliency factors in identifying candidates for early intervention. Although we lack a detailed understanding of the synergy between and among various risk factors at the present time, we know that some are generally more potent than others. Norris, Friedman, and Watson's (2002) assertion that we must, at present, treat risk factors as additive does not preclude prioritizing them as a function of potency. Regardless, attention to needs assessment and severity of distress will be a significant advance in early trauma intervention efforts. Assessing these factors is essential in conserving resources, ensuring treatment for truly needy individuals, and differentiating effective from ineffective interventions.

RANDOMIZED CLINICAL TRIALS AND TIMING
OF EARLY INTERVENTIONS

As noted previously, we have little definitive information about what interventions (if any) are helpful in the wake of trauma. Only methodologically rigorous clinical trials will be able to answer this question as well as the even more basic question of whether formal interventions within the first few weeks following traumatic exposure should be attempted at all. Although randomized allocation of participants to treatments is difficult following trauma (especially large-scale disasters), it is essential in answering these questions. Given that we have no firm basis for advocating any particular form of intervention, it is also an ethical imperative to employ RCTs to work toward discontinuing the routine administration of interventions proven to be ineffective and providing forms of treatment that have long-term beneficial impact.

In addition to the obvious question of whether early intervention should be provided (as evidenced by lower incidence rates and/or severity of psychopathology), there is the important question of the optimal time frame for intervening. This is an open empirical question that must be answered to ensure proper posttraumatic care. We argue that formal interventions should not be provided during the immediate impact phase, but it is unclear whether there is an optimal time frame for intervening after this initial 48-hour period. Although there are no compelling data addressing this question, it is interesting to note that interventions that are provided within hours or a few days of trauma (i.e., debriefing-based interventions) have not been shown to be especially helpful (Litz et al., 2002), whereas a couple of early interventions that have yielded positive outcomes were implemented an average of 10 or more days after the trauma occurred (Bryant et al., 1998; Foa et al., 1995). We propose that RCTs explicitly designed to answer the question of the best timing for an intervention should be conducted. In the context of mass violence and large-scale disasters, clinical resources are scarce; thus it is most often impossible to provide assistance to all who may need it in a timely fashion. In these instances, wait lists are invariably implemented. It would be just as easy to randomly assign participants to treatment waves such that the effects of the same intervention provided at different time points could be determined empirically.

Clearly, some individuals will be more distressed than others (and therefore more in need of professional assistance); thus it may seem intuitively obvious to triage victims in the event of limited clinical resources and to provide services to the most distressed individuals first. This ethical consideration would obviously disallow a randomized trial of intervention timing. We argue, however, that this "intuitively obvious" solution may not be appropriate, as this scenario is more complex than meets the eye. Specifically, this solution relies on the implicit assumption that the earlier intervention is provided, the less likely it is that chronic posttraumatic difficulties will ensue. Although RCTs of intervention timing have yet to be conducted, existing data are more consistent with the possibility that intervention is more helpful after some (unspecified) delay (as discussed earlier). These interventions differ from traditional, immediately delivered treatments on a number of dimensions, so their therapeutic effects cannot be fully attributed to their timing. Still, adopting a symptom-severity triage approach may seem to be the ethical high road, but this strategy begs the question of optimal timing and, if anything, is contrary to extant research findings. Only RCTs of interval timing can answer the question of *when* to intervene in addition to how to intervene after a trauma.

STANDARDIZED TREATMENT PROTOCOLS AND TREATMENT FIDELITY

Improvements in posttraumatic care are contingent upon explicit, detailed descriptions of interventions offered. The more detailed intervention descriptions are, the easier it will be for the scientific community to discern critical components and parametric features (e.g., timing and duration) which differentiate helpful from unhelpful interventions. To this end, we recommend that treatment innovators develop and disseminate detailed treatment manuals which fully delineate their interventions. It is insufficient to simply note that an intervention employed cognitive restructuring, *in vivo* exposure, or imaginal exposure, for instance. An apparently ineffective intervention may indeed be due to the inclusion of inappropriate or inert components. But it is often the case that effective treatment components are poorly timed or administered for an insufficient duration. It has been suggested, for instance, that debriefing-based interventions use a degree of exposure therapy but that the exposure is hasty and incomplete, which has the effect of exacerbating distress rather than abating it (Bisson, McFarlane, & Rose, 2000). Detailed depictions of the parameters of an intervention, rather than a brief listing of treatment components, permit early intervention researchers to revise potentially helpful interventions rather than summarily concluding that a treatment does not work.

Detailed manualized interventions also allow researchers to ascertain whether the intervention was administered properly. Routine assessments of treatment fidelity allow researchers to decide whether ineffectual treatments are indeed inert—or whether apparent treatment failures are attributable to poor implementation or administration of theoretically sound treatments. Similarly, evidence of high treatment integrity increases one's confidence in the outcome of a clinical trial. Unfortunately, even when detailed accounts of an intervention are provided in the literature, mention of manipulation checks or evaluation of treatment integrity is almost invariably absent. As noted by Kazdin (1998), assessment of treatment fidelity ensures that treatment conditions are distinct. For example, assume that trauma victims who have been deemed especially likely to develop chronic posttraumatic difficulties are randomly assigned to an early intervention which is anticipated to be quite beneficial (e.g., five sessions of cognitive-behavioral therapy), to a placebo/nonspecific factors, control condition (also five sessions) or to a no-treatment control condition. Assume also that at the end of the clinical trial, both active treatment conditions resulted in a 50% reduction in symptom severity relative to no-treatment control participants. In this situation, it would be tempting to conclude that the five sessions of cognitive-behavioral therapy (CBT; hypothesized to be especially helpful) promoted positive posttraumatic adjustment but not to a greater extent than nonspecific therapeutic factors such as basic empathy and support. That is, the unique components of the CBT intervention such as imaginal and *in vivo* exposure are not associated with incremental treatment gains above and beyond nonspecific therapeutic factors. Although this conclusion may be accurate, it is possible that the "nonspecific factors" condition included an exposure component. An evaluation of the integrity of the nonspecific factors condition may reveal that participants in that condition spent a good deal of time talking about the traumatic event in detail. In such a scenario, the condition would arguably be a variant of exposure rather than a proxy for professional therapeutic support. Without evaluating the fidelity with which all conditions were administered, one might hastily conclude that a truly helpful intervention is not particularly useful. The critical importance of developing and implementing effective treatments that can ameliorate the severe emotional distress that often accompanies trauma mandates that the scientific community provide more detailed accounts of early interventions and, more important, that we attend to, and document, the fidelity with which our interventions are delivered.

EVALUATION OF MULTIPLE OUTCOMES BY MULTIPLE INFORMANTS

Perhaps understandably, trauma researchers and responders have focused their efforts on the study and treatment of PTSD following traumatic events. However, this focus should not prevent researchers from attending to other forms of emotional and behavior distress. Norris, Friedman, Watson, et al. (2002) review varied and diverse difficulties that have been extensively documented in the wake of trauma. These difficulties include specific psychological problems (PTSD, major depressive disorder, panic disorder, and generalized anxiety disorder), nonspecific emotional distress, health problems, alcohol and substance abuse and dependency, occupational and financial stress, impairments of social supports and interpersonal relationships, and age-specific problems (e.g., temper tantrums, incontinence, and hyperactivity in children). Evaluating and documenting more diverse outcomes will allow investigators to determine the breadth of impact of their interventions and will also allow interventions with fairly specific effects to be modified in order to target more varied forms of psychopathology. For instance, it may become apparent that an explicit focus on maladaptive coping strategies (substance abuse) needs to be incorporated depending on the documented prevalence of this problem in specific populations and contexts. Although the immediate posttraumatic environment may not allow for comprehensive assessment of all possible difficulties, investigators can use the literature to inform the selection of outcome domains to be examined (e.g., complicated grief reactions in incidents of mass violence).

In addition to evaluating diverse outcome domains, investigators should, to the extent possible, use multiple informants in assessing treatment response. In addition to self-report measures (which is often the only means used to evaluate treatment response), investigators should consider using structured clinical interviews and, if possible, the reports or ratings of significant others. Clearly, if structured clinical interviews are employed, they should be conducted by individuals who are unaware of the participants' treatment condition status. Finally, instead of the traditional exclusive focus on differences between treatment conditions at the end of treatment, greater attention should be paid to the rate of recovery promoted by alternative interventions (Kenardy et al., 1996). That is, two seemingly equivalent interventions (as evidenced by end-state symptom levels) may, in fact, be quite different in terms of how precipitous the decrease of symptoms is in each condition. An intervention that achieves improvement more quickly is arguably a superior intervention, all other things being equal.

TIMING AND DURATION OF EVALUATIONS

It goes without saying that it is difficult to determine the impact of an intervention if measures of emotional and behavioral functioning are not administered prior to beginning treatment. Unfortunately, a surprising number of published reports attesting to the efficacy of a trauma intervention have relied exclusively on posttreatment evaluations, preventing definitive statements regarding the magnitude of symptom change. Precious few data are available to illuminate the persistence of treatment gains following effective interventions. Although it is often quite difficult to track trauma victims longitudinally, efforts to do so will afford information about the maintenance of treatment gains and may also provide information about benefits of treatment which are not immediately apparent. For instance, marital or occupational problems may increase significantly after a period of relative quiescence. One's spouse or employer may be understanding or especially accommodating of problems within the first few months of a traumatic event—but may be less accommodating thereafter. Conceivably, alterations in marital or employment status may not become known until well after a traumatic event. In such a scenario, the full benefit of a therapeutic intervention relative to a no-treatment or a nonspecific-factors control condition may go undetected if the participants are only followed for a few months after the traumatic event.

Finally, with respect to the timing of evaluations, periodic measurement of functioning and distress during the intervention period may be illuminating. Although this may not be appropriate or feasible for all or even most early intervention studies, periodic evaluation of functioning during treatment may help to elucidate which elements of multicomponent treatment packages are associated with greater improvements and may also help to identify possible process variables which are instrumental in promoting positive posttraumatic adjustment. There exists, for instance, a great deal of speculation that emotion-focused traumatic processing too soon after traumatic exposure may exacerbate rather than alleviate posttraumatic distress (Bisson et al., 2000). This may certainly be the case, but at present, there are no compelling data to substantiate or disconfirm this possibility. Associations between postintervention symptom status and peri-intervention negative affect and arousal would be required to empirically evaluate this possibility.

GREATER ATTENTION TO INDIVIDUAL DIFFERENCES

Given the limitations of our current knowledge about early intervention for trauma, it is not especially surprising that clinical trials to date have focused primarily on group-based outcomes. That is, interventions have been applied in a one-size-fits-all fashion, and investigators have understandably concerned themselves with the question whether the active treatment condition exhibits superior outcomes when compared to the group(s) not receiving the favored intervention. Clearly, individuals differ in their needs following trauma, their capacities to use formal interventions and informal supports effectively, their inclinations to discuss the trauma and associated difficulties with others, and so forth. As we have noted elsewhere (Litz et al., 2002), some individuals may benefit greatly from sharing their harrowing experience with supportive others whereas others may prefer to work out problems on their own and may therefore perceive encouragements to share their experiences as impositions. Conclusions about intervention effectiveness based on group-based statistics necessarily obscure individual differences in symptom course and do not speak to individual difference variables which are associated with differential outcomes. Accordingly, the inclusion of measures which may mediate responses to intervention (personality measures, coping indices, etc.) will enhance our ability to apply interventions selectively and appropriately and will allow clinicians to "troubleshoot" problems along the way by identifying individuals who are unlikely to benefit from standard interventions by tracking process variables known to be predictive of deleterious outcomes. Collecting data on individual differences and process variables will improve our understanding of the synergy between and among the resiliency and vulnerability factors reviewed above.

ATTENTION TO TRAUMA-SPECIFIC CHARACTERISTICS

When investigating and attempting to alleviate posttraumatic distress, it is necessary to consider issues unique to particular trauma types and contexts that may affect symptom expression and treatment.

Terrorism and Mass Violence

A recent review comparing the psychological impact of natural and man-made disasters found that intentional mass violence was the most distressing type of disaster (Norris, Friedman, Watson, et al., 2002). The specification of traumatic exposure includes the possibility of witnessing an event, a dead body, or body parts (American Psychiatric Association, 2000). Without the specification of in-person observation, the question of the extent to which witnessing events via live television coverage or video replay may result in significant posttraumatic distress arises. Schlenger et al. (2002) found that during the second month following the terrorist attacks of 9-11-01, the amount of television coverage watched and the number of different kinds of events that respondents reported seeing on television (live coverage of the planes as they impacted the buildings, people jumping or falling from the World Trade Center [WTC], people running to escape the buildings, replayed footage, etc.) were both significantly related to the prevalence of probable PTSD.

Moreover, one's proximity to a natural or technological disaster or mass violence event may have implications for mental health outcomes. Schlenger et al. (2002) also found the prevalence of probable PTSD was significantly related to the individual's geographic proximity to the WTC site on 9-11. Studies investigating the relationship between proximity to an incident of mass violence and subsequent distress have not produced uniform findings. For instance, although the prevalence rate in the Washington, DC area was slightly higher than the national prevalence rate, it was not statistically significant (Schlenger et al., 2002). Considering the incongruous findings, early intervention research in the context of mass violence should include information regarding both direct (e.g., first-person observation) and indirect (e.g., media coverage) exposure to the potentially traumatic event and, if applicable, should determine victims' relative proximity to the disaster epicenter. This variable may be important because it serves as a proxy for legitimate life threat or endangerment.

Compensation and Symptom Exaggeration

When the mental health and legal arenas coincide, research and anecdotal evidence illustrate the demand characteristics inherent in litigation and attest to the possibility of malingering. It has been suggested that as many as 20–30% of personal injury plaintiffs could be considered possible malingerers (Lees-Haley, 1997). Are PTSD symptoms exaggerated or falsely reported in an effort to establish grounds for a personal injury claim? Ehlers and Mayou (1998) assessed PTSD diagnosis and litigation status for individuals who had been involved in motor vehicle accidents (MVA). At 1-year post-MVA, 28.9% of those whose claims had not been settled reported symptoms that met criteria for PTSD. Those who had not filed a claim, had dropped a claim, or whose claim had been settled had a 10.4% PTSD incidence rate. This is not to say that all claimants embellish their symptoms. When an individual's primary goal is to alleviate his or her PTSD symptoms, malingering has been found to be less frequent (Kuch, Cox, & Evans, 1996). However, an individual's worker's compensation claim, Veterans Affairs benefits, or personal injury lawsuit may affect the severity and persistence of his or her reported symptomatology. To more accurately assess the veracity of symptom reporting, and to eliminate the possibility of responding biases affecting outcomes, researchers should consider assessing litigation status or compensations seeking as part of their protocol.

Symptom Minimization

It has been suggested that in some contexts, individuals may minimize symptom severity or be reluctant to endorse symptoms. Military personnel may prefer not to report symptoms while continuing to serve in the military (e.g., Wolfe, Erickson, Sharkansky, King, & King, 1999). Emergency service personnel (e.g., firefighters and police officers) may fear being viewed as "unfit" or having their duties restricted. Some trauma survivors may fear they will be stigmatized for seeking psychological services (Yehuda, 2002). As with screening for litigation, researchers should be aware of the impact that specific contexts or populations may have on veracity of reported distress.

Sexual Assault

Resick and Schnicke (1996) discuss the necessity of assessing for, and addressing, issues of trust and intimacy for survivors of sexual assault. Self-distrust may be manifest in thoughts of self-blame, second-guessing of choices, or difficulty with everyday decisions. Other people are often presumed untrustworthy. Family and friends may unwittingly reinforce this presumption through their own reactions. Sexual assault survivors may also avoid emotional intimacy with friends and family in an effort to avoid possible rejection or blame, thus depriving themselves of social support. Physical intimacy is rife with reminders of the assault, may trigger intense fear or flashbacks, and is, therefore, often avoided. Intimate relationships may suffer, further isolating the individual. In addition, the sexual assault survivor may not have any positive intimate experiences with which to counter the traumatic experience of the assault. The seemingly protective measures taken in an effort to avoid intimacy or violations of trust may ultimately be counterproductive during PTSD intervention. As such, early interventions for sexual assault need to be designed with these issues in mind. Moreover, explicit assessment of social support utilization may be more important in this particular posttraumatic context.

OVERVIEW OF RESEARCH "BEST PRACTICE" RECOMMENDATIONS

In this chapter, we have reviewed the ideal characteristics of early trauma intervention investigations. We recognize that no single study will likely adhere to all these recommendations because the early posttraumatic environment is fraught with a number of practical barriers. Optimal methods are, in many instances, simply impossible to employ due to practical and ethical issues and resource limitations. As a community of clinical scientists, however, we can collectively overcome the limitations of any single investigation by attending to and improving existing limitations of the literature in this area. Thus, although it may be impossible to implement all the suggestions advanced in this chapter in a single clinical trial, multiple clinical trials should be able to compensate for the methodological deficiencies of any particular trial. Moreover, single clinical trials will be particularly compelling to the extent that they are able to incorporate several of these features.

1. *RCTs must be employed to evaluate the efficacy of early interventions.* Because the present "standard of treatment" appears not to be superior to receiving no intervention whatsoever (Rose et al., 2001; Litz et al., 2002), there seems to be no ethical risk in using no-treatment control conditions and/or nonspecific-factor control groups. A state of clinical equipoise certainly exists, as we presently have no form of early posttraumatic intervention which has been shown, in the context of rigorous clinical trials, to be superior to receiving no treatment and which has been shown to be broadly applicable to varied posttraumatic populations and contexts. Although promising interventions are being developed, only large-scale RCTs using appropriate control conditions will determine whether they are superior to inefficacious debriefing-based interventions that have been the treatment standard to date.

2. *Researchers should seek to identify and treat only those individuals who bear some known risk for developing chronic posttraumatic difficulties.* As reviewed earlier, intervening only with individuals likely to develop chronic distress represents a judicious use of limited clinical resources. In addition, from a methodological standpoint, focusing our efforts on those who are unlikely to exhibit spontaneous symptom remission makes it easier to detect genuine treatment effects—effects which may be masked if treatment is supplied to all victims, as the vast majority of participants in all experimental conditions will experience pronounced symptom decreases in the months following traumatic exposure.

3. *Randomly assignment to varied timings of intervention will elucidate the optimal time frame for treating at-risk trauma victims.* Despite a great deal of speculation about the merits or dangers of providing formalized intervention at certain time points shortly after traumatic exposure, there are no compelling data that speak to the issue of timing. Promising interventions have been delivered approximately 1½ weeks after traumatic exposure and ineffective treatments are often provided within hours of the event. Yet these various interventions differ in a number of ways; thus differential efficacy cannot be fully attributed to differences in timing. This issue must be empirically evaluated in the context of subsequent clinical trials.

4. *Researchers should use detailed, manualized treatment protocols and should evaluate the fidelity with which interventions are implemented.* Dissemination, implementation, and evaluation of effective interventions require that other clinicians and research teams can replicate newly developed treatments. The mere listing of treatment components does not allow for advancement of the science. Moreover, hasty conclusions regarding treatment efficacy may be prevented to the extent that treatment integrity is formally evaluated.

5. *Researchers should evaluate multiple outcome and process variables and*

individual difference variables across diverse domains and should attempt to use multiple informants. Researchers are advised not only to include measures that assess diverse forms of emotional distress but also to include measures of functional impairment and relationship difficulties. Moreover, inclusion of measures of treatment process variables and individual difference measures will illuminate differential responses to (overall) effective interventions, which will allow clinicians to begin tailoring treatments to individuals based on unique constellations of risk and resiliency factors. Using multiple informants, rather than relying exclusively on self-report measures, will shed light on the strength and generality of reported treatment gains and will reduce the threat of expectancy effects and demand characteristics.

6. *Evaluations should be made frequently before, during, and after treatment.* The inclusion of a pretreatment evaluation is absolutely necessary if any firm conclusions about treatment efficacy are to be made. Longitudinal evaluation of functioning (i.e., well after the termination of treatment) will allow for the assessment of the persistence of treatment gains and will also allow researchers and clinicians to detect posttraumatic difficulties which may emerge well after traumatic exposure. In addition, evaluations during the course of treatment will allow researchers to empirically evaluate potentially important process variables of existing early interventions (e.g., premature emotion-focused processing of trauma as an indicator of deleterious outcomes).

7. *Finally, researchers should be mindful of unique characteristics of different trauma populations and contexts and should resist the temptation to apply effective interventions to different trauma populations without regard to necessary modifications.* Early intervention researchers should develop interventions geared to specific trauma contexts. Existing early interventions are often applied without regard for unique needs of different trauma populations and have not been shown to be especially helpful.

In summary, efforts to treat trauma victims soon after exposure have been largely ineffective. A sober examination of methodological and ethical issues germane to early intervention research reveals that attention to methodological rigor exposes seductive but inert treatments and will stimulate further efforts to develop more fruitful interventions. Waiting for chronic pathology to develop is counterintuitive, and innovated researchers are beginning to modify empirically validated treatment components for use in acute trauma intervention contexts. We are encouraged by recent early intervention innovations which will likely supplant traditional debriefing-based interventions. But we are more encouraged by the ever-increasing quality of early intervention research designs. Attention to the considerations and recommendations outlined in this chapter will allow us to better serve at-risk trauma victims and will ensure that our interventions continue to grow and evolve in order to meet the needs of traumatized populations.

REFERENCES

American Psychiatric Association. (1994). *Diagnostic and statistical manual of mental disorders* (4th ed.). Washington, DC: Author.

American Psychiatric Association. (2000). *Diagnostic and statistical manual of mental disorders* (4th ed., text revision). Washington, DC: Author.

American Red Cross. (1998). *Disaster mental health services,* No. 3043. Washington, DC: Author.

Bisson, J., Jenkins, P., Alexander, J., & Bannister, C. (1997). Randomized controlled trial of psychological debriefing for victims of acute burn trauma. *British Journal of Psychiatry, 171,* 78–81.

Bisson, J. I., McFarlane, A. C., & Rose, S. (2000). Psychological debriefing. In E. B. Foa, T. M. Keane, & M. J. Friedman (Eds.), *Effective treatments for PTSD* (pp. 39–59). New York: Guilford Press.

Breslau, N., Kessler, R., Chilcoat, H., Schultz, L., Davis, G., & Andreski, M. (1998). Trauma and posttraumatic stress disorder in the community: The 1996 Detroit area survey of trauma. *Archives of General Psychiatry, 55,* 626–632.

Bryant, R., Harvey, A., Dang, S., Sackville, T., & Basten, C. (1998). Treatment of acute stress disorder: A comparison of cognitive-behavioral therapy and supportive counseling. *Journal of Consulting and Clinical Psychology, 66,* 862–866.

Christianson, S. A. (1992). *The handbook of emotion and memory: Research and theory.* Mahwah, NJ: Erlbaum.

Ehlers, A., & Mayou, R. A. (1998). Psychological predictors of chronic post-traumatic stress disorder after motor-vehicle accidents. *Journal of Abnormal Psychology, 107,* 508–519.

Enkin, M. (2000). Clinical equipoise and not the uncertainty principle is the moral underpinning of the randomized clinical trial. (Against.) *British Medical Journal, 321,* 757–758.

Eysenck, M., & Calvo, M. (1992). Anxiety and performance: The processing efficiency theory. *Cognition and Emotion, 6,* 409–434.

Foa, E., Hearst-Ikeda, D., & Perry, K. (1995). Evaluation of a brief cognitive-behavioral program for the prevention of chronic PTSD in recent assault victims. *Journal of Consulting and Clinical Psychology, 63,* 955–978.

Freedman, B. (1987). Equipoise and the ethics of clinical research. *New England Journal of Medicine, 317,* 141–145.

Kazdin, A. E. (1998). *Research design in clinical psychology* (3rd ed.). Boston: Allyn & Bacon.

Kenardy, J., Webster, R., Lewin, T., Carr, V., Hazell, P., & Carter, G. (1996). Stress debriefing and patterns of recovery following a natural disaster. *Journal of Traumatic Stress, 9,* 37–49.

Kessler, R., Sonnega, A., Bromet, E., & Nelson, C. (1995). Posttraumatic stress disorder in the National Comorbidity Survey. *Archives of General Psychiatry, 52,* 1048–1060.

Kuch, K., Cox, B. J., & Evans, R. J. (1996). Post-traumatic stress disorder and motor-vehicle accidents. *Canadian Journal of Psychiatry, 41,* 429–432.

Lees-Haley, P.R. (1997). MMPI-2 baserates for 492 personal injury plaintiffs. *Journal of Clinical Psychology, 53,* 745–755.

Litz, B., Gray, M., Bryant, R., & Adler, A. (2002). Early intervention for trauma: Current status and future directions. *Clinical Psychology: Science and Practice, 9,* 112–134.

Mayou, R., Ehlers, A., & Hobbs, M. (2000). Psychological debriefing for road traffic accident victims. *British Journal of Psychiatry, 176,* 589–593.

Norris, F., Friedman, M., & Watson, P. (2002). 60,000 disaster victims speak: Part II. Summary and implications of the disaster mental health research. *Psychiatry, 65,* 240–260.

Norris, F., Friedman, M., Watson, P., Byrne, C., Diaz, E., & Kaniasty, K. (2002). 60,000 disaster victims speak: Part 1. An empirical review of the empirical literature, 1981–2001. *Psychiatry, 65,* 207–239.

Resick, P., & Schnicke, M. (1996). *Cognitive processing therapy for rape victims: A treatment manual.* Thousand Oaks, CA: Sage Publications.

Rose, S., Bisson, J., & Wesseley, S. (2001). Psychological debriefing for preventing post-traumatic stress disorder (PTSD). *Cochrane Database of Systematic Reviews* [Online version]. *www.update-software.com/abstracts/ab00560.htm*

Rose, S., Brewin, C., Andrews, B., & Kirk, M. (1999). A randomized controlled trial of individual psychological debriefing for victims of violent crime. *Psychological Medicine, 29,* 793–799.

Schlenger, W. E., Caddell, J. M., Ebert, L., Jordan, B. K., Rourke, K. M., & Wilson, D., Thalji, L., Dennis, J. M., Fairbank, J. A., & Kulka, R. A. (2002). Psychological reactions to terrorist attacks: Findings from the National Study of Americans' Reactions to September 11. *Journal of the American Medical Association, 288,* 581–588.

Steering Committee of the Physicians' Health Study Research Group. (1988). Preliminary report: Findings from the aspirin component of the ongoing physicians' health study. *New England Journal of Medicine, 318,* 262–264.

Weijer, C., Shapiro, S., & Glass, K. (2000). Clinical equipoise and not the uncertainty principle is the moral underpinning of the randomized controlled trial. (For). *British Medical Journal, 321,* 756–757.

Wolfe, J., Erickson, D. J., Sharkansky, E. J., King, D. W., & King, L. A. (1999). Course and predictors of posttraumatic stress disorder among Gulf War veterans: A perspective analysis. *Journal of Counseling and Clinical Psychology, 67,* 520–528.

Yehuda, R. (2002). Post-traumatic stress disorder. *New England Journal of Medicine, 346,* 108–114.

Young, S., Annable, L., & Stat, D. (2002). The ethics of placebo in clinical psychopharmacology: The urgent need for consistent regulation. *Journal of Psychiatry and Neuroscience, 27,* 319–321.

III
Special Topics

10

The Professional Response to the Aftermath of September 11, 2001, in New York City

Lessons Learned from Treating Victims of the World Trade Center Attacks

YUVAL NERIA
EUN JUNG SUH
RANDALL D. MARSHALL

On 9-11-01, terrorists took aim at the World Trade Center (WTC), a prominent symbol of the Western World, and shocked America and the world community. At 8:45 A.M. on a clear blue morning, a hijacked American Airlines Boeing 767 carrying 92 people crashed into the north tower of the WTC. Eighteen minutes later, a United Airlines Boeing 767 carrying 65 people crashed into the south tower, erasing any lingering doubt that the first crash was accidental. At 10:05 that morning, the south tower collapsed followed by the north tower at 10:28.

The intent of this devastating attack was to exact maximum physical and emotional damage by using passenger aircrafts as flying missiles to destroy vulnerable buildings in a densely populated business center. Two thousand, eight hundred and one people died in these attacks. The enormous loss of human lives, the crippling of a major economic center, and the nonstop, live media coverage provided unprecedented exposure to trauma and loss, making it difficult to predict the scale of mental health ramifications and needs. The mental health community in New York City was taken by surprise and was unprepared to respond to a disaster of such magnitude.

This chapter aims to describe the professional response of a team of clinicians and researchers at Columbia University and the New York State Psychiatric Institute (NYSPI). This team tried to meet the anticipated mental health needs of the community in the wake of the 9-11 disaster by providing trauma education and training to health care providers and treatment to traumatized individuals. The chapter is organized such that events unfold chronologically in order to give the reader an authentic, phase-by-phase, sense of what happened following the 9-11 disaster.

In the days and weeks following the WTC attack, we turned our attention to the possible psychological consequences of large-scale disasters. This chapter begins by highlighting an influential disaster research study conducted by Carol North et al. (1999). The second section of this chapter briefly discusses how we began to piece together the information gathered from the available research to anticipate the needs of general population in New York City. The third section of the chapter describes the mobilization of New York City mental health community, including clinicians, researchers, and educators at the Trauma Program of Columbia University and NYSPI to meet the psychosocial needs of the city. The fourth section discusses the dissemination of evidence-based trauma treatment undertaken by our trauma team through a series of training seminars aimed at rapidly educating community clinicians. This section also outlines the results of the evaluation research conducted on our training seminars. In the fifth section of this chapter we discuss the findings from the epidemiological surveys conducted in New York City and nationally since September 11, 2001, examining the question whether the findings give support to our assumptions. In the last section we attempt to reflect on what has been done so far and to lay out directions for future preparedness.

PHASE I (SEPTEMBER 2001): POSSIBLE CONSEQUENCES FOLLOWING DISASTERS—EPIDEMIOLOGICAL RESEARCH

In the days following the attack, the mental health community in the Greater New York area began bracing itself for a widely anticipated increase in the need for mental health services. The scope of these needs, however, was unknown. A careful review of the existing literature revealed a paucity of well-executed studies conducted after terrorist attacks, despite the frequency of these attacks around the world. Specifically, there were no studies delineating the immediate needs of urban communities in the wake of this type of exposure.

Prevalence studies of posttraumatic stress disorder (PTSD), not related to intentional terrorist attacks, demonstrated that, on average, 5–6% of men and 10–14% of women in the United States have had PTSD at some time in their lives (Breslau, Davis, Andreski, & Peterson, 1991; Breslau, Davis, Peterson, & Schultz, 1997; Kessler et al., 1995). These figures mark PTSD as the fourth most common psychiatric disorder in the United States. However, as the stressor criterion (Criterion A) of the PTSD definition (DSM-IV; American Psychiatric Association, 1994) is highly heterogeneous, rates of PTSD after severe trauma can vary from as low as 1.4% to as high as 65% (Yehuda 2002). This range is generally interpreted as support for the assertion that traumatic events vary considerably in type, characteristics, and severity (e.g., single vs. multiple assailants, proximity to event, witnessing of graphic or gruesome sights). For example, events that involve interpersonal violence are associated with higher rates of PTSD (46% for women; 65% for men) than events such as natural disaster (5.4% for women; 3.7% for men) (Kessler, Sonnega, Bromet, & Nelson, 1995). Given the large numbers of people exposed on 9-11-01, the question whether such exposure would produce PTSD in 5% or 50% of eyewitnesses had immediate public health consequences and treatment implications.

North et al. (1999) conducted one of the few studies investigating the long-term effects of a deliberate act of terrorism prior to 9-11. They surveyed a random sample of 182 adults from a registry of individuals who had been directly exposed to the bombing of the Murrah Federal Building on April 19, 1995. This blast resulted in 168 deaths and 684 injuries. The authors conducted this survey approximately 6 months after the bombing. They had a cooperation rate of 71%, and found that those who refused to be interviewed (14%, $n = 35$) had significantly less exposure than those who agreed to participate. Most (87%) of those interviewed sustained physical injuries related to the blast.

Participants were evaluated for the presence of eight major psychiatric disorders (PTSD, major depression, panic, generalized anxiety, somatization, alcohol, drug use, and antisocial personality disorders). In addition, demographics, as well as data on level of functioning and treatment received, were also collected. Nearly half (45%) of the respondents met current criteria for at least one psychiatric disorder, while 34% met criteria for PTSD, and 22.5% of the sample were diagnosed with major depressive disorder (MDD). Consistent with other studies, rates of PTSD and MDD were higher in women than men (45% vs. 23%; 32% vs. 13%, respectively). Rates of prebombing diagnoses were relatively high (43% had at least one predisaster diagnosis), but the majority of illnesses initially occurred after the exposure. As in other epidemiological studies, individuals with prior psychiatric histories were more likely to develop PTSD (45% vs. 26%). In fact, for all disorders detected, a diagnosis after the bombing was associated with a predisaster diagnosis. These findings support the conclusions of previous research, which has suggested that after a severe community trauma, both relapse/exacerbation of previous illness and new disorders that develop after the trauma must be considered. Moreover, in these samples, all cases of PTSD followed the acute-onset pattern, with 94% of individuals developing symptoms within the first week. At 6 months posttrauma, 63% of participants reported some disaster-related symptoms (including subthreshold symptomatology). This finding was consistent with recent research on subthreshold PTSD as a source of disability (Marshall et al., 2001; Stein, Walker, Hazen, & Forde, 1997; Weiss et al., 1992). In addition, reported functional impairment in this sample was high, with 75% of those diagnosed with PTSD acknowledging negative changes in their relationships, compared to 27% of those without PTSD. Not surprisingly, PTSD patients were also likely to report that their symptoms interfered with daily functioning.

PHASE II (OCTOBER 2001): ATTEMPT TO CREATE A RATIONALE FOR APPROPRIATE RESPONSE

Extrapolating from the Oklahoma Bombing studies, we anticipated that the larger scale of loss and destruction from the 9-11 attacks, as well as the greater number of direct and indirect witnesses, would produce a significant and enduring impact on both the physical and mental health of the general population. Prior research suggested that evacuees, rescue personnel, clean-up workers, and the traumatically bereaved would be at higher risk for long-term mental health consequences (Kessler et al., 1995; Kulka et al., 1990; North et al., 1999). We anticipated that there would be at least four major categories of individuals more likely to be in need of therapeutic intervention: (1) those with new-onset psychiatric disorder due to exposure to the attack, including, but not limited to, PTSD (see Neria & Bromet, 2000); (2) those suffering a relapse of a preexisting psychiatric disorder (e.g., major depression, panic disorder, substance abuse, and PTSD); (3) those experiencing relapse/new-onset psychiatric disorder related to secondary consequences of the attack (e.g., protracted unemployment, relocation, and ongoing stressors related to living and/or working in lower Manhattan); and (4) those with widespread, subthreshold symptoms related to various levels of functional impairment (see Marshall et al., 2001).

Although mental health professionals would generally agree that early preventive intervention for trauma is both necessary and important, there is no consensus about who should receive interventions, when they should be conducted, or what the best interventions are (Litz, Gray, Bryant, & Adler, 2002). In the years before the 9-11 attacks, accumulated evidence suggested that early interventions such as *critical incident stress debriefing* (CISD; Mitchell, 1981), which had been perceived for years as the state-of-the-art intervention following trauma exposure and adopted by prominent organizations such as FEMA (Federal Emergency Management Agency) and the Red Cross, was not only limited in its capacity to cure trauma residues but also potentially harmful, especially if conducted indiscriminately (Litz et al., 2002). We argue that any group-based, brief format for all those exposed, without pre- and/or postintervention evaluation, might potentially be harmful for certain symptomatic trauma survivors (Neria, Solomon, & Ginzburg, 2000).

To date, multiple, well-controlled studies conducted with a variety of trauma victims, including war veterans (Cooper & Clum, 1989; Glynn et al., 1999; Keane, Fairbank, Caddell, & Zimmering, 1989), female victims of assault (Foa, Rothbaum, Riggs, & Marks, 1991; Foa et al., 1999; Resick, Jordan, Girelli, Hutter, & Marhoefer-Dvorak, 1988), and mixed trauma populations (Marks, Lovell, Noshirvani, Livanou, & Thrasher, 1998; Tarrier et al., 1999) have found cognitive-behavioral therapy (CBT) modalities to be highly effective in the treatment of PTSD. Among the CBT programs, exposure therapy has the most empirical support for its high efficacy and efficiency in different populations of trauma victims with PTSD.

PHASE III (NOVEMBER 2001): COMING TOGETHER

The National Center for PTSD, located within the Department of Veterans Affairs (National Center for PTSD website, accessed 2002) states that interventions conducted postdisaster are best understood within the context of when, where, and with whom interventions take place. With this in mind, the New York City Consortium for Effective Trauma Treatment was created to use existing expertise and resources available to the mental health professionals in the New York City area to meet the needs of New Yorkers suffering from posttrauma sequelae. The New York City Consortium was a collaboration of four trauma centers in Manhattan: Columbia/NYSPI, Mount Sinai, Cornell, and Saint Vincent's Hospital. The goals of the New York City Consortium were twofold: (1) to address the mental health care needs of adults, children, and families following the WTC disaster, and (2) to organize the deployment of well-trained clinicians by creating an infrastructure for ongoing training, provision of evidence-based treatment, and follow-up studies to monitor the effectiveness and quality of our treatment and training courses. The Consortium mobilized in time to respond during the 8th to 12th week following the disaster, typically referred to as the *restoration phase,* during which long-term recovery programs are generally implemented. As mental health professionals working in a hospital setting, clinicians from the Consortium treated clients off-site at the clinic and hospitals rather than at ground zero. The groups we focused on were adult and child survivors as well as the helpers in the community.

Efficacious treatments for PTSD such as CBT and prolonged exposure are a relatively new and highly specialized area of treatment and research. As few clinicians had the experience necessary to provide such treatments, our trauma center at Columbia University/New York State Psychiatric Institute was inundated with requests for education and training for clinicians. To meet this demand, the New York City Consortium for Effective Trauma Treatment held a series of intensive training seminars conducted by experts from around the world for a group of experienced clinicians who would, in turn, be providing treatment, at no cost, to victims of 9-11. In addition, these experts were to hold lectures and trainings for the community in the year following 9-11 (2001–2002). Within weeks after 9-11, the Consortium received the first year of funding for these efforts from the New York Times Foundation and the Surdna Foundation.

PHASE IV (NOVEMBER 2001–DECEMBER 2002): TRAINING TRAUMA THERAPISTS

There is a considerable literature indicating that merely listening to a series of lectures (such as is done with continuing medical education programs) does not result in changes in clinical practice (see Fishbein, 1995). This is especially true when the clinicians are being asked to shift clinical paradigms (e.g., from a psychodynamic to a cognitive-behavioral approach and from an unstructured therapeutic encounter to a manualized treatment). In these circumstances the "training" needs to be closer to a behavioral change intervention than to a mere sharing of information. According to the theory of reasoned action (Fishbein & Ajzen, 1975), behavioral change will depend on (1) therapists' outcome expectations, (2) therapists' norm perceptions, and (3) beliefs about professional effectiveness. The latter is closely related to the anticipation of barriers in conducting the new treatment and to the availability of strategies to overcome them. The training we have designed, in collaboration with Drs. Laurence Amsel and Peter Jensen, addresses a number of these issues through the use of multiple demonstrations, discussion sessions, and small-group supervised practice sessions (which enhanced self-efficacy while establishing clinical practice norms).

Moreover, because evaluation of these trainings is integral to the model we are using, an evaluation component was designed to ascertain not only what was learned during the training but also what changes in attitude, behavior, and self-efficacy might have occurred. If the investment in training is to have a meaningful effect on clinician behavior, this type of evaluation is essential to track and document changes brought about by training in order to help guide future course development. It should be noted that extensive clinician training on this scale is relatively unprecedented and serves as an opportunity to better understand the training process and its relationship to desired clinical behavior change.

Over the last 12 months our team has conducted 4-day training courses for more than 500 clinicians. The goal of these training courses was to educate community clinicians in evidence-based treatment for PTSD as efficiently as possible. The manualized CBT, prolonged exposure (PE) treatment program for PTSD (Foa & Rothbaum, 1998) was initially selected to disseminate, based on research demonstrating the efficacy of CBT–PE treatment (e.g., Foa et al., 1991; Foa et al., 1999; Marks et al., 1998) and due to the preexisting expertise in CBT–PE treatment of the training clinicians at the Columbia University and NYSPI Trauma Studies and Services Program. A variety of educational strategies, including lectures and discussion, clinical case demonstrations, and individual role play, were implemented in order to maximize trainees' knowledge-acquisition as well as clinical behavioral changes.

The preliminary results from our training evaluations (Amsel, Jensen, & Marshall, 2002) are based on a sample size of 104 trainees who participated in the first few seminars. The trainees were qualified, licensed clinicians with many years of clinical experience (average number of years in practice was 17 years; 70% of trainees had greater than 10 years of clinical experience). Approximately 60% of the trainees were social workers (MSW), 20% were psychologists (PhD), and 10% were psychiatrists (MD). Findings from this study suggested that clinical case demonstration was significantly superior to formal slide presentation and to role play in fostering positive change in beliefs and attitudes about CBT. In addition, role play showed a trend toward being superior to slide presentation lectures. Interestingly, contrary to predictions based on the theoretical model, case demonstration was significantly superior to role play in fostering self-reported change in perceived skill level (self-efficacy). As expected, clinical demonstration was superior to slide presentation on this outcome measure. Also, as predicted, role play was superior to slide presentation for skill building. Surprisingly, clinical case demonstration was also rated significantly better than slide presentation in conveying theoretical basis and methodological details of the therapy (i.e., the informational content). Clinical demonstration was also rated better than role play in these areas. As expected, slide presentation was superior to role play in conveying the theoretical information. However, slide presentations were not rated as significantly better than role play in conveying details of methodology.

These results suggest that, in general, clinical case demonstration was perceived by the trainees as the most valuable training mode, followed by role play, with lectures being rated as least valuable. However, these findings do not necessarily nullify the importance of each teaching strategy, including the slide presentation lectures. Rather, these results underscore the need to further develop a more comprehensive and meaningful clinical case material, as it may be the most effective modality for many clinicians. In addition, ongoing supervision in group settings, where it is possible to discuss clinical case material in great detail, would likely increase the knowledge acquired from case demonstrations. Further research is needed to determine how well actual clinical behavior change is predicted by self-reported knowledge and skill changes.

PHASE V (DECEMBER 2002): ONE YEAR LATER: DO EPIDEMIOLOGICAL FINDINGS FROM THE SEPTEMBER 11 AFTERMATH SUPPORT OUR ASSUMPTIONS AND RATIONALE?

Since September 11, 2001, a number of general population surveys have been conducted in New York City. Galea et al. (2002) conducted a random-digit telephone survey focused on New Yorkers who reside below 110th Street in Manhattan, 4–8 weeks after the attacks. The sample consisted of 988 adults. The study assessed the relationship between severity of exposure and PTSD and depression. Among respondents, 7.5% reported symptoms consistent with a diagnosis of current PTSD related to the attacks, and 9.7% reported symptoms consistent with current depression. Criteria for either disorder were met by 13.6%, while 3.7% met criteria for both. Within the surveyed area, it was estimated that 67,000 people had PTSD and 87,000 had depression during the time of the study.

Predictors for PTSD in a multivariate model were Hispanic ethnicity (odds ratio [OR] = 2.6); history of two or more stressors preceding 9-11 (OR = 5.5); experience of a panic attack during or immediately after the event (OR = 7.6); residence below Canal Street (in lower Manhattan; OR = 2.9); and loss of possessions (OR = 5.6). Predictors for depression in multivariate analysis were Hispanic ethnicity, two or more prior stressors, a panic attack during or immediately postattack, a low level of social support, the death of a friend or relative during the attacks, and loss of a job due to the attacks. Ten percent of the respondents reported an increase in frequency of visits to a mental health professional in the month following 9-11 (compared to the month before) and 3.4% reported using new psychiatric medications during that time period (Galea, Boscarino, Resnick, & Vlahov, in press).

Results from the same survey also showed significant increases in tobacco, alcohol, and marijuana use (Vlahov et al., 2002) after the event. Specifically, 28.8% reported an increase in use of one of the three substances, 9.7% reported an increase in smoking, 24.6% in alcohol consumption, and 3.2% in marijuana use. Current PTSD was more prevalent in individuals who reported increase in use of cigarettes (24.2% versus 5.6%, $p = .001$) and of marijuana (36.6% versus 6.6%, $p = .05$). Frequency of PTSD, however, was similar among those who increased alcohol consumption and those who did not. Depression was also more frequent in people who increased use of cigarettes (22.1% versus 8.2%, $p = .004$), marijuana (22.3% versus 9.4%, $p = .05$), and alcohol (15.5% versus 8.3%, $p = .01$). In multivariate models, an increase in cigarette smoking was found to be strongly related to proximity to the site of the attacks, previous life stressors, and panic attacks in the first few hours after the attacks. Alcohol consumption was found to be related to high media exposure, while increased marijuana smoking was related to younger age, low household income, being single or divorced, and having a panic attack close to the time of the attack (Vlahov et al., 2002).

Vlahov and his colleagues predicted that the ongoing threats of terrorist attacks and high rates of unemployment, as well as ongoing clean-up efforts at the WTC area, would contribute to both severity and persistence of symptomatology. A second wave of their survey was conducted about 4 months after 9-11 (Galea et al., in press). Manhattan residents living south of 110th Street were oversampled to allow for comparison with the initial study waves. Response rate for the second wave was 60%. The prevalence of current PTSD and depression had dropped to 2.9% and 4.3%, respectively, suggesting a decrease by about 66% for PTSD and 60% for depression since the initial survey. Such decline in prevalence is consistent with findings from previous studies (Kessler et al., 1995; Shalev et al., 1998).

A web-based survey (Schlenger et al., 2002) conducted 1–2 months after the 9-11 attacks on a national sample ($n = 2,733$) found the prevalence of current PTSD due to 9-11 to be higher in the New York City metropolitan area (11.2%) than in Washington, DC (4.0%), and the rest of the country (4.0%). Schlenger and colleagues also found that PTSD was strongly related to number of hours of TV coverage of the attacks viewed on and in the days following 9-11. Being in the New York City area on the day of the attacks was associated with a 2.9-fold increase in the likelihood of PTSD. Among New Yorkers ($n = 691$), younger age, female gender, being at the WTC on 9-11, and media exposure were all found to be related to PTSD. The authors suggest that the low prevalence of PTSD in Washington, DC might be accounted for by differences in the nature of the attacks. The Pentagon site is a much more isolated one than the WTC and perceived as a military base by citizens. In addition, the attack on the WTC might have caused a stronger sense of vulnerability among New Yorkers. Furthermore, the WTC attack was viewed directly by a much larger number of people and received much broader media coverage.

The finding regarding relationship between number of daily hours of TV exposure and PTSD symptomatology is intriguing. DSM-IV does not explicitly mention media exposure (American Psychiatric Association, 1994), but insofar as it evokes fear, helplessness, or horror, media exposure can theoretically fulfill criterion A (Marshall, Galea, & Kilpatrick, 2002). Various competing explanations for this association have been suggested: TV exposure contributed to symptoms or alternatively, persons with 9-11 related symptoms were watching more TV, perhaps as a way of coping. Yet another possible explanation is that individuals who are more vulnerable to PTSD are more likely to seek exposure to the news.

The only published, longitudinal, nationwide study on record was aimed at a prospective investigation of a wide range of mental health consequences of the 9-11 attacks (Silver, Holman, McIntosh, Poulin, & Gil-Rivas, 2002). The researchers examined the degree to which various demographic and clinical factors predict psychological outcomes over time. Similar to Schlenger's study, the sample was also assembled by means of a web-based survey. Two months after the attack, 17% of the population outside New York City experienced acute or posttraumatic stress symptoms. Six months after the attacks, prevalence declined to 5.8%.

As can be seen, the studies are somewhat inconsistent, although well within expected confidence intervals. Each used different instruments to measure PTSD, with different psychometric properties and somewhat different time frames for the symptoms being assessed. In addition, study instruments were administered differently. The validity of a telephone interview may be limited by social expectation bias and by level of training of the interviewers. A web-based study insures anonymity but may be limited by other sources of invalidity, which have yet to be systematically examined.

CURRENT PHASE (DECEMBER 2002): REFLECTIONS ON WHAT HAS BEEN DONE AND PREPARATIONS FOR THE FUTURE

Following 9-11-01, there was an unprecedented need for the mental health community to mobilize and collectively respond to the psychosocial needs of those suffering from the terrorist attacks. Many mental health professionals put forth their time and expertise in an effort to best meet the needs of the people across the nation. Now, over 2 years later, it is necessary and timely to reflect on how we have responded, the lessons learned from our actions, what more needs to be done, and how to prepare resources and improve resilience for the future.

The aforementioned surveys together document the initial and intermediate clinically significant responses among individuals in the New York area. Comparison of the findings is limited by differences in sampling frames and the interval between the event and the assessment. However, these surveys clearly indicate the presence of significant stress reactions following the terrorist attacks of 9-11, both among residents of New York City and nationwide. It is also clear that there has been a significant need for treatment intervention in the community, especially in the New York City area. It was necessary to prepare to serve as many as possible, especially vulnerable populations such as those with comorbid disorders, those who were in close proximity to the disaster, those with greater severity of trauma exposure, and those who suffered the loss of a loved one.

It is clear that conducting clinical and epidemiological studies with state-of-the-art methodology is a difficult challenge when the study site is almost always chaotic (see also Norris, 2002; North & Pfefferbaum, 2002). Similarly, well-studied therapeutic interventions in the acute phase attempting to address the initial posttrauma and grief responses, although highly recommended (National Institute of Mental Health, 2002), are rare due to funding shortages (Pfefferbaum, North, Flynn, Norris, & Demartino, 2002), technical difficulties, and ethical concerns. However, *reliable* and *credible findings* based on strong study design, with pre-, during-, and follow-up evaluation and with scientifically sound comparison methodology, provided by experienced researchers and clinicians are essential for responding professionally to trauma victims and addressing their acute and long-term needs. Reasonable response rates, eligible comparison groups, gold standard measures, and especially longitudinal data collection can support generalization of findings, help reconcile results from different studies, and guide the community of clinicians who seek trauma education (North & Pfefferbaum, 2002; Yehuda, 2002).

Investigators (e.g., Duffy, 1988) have pointed out that most human-made and natural disasters go through several, sometimes overlapping, stages of recovery, including the "heroic stage" characterized by altruistic actions directed at saving lives and property at the time of and shortly after the disaster; the "honeymoon period," usually lasting for several months after the disaster and characterized by solidarity and expectations of massive assistance; the "disillusionment" phase, lasting from several months to several years in which people become disillusioned over subsequent delays in hoped for and promised aid; and the "reconstruction" period during which victims assume a role in, and responsibility for, their own recovery and new programs, including the physical construction of new environments. We need to recognize the specific challenges and stressors faced by the victims of 9-11 as they try to cope with their lives during the current "disillusionment" and "restoration" phases.

Coordination, collaboration, and communication among various professional communities are essential elements toward disaster preparedness. Different service groups such as mental health providers, primary health care physicians, rescue workers, and other professionals who are most likely to have initial contact with victims of disasters need to integrate their efforts to maximize efficiency and effectiveness. Health care professionals also need to coordinate their efforts with local religious and community leaders to best meet the specific needs of the community by providing assessment and interventions appropriately adapted for particular individuals. Through these integrative approaches, we hope not only to discern the most effective trauma interventions but also to discover how best to strengthen resilience and coping in the community.

An important consequence of our program to date has been the creation of a potential long-term resource for the community. The disaster research literature suggests that the primary and secondary consequences of a disaster of this scale will continue over a period of several years. One main objective of our trauma center is to continue to provide evidence-based treatments for trauma and traumatic loss for the community. Another main goal is to continue providing education training and supervision to mental health clinicians in the greater New York City area. Finally, it is our aim to continue advancing our knowledge in the area of trauma-related interventions as well as refining our ability to effectively educate clinicians in the community through rigorous research studies.

ACKNOWLEDGMENTS

The New York Times Foundation and the Surdna Foundation supported the work described in this chapter.

We thank the NYSPI trauma-team members: Laurence Amsel, Alana Balaban, Jaime Carcamo, Sapana Patel, Steve Rudin, Arturo Sanchez-LaCay, Franklin Schneier, Gretchen Seirmarco, Kim Thompson, and Donna Vermes.

REFERENCES

American Psychiatric Association. (1994). *Diagnostic and statistical manual of mental disorders* (4th ed.). Washington, DC: Author.

Breslau, N., Davis, G. C., Andreski, P., & Peterson, E. (1991). Traumatic events and posttraumatic stress disorder in an urban population of young adults. *Archives of General Psychiatry, 48,* 216–222.

Breslau, N., Davis, G. C., Peterson, E., & Schultz L. (1997). Psychiatric sequelae of post-traumatic stress diorder in women. *Archives of General Psychiatry, 54,* 81–87.

Cooper, N. A., & Clum, G. A. (1989). Imaginal flooding as a supplementary treatment for PTSD in combat veterans: A controlled study. *Behavior Therapy, 3,* 381–391.

Duffy, J. C. (1988). The Porter lecture: Common psychological themes in societies' reaction to terrorism and disasters. *Military Medicine, 153*(8), 387–390.

Fishbein, M. (1995). Developing effective behaviour change intervention: Some lessons learned from behavioural research. In T. E. Backer, S. L. David, & G. Saucy (Eds.), *Reviewing the behavioural science knowledge base on technology transfer* (pp. 246–261). Rockville, MD: National Institute on Drug Abuse.

Fishbein, M., & Ajzen, I. (1975), *Belief, attitude, intention and behavior: An introduction to theory and research.* Reading, MA: Addison-Wesley.

Foa, E. B., Dancu, C. V., Hembree, E. A., Jaycox, L. H., Meadows, E. A., & Street, G. P. (1999). A comparison of exposure therapy, stress inoculation training, and their combination for reducing posttraumatic stress disorder in female assault victims. *Journal of Consulting and Clinical Psychology, 67*(2), 194–200.

Foa, E. B., & Rothbaum, B. O. (1998). *Treating the trauma of rape: A cognitive-behavioral therapy for PTSD.* New York: Guilford Press.

Foa, E. B., Rothbaum, B. O., Riggs, D., & Murdock, T. (1991). Treatment of post-traumatic stress disorder in rape victims: A comparison between cognitive-behavioral procedures and counseling. *Journal of Consulting and Clinical Psychology, 59,* 715–723.

Galea, S., Ahern, J., Resnick, H., Kilpatrick, D., Bucuvalas, M., Gold, J., & Vlahov, D. (2002) Psychological sequelae of the September 11 terrorist attacks in New York City. *New England Journal of Medicine, 346,* 982–987.

Galea, S., Boscarino, J., Resnick, H., & Vlahov, D. (in press). Mental health in New York City after the September 11 terrorist attacks: Results from two population surveys. *Mental Health Year Book 2001.*

Glynn, S. M., Eth, S., Randolph, E. T., Foy, D. W., Urbatis, M., Boxer, L., Paz, G. B., Leong, G. B., Firman, G., Salk, J. D., Katzman, J. W., & Crothers, J. (1999). A test of behavioral family therapy to augment exposure for combat-related PTSD. *Journal of Consulting and Clinical Psychology, 67,* 243–251.

Keane, T. M., Fairbank, J. A., Caddell, J. M., & Zimmering, R. T. (1989). Implosive (flooding) therapy reduces symptoms of PTSD in Vietnam combat veterans. *Behavior Therapy, 20,* 245–260.

Kessler, R. C., Sonnega, A., Bromet, E., & Nelson, C. B. (1995). Posttraumatic stress disorder in the National Comorbidity Survey. *Archives of General Psychiatry, 52,* 1048–1060.

Kulka, R. A., Schlenger, W. E., Fairbank, J. A., Hough, R. L., Jordan, B. K., Marmar, C. R., & Weiss, D. A. (1990). *Trauma and the Vietnam War generation.* New York: Brunner/Mazel.

Litz, B. T., Gray, M. J., Bryant, R. A., & Adler, A. B. (2002). Early intervention for trauma: Current status and future directions. *Clinical Psychology: Science and Practice, 9,* 112–134.

Marks, I., Lovell, K., Noshirvani, H., Livanou, M., & Thrasher, S. (1998). Treatment of post-traumatic stress disorder by exposure and/or cognitive restructuring: A controlled study. *Archives of General Psychiatry, 55,* 317–325.

Marshall, D. M., Galea, S., & Kilpatrick, D. (2002). Letter to the editor. *Journal of the American Medical Association, 288,* 2683–2684.

Marshall, R. D., Olfson, M., Hellman, F., Blanco, C., Guardino, M., & Struening, E. (2001). Comorbidity, impairment, and suicidality in subthreshold PTSD. *American Journal Psychiatry, 158,* 1467–1473.

Mitchell, J. T. (1981). *Emergency response to crisis: A crisis intervention guidebook of emergency service personnel.* Bowie, MD: Brady.

National Institute of Mental Health. (2002). *Mental health and mass violence: Evidence-based early psychological intervention for victims/survivors of mass violence: A workshop to reach consensus on best practices.* (NIH Publication No. 02-5138). Washington, DC: U.S. Government Printing Office.

Neria, Y., & Bromet, E. (2000). Comorbidity of PTSD and depression: Linked or separate incidence. *Biological Psychiatry, 48,* 878–880.

Neria, Y., Solomon, Z., & Ginzburg, K. (2000). Posttraumatic and bereavement reactions among POWs following release from captivity: The interplay of trauma and loss. In R. Malkinson, S. S. Rubin, & E. Witztum (Eds.), *Traumatic and non traumatic loss and bereavement: Clinical theory and practice* (pp. 91–111). Madison, CT: Psychosocial Press.

Norris, F. H. (2002). Psychosocial consequences of disasters. *PTSD Research Quarterly, 13,* 1–7.

North, C. S., Nixon, S. J., Shariat, S., Mallonee, S., McMillen, J. C., Spitz-Nagel, E. L., & Smith, E. M. (1999). Psychiatric disorders among survivors of the Oklahoma City bombing. *Journal of the American Medical Association, 282,* 755–762.

North, C. S., & Pfefferbaum, B. (2002). Research on the mental health effects of terrorism. *Journal of the American Medical Association, 288,* 633–636.

Pfefferbaum, B., North, C., Flynn, B., Norris, F., & Demartino, R. (2002). Disaster mental health services following the 1995 Oklahoma City Bombing: Modifying approaches to address terrorism. *CNS Spectrums, 7,* 575–579.

Resick, P. A., Jordan, C. G., Girelli, S. A., Hutter, C. K., & Marhoefer-Dvorak, S. (1988). A comparative victim study of behavior group therapy for sexual assault victims. *Behavior Therapy, 19,* 385–401.

Schlenger, W. E., Caddell, J. M., Ebert, L., Jordan, B. K., Rourke, K. M., Wilson, D., Thalji, L., Dennis, J. M., Fairband, J. A., & Kulka, R. A. (2002). Psychological reactions to terrorist attacks: Findings from the national study of Americans' reactions to September 11. *Journal of the American Medical Association, 288,* 581–588.

Shalev, A. Y., Freedman, S., Pero, T., Brandes, D., Sahar, T., Orr, S. P., & Pitman, R. K. (1998). Prospective study of posttraumatic stress disorder and depression following trauma. *American Journal of Psychiatry, 155,* 630–637.

Silver, R. C., Holman, E. A., McIntosh, D. M., Poulin, M., & Gil-Rivas, V. (2002). Nationwide longitudinal study of psychological responses to September. *Journal of the American Medical Association, 288,* 1235–1244.

Stein, M. B., Walker, J. R., Hazen, A. L., & Forde, D. R. (1997). Full and partial Posttraumatic Stress Disorder: Findings from a community survey. *American Journal of Psychiatry, 154,* 1114–1119.

Tarrier, N., Pilgrim, H., Sommerfield, C., Faragher, B., Reynolds, M., Graham, E., & Barrowclough, C. (1999). A randomized trial of cognitive therapy and imaginal exposure in the treatment of chronic post traumatic stress disorder. *Journal of Consulting and Clinical Psychology, 67,* 13–18.

Vlahov, D., Galea, S., Resnick, H., Ahern, J., Boscarino, J. A., Bucuvalas, M., Gold, J., & Kilpatrick, D. (2002). Increased use of cigarettes, alcohol, and marijuana among Manhattan, New York, residents after the September 11th terrorist attacks. *American Journal of Epidemiology, 155,* 988–996.

Weiss, D. S., Marmar, C. R., Schlenger, W. E., Fairbank, J. A., Jordan, B. K., Hough, R. L., & Kulka, R. A. (1992). The prevalence of lifetime and partial post-traumatic stress disorder in Vietnam theater veterans. *Journal of Traumatic Stress,* 365–376.

Yehuda R. (2002). Posttraumatic stress disorder. *New England Journal of Medicine, 346,* 130–132.

11

Sexual Trauma

Impact and Recovery

SHEILA A. M. RAUCH
EDNA B. FOA

Prevalence estimates of sexual assault vary due to differences in assessment and data collection. Crime statistics tend to underestimate the rates of sexual assault as most rapes go unreported (Kilpatrick, Saunders, Veronen, Best, & Von, 1987). Epidemiological studies help to approach accurate estimates, but different methods of interviewing result in large differences in rates (e.g., Resnick, Kilpatrick, Dansky, Saunders, & Best, 1993; Spitzberg, 1999). Lifetime prevalence of rape ranges from 9% to 18% for women and less than 1% to 3% for men (Kessler, Sonnega, Bromet, Hughes, & Nelson, 1995; Norris, 1992; Resnick et al., 1993; Tjaden & Thoennes, 2000). The National Crime Victimization Survey (NCVS) reported 1-year incidence rates for sexual assault/rape of 0.2 for men and 1.9 for women per 1,000 persons 12 or older (Rennison, 2002) with rape rates almost 10 times higher for women than men (Bachman & Saltzman, 1995). In a review of 120 studies, Spitzberg (1999) reported a rape prevalence of 13% for women and 3% for men. The National Violence Against Women Survey (NVAW) found that physical assault was common with rape (41.4% for men; 33.9% for women: Tjaden & Thoennes, 2000). Controversy over how to assess sexual assault and rape continues (e.g., Fisher & Cullen,

2000; Kelley, 2002; Russell & Bolen, 2002); however, research supports that sexual assault is a prominent social problem in the United States that affects women more than men and often co-occurs with physical violence. Data from other countries find that this problem is not limited to the United States (see Weldon, 2002, for a summary).

This chapter aims to examine sexual assault in adulthood and its impact on survivors and society. Given the higher rates of sexual trauma in women compared to men, much of the research examining the impact of sexual trauma has focused on women. Thus, much of the research presented in this chapter focuses on women. In the aftermath of sexual trauma, the survivor is confronted with many decisions (whether to report the crime, whether to seek medical attention, etc.) that can heavily influence the impact and resolution of the trauma. We begin with a discussion of issues related to these decisions, including rates of reporting to police and health professionals. We then summarize the short- and long-term physical and mental health impact of sexual trauma on survivors and how social support affects adjustment. We then discuss the development of psychiatric disorders (posttraumatic stress disorder, panic disorder, etc.) following sexual traumatization. We end with a summary of early interventions for the prevention of posttraumatic stress disorder (PTSD) after sexual trauma, suggestions for professionals who provide services to sexual trauma survivors, and future research directions.

IMPACT ON SURVIVORS OF SEXUAL ASSAULT

For many survivors, sexual assault generates specific problems that require immediate attention. Decisions following sexual assault, such as whether to report it to police, medical personnel, family, or peers, hold many implications for the survivor. Unfortunately, many survivors do not seek professional assistance. In a study examining support-seeking postsexual assault from a media-recruited sample, 87% of survivors had told someone about the assault in the past. Of those who told someone about the sexual assault, 94% told friends/relatives, 26% told police, 27% told medical personnel, and 52% told mental health professionals (Ullman & Filipas, 2001). Thus, informal supports were favored over professional assistance. Similar rates were found in a representative sample of urban rape survivors: 39% reported the crime to the criminal justice system, 43% sought medical care, and 39% obtained mental health services (Campbell, Wasco, Ahrens, Sefl, & Barnes, 2001). Women who experienced sexual assaults that were in line with common cultural beliefs about rape (i.e., raped by a stranger and incurred physical injuries) are more likely to report the rape to professionals (e.g., police and medical personnel; Campbell,

Wasco, et al., 2001; Ullman & Filipas, 2001). Additional fears about insensitivity and homophobia are found among male survivors (Gregory & Lees, 1999), and these may lead to lower rates of reporting following assault.

Police, Legal, and Social Services after Sexual Trauma

Kilpatrick et al. (1987) found that sexual assault has the lowest reporting rate (7.1%) of any of the crimes reported to the police. Women who are raped by strangers are more likely to report it to police and medical care than women with known assailants (Campbell, Wasco, et al., 2001). Even after a survivor reports the crime to authorities, attrition of sexual assault cases between reporting and conviction is high. Frazier and Haney (1996) found that 25% of reported sexual assaults are prosecuted, 12% of defendants are found guilty, and 7% of cases result in a prison term. Dumont and Myhr (2000) found an overall conviction rate of 17% for reported sexual assaults. Similarly low rates of conviction are found in other countries (e.g., Dumont & Myhr, 2000; Statistics Canada, 1993).

Unfortunately, many reported sexual assaults were classified by the police as unfounded and, therefore, were not followed up: 68% were dropped because the allegation was perceived as noncredible (e.g., survivor's use of drugs) or the victim was unable to be reached and 33% due to insufficient evidence (Gregory & Lees, 1999). Having a reported rape classified as unfounded by the police is likely to be extremely frustrating and marginalizing for survivors. Reports that involve allegations of vaginal penetration are perceived as more unfounded than reports of other sexual acts. Reports involving survivors' alcohol consumption during the rape are also more likely to be classified as unfounded (Bouffard, 2000; Schuller & Stewart, 2000). Factors associated with a higher follow-up rate include being raped by an acquaintance rather than a stranger, a completed sexual assault exam, the perception of the survivor as credible, and police belief that the perpetrator will be found guilty (Bouffard, 2000; Dumont & Myhr, 2000; Schuller & Stewart, 2000).

Once the report is founded, prosecutors must decide whether or not to prosecute. Alksnis (2001) found three primary reasons cases are not prosecuted: (1) presence of a relationship between the survivor and perpetrator, (2) lack of physical harm to the survivor, and (3) no prior criminal record of the accused. Assaults that fit the classic definition of rape (i.e., stranger rape, physical injury, and weapon threat) are more likely to be prosecuted (Campbell, Wasco, et al., 2001; Frazier & Haney, 1996). Indeed, stranger rapes are almost twice as likely to go to trial as nonstranger rapes (34% vs. 18%; Kingsworth, MacIntosh, & Wenworth, 1999). Some of the factors that increase the likelihood that a case is founded decrease the chances of prosecution and vice versa.

For instance, although a prior relationship between the survivor and assailant decreased unfounding (possibly due to ease identifying and arresting the perpetrator), it increased the likelihood that the case is not prosecuted (Bouffard, 2000).

Predictors of whether a case went to trial are different for stranger versus nonstranger sexual assault (Kingsworth et al., 1999). In instances of rape by strangers, prior felonies of the accused, survivor cooperation with prosecution, and witness support are related to higher rates of full prosecution. For rape by nonstrangers, injury severity, incriminating remarks made by the accused, arrest charges, quick reporting of the crime, survivor cooperation with prosecution, witness support, and younger survivor age are all related to full prosecution (Kingsworth et al., 1999). Thus, when the sexual assault coincided with cultural beliefs about rape being perpetrated by a stranger, fewer factors related to the survivor's behavior influence prosecution than in sexual assault where the survivor and assailant had a relationship. The effect of race on prosecution is unclear. Although Campbell, Wasco, et al. (2001) found higher rates for prosecution for sexual assaults of white women, other studies have not found a difference in prosecution rates based on race/ethnicity (e.g., Bouffard, 2000).

Once prosecuted, conviction and sentencing are uncertain. Increased use of physical force is related to higher rates of conviction (Dumont & Myhr, 2000). Rates of conviction varied with survivor–perpetrator relationship [stranger (45%), acquaintance (24%), intimate (0%; Gregory & Lees, 1999]. When found guilty, strangers are more likely to receive a prison term (82% vs. 50%) and, on average, the sentence received is more than twice as long (203.6 vs. 93.1 months; Kingsworth et al., 1999; Frazier & Haney, 1996). Though stranger assaults in this study tended to be more severe (i.e., more accomplices, more arrest charges and felony counts, more convicted counts, and weapon use) and were reported more quickly than nonstranger sexual assaults, this disturbing trend is in need of closer examination. When survivors exhibit characteristics that coincide with commonly held rape myths (use of alcohol, past involvement in prostitution, being out alone at night, etc.), sentences are, on average, reduced about 17 months for each characteristic (Kingsworth et al., 1999).

Thus, at each stage of interaction with the criminal justice system, sexual assault survivors are confronted with a system reflecting cultural biases and skepticism (Hodgson & Kelley, 2002). They are often subjected to examination of the most intimate areas of their own behavior and life and are forced to prove that both a crime occurred and injury resulted. The impact of this experience with the criminal justice system can be detrimental. Roughly half the women who report sexual assault to the criminal justice system experience the interaction as hurtful or unsatisfying (Campbell, Wasco, et al., 2001; Jordan, 2001). Their satisfaction with the criminal justice system is related to their desire for more professionalism, sensitivity, and belief in their report from police (Jordan, 2001). Women whose sexual assaults did not fit with common rape myths (i.e., raped by a partner) report less satisfaction with police officers, prosecutors, victim's assistance staff, and judges than nonpartner assault survivors (Byrne, Kilpatrick, Howley, & Beatty, 1999). Women who do not have their case prosecuted and those who rate their interactions with the legal system as hurtful have more physical and psychological distress (Campbell, Wasco, et al., 2001).

The justice systems of the United States and many other countries are based on the premise that the prosecutor has a dual responsibility to protect the interest of society as well as the rights of the accused (Murphy, 2001). Thus, as prosecutors do not represent sexual assault survivors, they have no duty to protect the rights of survivors (Murphy, 2001). Konradi (2001) found that survivors often experience little or no preparation for legal proceedings, and, when preparation occurs, it focuses primarily on prosecutor needs (how to dress, general orienting information, emotional display of injury, getting the story straight, etc.) with no attention paid to the impact of the legal process on survivors. Such experiences disempower survivors and contribute to increased distress. In cases in which the survivor's privacy or rights may impede prosecution of the case, the survivor may not be informed of his or her rights. In addition, his or her rights may be violated in the interest of obtaining a conviction. Another primary actor in the court, the judge has a primary interest in upholding the rights of the accused to prevent the ruling from being overturned on appeal. Here the survivor's interests are left unrepresented in the legal process. Legal representation and/or survivor advocates would fill this hole in the current system and assert survivors' rights and needs (Alksnis, 2001; Konradi, 2001; Murphy, 2001). In fact, Campbell and Martin (2001), when reviewing the impact of rape crisis centers, reported that although interactions with the legal system tend to result in increased distress, working with rape crisis center advocates reduces the distress.

The past 35 years have seen great strides in the passage of laws and changes in policies and procedures to address injustice done to survivors. Although sexual violence has become more visible, the success of these policies has been variable (Bernat, 2002; Del Bove & Stermac, 2002; Lord & Rassel, 2002). For a review of worldwide policy responses to violence against women, see Weldon (2002). The reforms have largely centered around five areas: (1) broadening of the definition of sexual assault to include more than penile/vaginal contact, (2) allowance for nonfemale survivors, (3) removal of the spousal exemption, (4) changing the wording of the law to reflect violence rather than sexual gratification, and (5) shield laws to protect the privacy of survivors (Bernat, 2002). When states are divided based on implementation of reforms, survivor satisfaction ratings for criminal justice interactions significantly differ between partner versus nonpartner assault survivors only in those states in which few reforms are implemented (Byrne et al., 1999). Specifically, in states with few reforms, women assaulted by partners report significantly lower satisfaction with court procedures than women assaulted by strangers. No significant differences are found in states in which reforms are in place. Given these variations in law and policy, survivors experience large variations in their treatment and the criminal justice environment simply depending on the police department where they reported the crime. Departments with closer contact to rape crisis centers (through training, provision of survivor advocates, etc.) are more likely to have implemented the reforms (Lord & Rassel, 2002).

By 1985, all but two states had passed rape shield laws designed to protect sexual assault survivors from admission of past sexual behavior into the legal proceedings. Variation in the strength of these laws, specifically the degree that judges have discretion to override the law, result in distinct differences in effectiveness (Bernat, 2002). As a result, the common defense tactic of discrediting the survivor in sexual assault trials continues to be used and often results in perception of harassment and intimidation of the survivor. Personal information about the survivor is still presented in courts in order to discredit them (e.g., Bernat, 2002). Such information includes anything from the use of food stamps and medical or psychiatric history to religious views and vague innuendoes (Del Bove & Stermac, 2002). Further, this information was most often sought by the defense counsel, with little or no proof needed to obtain and present confidential records at trial (i.e., even unsubstantiated comments about the complainant's mental health status were sufficient; Del Bove & Stermac, 2002).

Medical/Health Impact

The health impact of sexual trauma on survivors often begins with the physical trauma experienced from the sexual assault. Sexual assault survivors experience vaginal and/or anal tearing, urinary tract infections, sexually transmitted diseases, pelvic pain, other vaginal or perineal trauma, and other acute physical injuries (Campbell & Alford, 1989; Geist, 1988; Harlow, 1989; Koss & Heslet, 1992; Tjaden & Thoennes, 2000). As mentioned in the introduction, many sexual assaults also involve physical assault (Tjaden & Thoennes, 2000). The NVAW reported that 21% of physical injuries incurred with sexual assault are severe (i.e., broken bones, dislocated joints, and spinal cord or head injury; Tjaden & Thoennes, 2000).

In addition to physical injuries, about 5% of rapes of women of child-bearing age result in pregnancy (e.g., Holmes, Resnick, Kilpatrick, & Best, 1996). This additional stressor adds to the survivor's distress. In one study, it was found that 32% of sexual assault survivors kept the infant, 50% underwent an abortion, 12% spontaneously aborted, and 6% gave up their infant for adoption (Holmes et al., 1996).

The fear of contracting sexually transmitted diseases (STDs), including HIV, after sexual assault is realistic: up to 43% of rape survivors develop STDs as a result of their sexual assault (Harlow, 1989). Given the high rates of sexual assaults of incarcerated men, (Nacci & Kane, 1982) and the high rates of HIV and other STDs in prisons (Maruschak, 2002), incarcerated men are at even higher risk. Early detection of possible contact with certain STDs may be critical for prevention of infection in sexual assault survivors. However, legal and medical issues surrounding mandated testing of those accused of sexual assault in order to assist in the medical care of the sexual assault survivors remains an issue of controversy (for discussion, see Gostin et al., 1994).

Despite the high rates of medical concerns and problems among sexual assault survivors, most do not present in medical settings for the acute trauma (e.g., Campbell, Wasco, et al., 2001; Holmes et al., 1996). Only 17% of rape cases from a national representative sample of rape survivors had a medical exam postassault (Kilpatrick, Edmunds, & Seymour, 1992). Similarly, in a national sample of women, only 36% of women received medical care for their most recent rape (Tjaden & Thoennes, 2000). Most (82%) of this medical care occurred in a hospital setting (Tjaden & Thoennes, 2000). At 1 year postassault, women who survived sexual assault still used medical services more than women without this history (Kimerling & Calhoun, 1994). Surprisingly, they did not have higher levels of mental health service utilization. Although 73% of the women sought medical treatment, only 19% sought mental health treatment (Kimerling & Calhoun, 1994). Nearly one-third of women who reported the sexual assault to medical professionals experienced the interaction as hurtful (Campbell, Wasco, et al., 2001). Women who rated the interaction as hurtful had more physical and psychological distress than did women who did not rate the interaction as hurtful (Campbell, Wasco, et al., 2001).

In addition to acute physical problems related to the sexual trauma, survivors also experience higher rates of chronic health problems and lower perceptions of physical health, even years after a sexual trauma. Survivors of sexual assault have more chronic pelvic pain, general pain, chronic headaches, musculoskeletal symptoms (e.g., muscle aches and headaches), genitorurinary symptoms (e.g., vaginal discharge, low sexual desire, and painful intercourse), skin rashes and itching, gastrointestinal symptoms, sexual dysfunction, disability days, more surgeries, as well as decreased functional status, excessive menstrual bleeding, genital burning, painful intercourse, lack of sexual pleasure, menstrual irregularities, and dysmenorrhea (Campbell & Alford, 1989; Golding, 1996a, 1996b, 1999a, 1999b; Leserman, Drossman, & Hu, 1998; Letourneau, Resnick, Kilpatrick, Saunders, & Best, 1996). Sexual assault survivors are more likely to have hypertension, smoke cigarettes, have high cholesterol, and be obese. In addition, they are more likely to perceive their health as poor, both in general and within the past month. (Cloutier, Martin, & Poole, 2002; Golding, Cooper, & George, 1997; Kimerling & Calhoun, 1994). In older women, a lifetime history of sexual assault is related to increased risk of arthritis and breast cancer (Stein & Barrett-Conner, 2000). In older men, a history of sexual assault is related to increased odds of developing thyroid disease (Stein & Barrett-Conner, 2000).

Women who experience both sexual and physical trauma have worse physical health outcomes (Campbell & Soeken, 1999; Leserman et al., 1996; Sadler, Booth, Nielson, & Doebbeling, 2000). Indeed, these women report worse health impairment than do women with recent myocardial infarction or diabetes mellitus type II and similar to those with advanced Parkinson's disease (Sadler et al., 2000).

Completed sexual assaults have more detrimental physical and mental health effects than sexual assaults that are not completed (Golding, 1996a, 1999b; Leserman et al., 1996). Repeated assaults, spousal or stranger assaults, and physically threatening assaults are more strongly related to functional impairment and odds of developing certain chronic conditions than sexual assaults without these characteristics (Golding, 1996a; Golding et al., 1997). Also, in the previously mentioned study with older adults, repeated sexual assaults increased the likelihood of developing arthritis and breast cancer in women and thyroid disease in men more than did single incidents (Stein & Barrett-Conner, 2000). Abuse severity, physical symptoms, and functional disability predicted 30% of the variance in health care visits in the year the study was conducted (Leserman et al., 1998).

In a prospective study, women who were sexually assaulted had more somatic complaints, poorer perceived health status, and more psychological symptoms at 1 month postassault than women who were not assaulted (Kimerling & Calhoun, 1994). At 1 year postassault, physical symptoms and perceived health status were no longer significantly elevated, but survivors continued to report more psychological symptoms and had more physician visits than did women who were not assaulted. Specifically, after controlling for prior victimization history, assault severity, and physical reactions during the assault, symptoms of PTSD and depression were significantly related to global health perceptions and severity of reported health symptoms (Clum, Calhoun, & Kimerling, 2000). However, PTSD but not depression was related to reproductive health symptoms (Clum et al., 2000). In another study, after controlling for negative life events, anger, and depression, PTSD predicted self-reported physical symptoms (Zoellner, Goodwin, & Foa, 2000).

Together, the research on health and sexual trauma suggests that a variety of health problems occur after sexual assault (Golding, 1999b) and that PTSD symptoms may mediate the relationship between trauma/sexual assault and physical health (Friedman & Schnurr, 1995; Resnick, Acierno, & Kilpatrick, 1997). The mechanisms underlying the relationship between health problems and sexual assault remain unclear. Although some researchers have suggested a direct relationship, others suggested that the relationship is mediated by increased negative health behaviors after the assault (e.g., Clum et al., 2000; Kimerling, Clum, & Wolfe, 2000; Resnick et al., 1997).

Psychological Adjustment

In addition to medical difficulties, many sexual assault survivors suffer from psychological difficulties such as PTSD and depression. Acquaintance, spousal, and stranger rapes are all related to mental health problems (e.g., Culbertson & Dehle, 2001; Kilpatrick, Best, Saunders, & Veronen, 1988). Although PTSD may occur following many types of traumatic experiences, epidemiological studies have suggested that the prevalence of PTSD following sexual assault is particularly high compared to other traumas (e.g., Breslau et al., 1998; Kilpatrick et al., 1987). In a prospective study following sexual assault survivors from within 2 weeks of the assault to 12 weeks postassault, Rothbaum, Foa, Riggs, Murdock, and Walsh (1992) found that 94% of the women met symptom criteria for PTSD (except duration) within 2 weeks of the assault (Figure 11.1). By 12 weeks postassault, 47% of these women still met criteria for PTSD. From Figure 11.1, it is apparent that although many women recovered following sexual assault, a large minority developed chronic PTSD.

Kimerling and Calhoun (1994) found that sexual assault survivors had more psychological symptoms a year after the assault compared to women who had not been assaulted but did not use more mental health services. In fact, survivors used more medical services than mental health services (73% vs. 19%). Because these women were recruited through presentation in a medical setting postassault, the sample may be biased in that it may include women who are likely to use medical care. However, other studies have also found low rates of mental health care utilization (Campbell, Wasco, et al., 2001; Mahoney, 1999). Among nonwhite women, rates of seeking mental health care following sexual assault are even lower than for white women (Campbell, Wasco, et al., 2001).

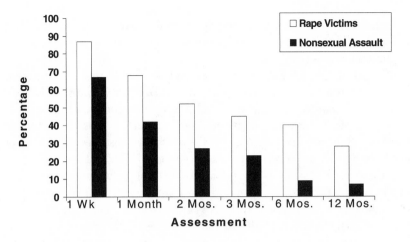

FIGURE 11.1. Percentage of sexual assault survivors with PTSD.

Even among people with PTSD, rates of mental health care utilization are low. Kessler (2000) reported that only 38% of people with PTSD were in treatment in a given year. Of those in treatment, 58% were seeing a psychiatrist, clinical psychologist, or other mental health professional. Kessler noted that usage was comparable to the rates of usage in depression but higher than other anxiety disorders. In this sample, the most common reason for not seeking treatment was the perception, even among those reporting significant impairment, that they do not have a problem requiring treatment.

Several factors are related to increased psychological distress following sexual trauma. In a sample of active-duty military men and women who experienced sexual or nonsexual trauma, lower education, female gender, more personal exposure to trauma (including sexual assault and rape), and lower perceived military unit cohesion were related to more psychological symptoms. Further, under low leadership support, the impact of multiple trauma exposure was stronger than under higher leadership support (Martin, Rosen, Durand, Knudson, & Stretch, 2000).

Besides PTSD, many survivors of physical and sexual assault report increased depressive symptoms, including suicidal ideation and attempts (e.g., Boudreaux, Kilpatrick, Resnick, Best, & Saunders, 1998; Golding, 1996a; Kessler, 2000; Kilpatrick, et al., 1992; Krakow et al., 2000). As with physical health, dually victimized survivors report more depressive symptoms than those who experience physical assault only (Campbell & Soeken, 1999). Among survivors with PTSD, rates of panic disorder are also elevated (Boudreaux et al., 1998). Leserman et al. (1998) found that women who survived child and/or adult sexual and physical abuse were two to two and a half times more likely to report panic-like symptoms (blurred vision, numbness/tingling, shortness of breath, etc.).

Winfield, George, Swartz, and Blazer (1990) found that sexual assault history was most strongly associated with PTSD, panic disorder, obsessive-compulsive disorder (OCD), and alcohol/drug abuse or dependence. Although the study was retrospective, it suggested that sexual assault either coincided with or preceded the onset of the psychiatric disorder. Boudreaux et al. (1998) found that crime survivors were more likely to suffer from PTSD, major depressive episode, agoraphobia, OCD, social phobia, and simple phobia. Further, PTSD was the strongest and most consistent predictor of psychopathology beyond demographics and crime-related factors (Boudreaux et al., 1998). Higher rates of disordered eating were also found in adolescents who experienced dating violence and date rape (Ackard & Neumark-Sztainer, 2002).

Substance use and abuse also increase following sexual assault (Kilpatrick, Acierno, Resnick, Saunders, & Best, 1997). In a 2-year longitudinal study examining directionality of the relationship between physical/sexual assault and alcohol and substance use in women, Kilpatrick et al. (1997) found that use of drugs, but not alcohol, increased the odds of experiencing a new assault in the 2 years following the incident. After a new assault, odds of both alcohol abuse and substance use increased significantly, even among women who had no prior history of use or assault. Thus, although alcohol abuse appeared to develop after an assault, drug use appeared to occur in a vicious cycle when use increased risk of assault and assault increased use.

Interpersonal Adjustment

Social support has been proposed as a possible factor contributing to adjustment postassault. In the previously described study, Kimerling and Calhoun (1994) found that higher social support (i.e., more people in whom to confide) was associated with better health and better perceptions of health. Further, lower levels of social support immediately after sexual assault were predictive of higher levels of medical service utilization at 1 year postrape. However, several studies found no relationship between positive social reactions and recovery or posttrauma distress (e.g., Feehan, Nada-Raja, Martin, & Langley, 2001). Ullman (1999) suggested that the inconsistencies between studies may be due to differing assessment measures and procedures used in various studies. Another contributing factor may be that social support may not be a homogeneous construct. In fact, in her review, Ullman (1999) noted that negative social reactions have been consistently related to less positive psychological adjustment postrape. Positive social reactions have been less consistently related. In a series of studies, Ullman and colleagues found that the type of person providing the support had an impact on the amount of support received (friends provided more support than professionals and physicians and police provided more negative reactions than other sources; Ullman, 1996c). Finally, support from friends was more predictive of recovery than support from any other source (Ullman, 1996c). Negative social reactions were strongly related to delayed recovery, physical symptoms, and poorer perceptions of physical health (Ullman, 1996b; Ullman & Siegel, 1995). Negative social reactions (e.g., being told they were irresponsible, being patronized, wanting revenge, being told to get on with their life, and trying to control decisions) predicted PTSD, depression, and physical health symptoms regardless of severity or time since the assault (Campbell, Ahrens, Sefl, Wasco, & Barnes, 2001). Another critical finding of this study was that receiving no support is better for survivor recovery than negative reactions. Thus, encouraging survivors to seek positive support, and, more important, avoid negative support, through selective disclosure may be critical for the recovery of sexual trauma survivors (Campbell, Ahrens, et al., 2001).

Overall, positive social responses have not been found to predict better adjustment postrape; however, two specific types of positive responses have been related to better adjustment (Campbell, Ahrens, et al., 2001). Specifically, regardless of time since, or severity of, the assault, survivors who felt validated and survivors who talked to others about the trauma reported significantly lower PTSD, depressive symptoms, and fewer health problems. The degree of interpersonal friction shortly after assault predicted PTSD 3 months postassault, but degree of positive social support was not related to PTSD. Interestingly, survivors who experienced less physical injury, self-blame, and postassault distress received more positive social support (Ullman, 1996a). Although these results suggested an area in need of closer empirical examination, the retrospective nature of this study does not allow for a causal interpretation. Thus, those women who had the most severe sexual assaults and may be most in need of assistance may receive less positive social support. Alternatively, these findings may simply reflect the fact that women who received less social support may be more likely to experience distress.

SOCIETAL IMPACT OF SEXUAL ASSAULT

Given the negative impact of sexual trauma on survivors, it is not surprising that the societal costs of sexual assault are high. Miller, Cohen, and Weirsema (1996) estimated the annual cost of rape and sexual assault in the United States at $127 billion. As reviewed earlier, the increased physical and mental health difficulties following sexual trauma adds to the societal expense associated with this crime and can severely affect the health care system and society as a whole (e.g., Solomon & Davidson, 1997). In a sample taken from a longitudinal study of men and women who survived physical and sexual assault (33% of women and 6% of men reported a sexual component to the assault), unemployment was strongly related to psychological distress postassault after controlling for the presence of previous assaults and demographic characteristics (i.e., poor education and financial hardship; Feehan et al., 2001). Because the majority of the assaults were nonsexual, the relationship between sexual assault and unemployment cannot be discerned.

Cost estimates for PTSD, one possible negative outcome of sexual trauma, also sheds light on the price of sexual assault. Brunello et al. (2001) estimated over $3 billion of annual productivity loss in the United States. This estimate does not include lost productivity due to chronic functional impairment but only deviation from an individual's daily functioning. For instance, survivors of sexual assault have lower educational attainment than do nonassaulted women (Sadler et al., 2000). The impact that lower education may have on earning potential is not included in this cost estimate. In a series of analyses with the National Comorbidity Survey, people with PTSD and anxiety disorders had increased probabilities of high school and college failure, teenage childbearing, marital instability, days of work lost, and current unemployment than do people without anxiety disorders (Ettner, Frank, & Kessler, 1997; Kessler et al., 1997; Kessler, Foster, Saunders, & Stang, 1995; Kessler & Frank, 1997; Kessler, Walters, & Forthofer, 1998). Thus, Brunello et al. (2001) may have underestimated total societal costs for both PTSD and sexual assault. Kessler (2000) concluded that although the costs of PTSD are substantial in the United States, these costs are likely higher in developing countries where exposure to high-risk repetitive trauma (war, torture, etc.) is more common and access to treatment resources is scarce.

DEVELOPMENT OF POSTTRAUMATIC STRESS DISORDER

One common negative outcome of sexual assault that has a severe impact on the functioning of survivors is PTSD. The lifetime rate of PTSD following sexual assault is approximately 50% (e.g., Breslau et al., 1998; Kessler et al., 1995; Rothbaum et al., 1992). In many studies, rape has been shown to have the highest conditional probability of PTSD compared to other types of traumas (e.g., Breslau, Davis, Andreski, & Peterson, 1991; Norris, 1992).

Predictors/Risk Factors of Posttraumatic Stress Disorder in Sexual Assault Survivors

Many studies have examined predictors for the development of PTSD following trauma. On the basis of a meta-analysis of predictor studies, Brewin, Andrews, and Valentine (2000) concluded that there are three categories of predictors: (1) factors that predict PTSD in some but not all populations (i.e., gender, age at trauma, and race), (2) factors that predict PTSD in many populations with some variation across populations and methods (i.e., education, previous trauma, and childhood adversity), and (3) factors that predict PTSD across studies and populations (i.e., psychiatric history, childhood abuse, and family psychiatry history). Factors that operate peritraumatically and posttrauma, such as trauma severity, lack of social support, and life stress, tended to have larger effects on PTSD than pretrauma factors (Brewin, et al., 2000).

Trauma severity, measured as proximity to the trauma and physical injury, has been examined as a predictor of PTSD following sexual trauma. Personally experienced trauma results in longer symptom duration than indirectly experienced trauma (48 months vs. 12 months; Breslau et al., 1998). Similarly, direct threat to life and personal injury predicted PTSD in a national sample of women (Resnick et al., 1993). Completed rape, life threat, and injury predicted PTSD and other psychopathology (depression, agoraphobia, OCD, etc.) in a sample of crime survivors (Boudreaux et al., 1998; Kilpatrick et al., 1989). Experiencing multiple traumas and more frequent trauma has been associated with higher risk of PTSD posttrauma (e.g., Bernat, Ronfeldt, Calhoun, & Arias, 1998; Green et al., 2000; Nishith, Mechanic, & Resick, 2000; Resnick et al., 1993).

Some individual difference factors are associated with vulnerability for PTSD following trauma. Specifically, early separation from parents, neuroticism, pretrauma anxiety and depression, family history of anxiety, job instability, parental poverty, child abuse, early behavioral problems, other psychopathology, and lower social support were related to higher rates of PTSD posttrauma (Breslau et al., 1991; Brewin et al., 2000; Davidson, Hughes, Blazer, & George, 1991; Helzer, Robine, & McEvoy, 1987). However, the retrospective nature of these studies does not allow for causal attributions and suggests caution in interpretation of these results.

Several peritraumatic factors have been found associated with development of PTSD postsexual trauma. For instance, women with delayed peak reactions in PTSD, depression, and anxiety immediately following sexual assault reported more symptoms at 12 weeks postassault than did women with early peak reactions (Gilboa-Schetchman & Foa, 2001). Similarly, dissociation within 2 weeks of physical assault was predictive of PTSD at 3 months postassault in non-sexual assault survivors but not sexual assault survivors (Dancu, Riggs, Hearst-Ikeda, & Shoyer, 1996). Dissociation, negative emotional reactions, and panic symptoms during trauma were associated with more severe PTSD symptoms (Bernat et al., 1998). Diagnosis of acute stress disorder and high levels of reexperiencing and arousal symptoms in the first month following exposure to crime predicted PTSD at 6 months (Brewin, Andrews, Rose, & Kirk, 1999). Anger, wishful thinking, self-blame, and shame in the weeks following assault have also been implicated in the development of PTSD (Andrews, Brewin, Rose, & Kirk, 2000; Feeny, Zoellner, & Foa, 2000; Koss, Figueredo, & Prince, 2002; Valentiner, Foa, Riggs, & Gershuny, 1996). Negative thoughts about self, the world, and self-blame have also been found to discriminate between trauma survivors with and without PTSD (Foa, Ehlers, Clark, Tolin, & Orsillo, 1999).

PREVENTIVE INTERVENTIONS FOR SEXUAL TRAUMA

In primary prevention, interventions aim to prevent a certain negative event or outcome prior to its occurrence. Preventing sexual trauma from occurring would be the most desirable way to prevent its negative physical and mental health outcomes. Though discussion of sexual trauma prevention is beyond the scope of this chapter, it is important to mention that Bachar and Koss (2001) concluded that the effectiveness of prevention programs was largely unproven, especially outside college populations. Further development and evaluation of sexual assault prevention programs are critical components of any effort to reduce the impact of sexual trauma.

In secondary prevention, the interventions aim to prevent negative outcomes following an event, such as prevention of chronic PTSD following sexual trauma. Several interventions have been developed for sexual trauma survivors with mixed results (See Litz, Gray, Bryant, & Adler, 2002; Rauch, Hembree, & Foa, 2001). The review that follows focuses on cognitive-behavioral interventions which have been examined in controlled trials.

A brief behavioral intervention program was developed for use within 3 weeks of a sexual assault (Kilpatrick & Veronen, 1984). This program was composed of 4–6 hours of clinical contact and included (1) an induced affect interview about the rape, (2) psychoeducation about common reactions to the trauma, (3) discussion of guilt and blame about the rape, and (4) coping skills training. Half the participants received relaxation training instead of the induced affect interview. At 3 months postassault, no significant differences were found between women who received the intervention and women who received no intervention. Given the small sample and the change in the intervention during the study, these results were difficult to interpret.

Foa, Hearst-Ikeda, and Perry (1995) developed a brief prevention (BP) program which involved four, weekly 2-hour, sessions and included (1) pychoeducation about common reactions to trauma; (2) breathing and relaxation training; (3) confronting feared, but objectively safe, situations (*in vivo* exposure); (4) reliving the assault (imaginal exposure); and (5) cognitive restructuring. BP was provided within the first month postsexual or physical assault, with most participants receiving the intervention less than 2 weeks postassault. Survivors who received BP had lower rates of PTSD at 2 months (10%) than the assessment control condition (70%). However, at 5.5 months, the rates of PTSD diagnosis no longer differed. Therefore, the BP program may have accelerated natural recovery rather than preventing chronic PTSD. In a larger study of a modification of the BP program with the same components as the foregoing study, preliminary analyses suggest similar benefits for sexual assault survivors (Foa, Zoellner, & Feeny, 2003).

Resnick, Acierno, Holmes, Kilpatrick, and Jager (1999) evaluated the effectiveness of a prevention program for sexual assault survivors that was implemented in the emergency care center. The program included a brief meeting with a rape crisis counselor, a 17-minute video with two parts, and a forensic rape exam. The first part of the video described and explained the exam procedures. The second part of the video presented self-directed exposure exercises, methods to recognize and stop avoidance, and coping strategies. In a study examining the effectiveness of this 17-minute video to prevent PTSD, depression, and panic symptoms compared to standard care, including meeting with a rape crisis counselor and a forensic exam, preliminary analyses suggested that women who watched the video reported less anxiety following the forensic exam than women who did not watch the video.

Thus, preventive interventions following sexual assault have shown promising results for the prevention of PTSD and other psychopathology. In addition, some suggestions for more beneficial treatment of sexual trauma survivors can be made. Resnick, Acierno, Holmes, Dammeyer, and Kilpatrick (2000) provided guidelines for care of survivors of interpersonal violence (including sexual assault) in emergency and other medical settings. First, violence screening is recommended as a routine clinical practice in medical settings because survivors may not identify their experience as abuse or assault or, even if identified as abuse/assault, may be reluctant to disclose. They recommend that face-to-face assessment with behaviorally specific, closed-ended questions, rather than written assessment, occur as a part of history taking as literacy cannot be assumed. Further, patient safety and confidentiality must be protected. See Resnick et al. (2000) for a discussion of the merits of available measures for this purpose. Second, in cases in which recent sexual assault was identified, the survivor should be informed that quickly reporting the crime and completing a forensic medical exam would maximize the quality of evidence collected. The clinician should be knowledgeable about the local legal and reporting requirements in order to assist the patient in complying with requirements to maximize successful prosecution. Survivors must be informed not to bathe, shower, wash hands, urinate, brush their teeth, or any other activity that may degrade potential evidence of the crime prior to the exam. Immediate medical care is also necessary in order to provide prophylactic care to prevent STDs and possible pregnancy (if the survivor desires) and address any physical injuries that may have resulted from the sexual assault. Examination of a sexual assault survivor who reported the crime, even several days later, should still be conducted in order to attempt to collect any evidence that has not degraded. Safety of the survivor should be assessed prior to leaving the medical setting. The exam should also include counseling and referrals for continued assistance when necessary. They recommend that the survivor also be provided information about postrape testing to address any ongoing medical concerns prior to leaving the exam.

One key experience for many sexual assault survivors is the forensic medical exam. As previously discussed, the nature of the interactions with medical personnel can influence recovery. In a study examining the survivors' interactions with medical care staff following assault, women expressed a need for privacy, safety, respect, and sensitivity during the forensic exam (Jordan, 2001). The recognition of the special needs of sexual assault survivors has led to the development of Sexual Assault Nurse Examiner (SANE) model. This model provides guidelines for timely, sensitive, and comprehensive medical care and forensic evidence collection with sexual assault survivors. These programs often work in coordination with the police and rape crisis centers to provide a continuity of care for the survivor (Ledray, 2001). While SANE and similar programs have existed since the 1970s, medical personnel who lack specific training and expertise with sexual trauma survivors complete many forensic medical examinations. In a survey of sexual assault survivor services in Georgia, only 20% of medical exams following sexual assault were preformed by SANEs (Meredith, Speir, & Johnson, 2000).

In summary, preventive interventions for sexual trauma survivors have demonstrated some potential benefits in reducing the duration and severity of negative reactions following sexual trauma. More research is needed to clarify the types of programs or components that are most beneficial. In addition, maximizing survivor privacy, autonomy, social support, and control while minimizing negative social reactions are important factors to minimize the negative impact of sexual trauma on survivors.

FUTURE RESEARCH DIRECTIONS

Many areas remain in need of further research. First, clarification of the causes of sexual assault perpetration and development of effective interventions to prevent its occurrence are priorities. In addition, continued efforts to provide survivor protections through law and policy to minimize the negative impact of sexual trauma is imperative. These would include policies regarding guidelines for the medical care and legal empowerment of sexual trauma survivors. Significant knowledge has accumulated about the impact of sexual assault, but continued examination of the specific factors and interactions that predict satisfactory recovery is needed. Once such factors are identified, they may be used to develop more effective early interventions for sexual assault survivors. Finally, although we know that sexual trauma is related to physical and mental health difficulties, the specific mechanism of this relationship is still unclear and needs to be elucidated.

ACKNOWLEDGMENTS

Preparation of this chapter was partially supported by National Institute of Mental Health Grant Nos. MH52272 and MH42178 awarded to Dr. Edna B. Foa.

REFERENCES

Ackard, D. M., & Neumark-Sztainer, D. (2002). Date violence and date rape among adolescents: Associations with disordered eating behaviors and psychological health. *Child Abuse and Neglect, 26,* 455–473.

Alksnis, C. (2001). Fundamental justice is the issue: Extending full equality of the law to women and children. *Journal of Social Distress and the Homeless, 10*(1), 69–86.

Andrews, B., Brewin, C. R., Rose, S., & Kirk, M. (2000). Predicting PTSD symptoms in victims of violent crime: The role of shame, anger, and childhood abuse. *Journal of Abnormal Psychology, 109*(1), 69–73.

Bachar, K., & Koss, M. P. (2001). From prevalence to prevention: Closing the gap between what we know about rape and what we do. In C. M. Renzetti, J. L. Edleson, & R. K. Bergen (Eds.), *Sourcebook on violence against women* (pp. 117–142). Thousand Oaks, CA: Sage.

Bachman, R., & Saltzman, L. E. (1995, August). *Violence against women estimates from the redesigned survey* (NCJ-154348). Washington, DC: Bureau of Justice Statistics.

Bernat, F. P. (2002). Rape law reform. In J. F. Hodgson & D. S. Kelley (Eds.), *Sexual violence: Policies, practices, and challenges in the United States and Canada* (pp. 85–99). Westport, CT: Praeger.

Bernat, J. A., Ronfeldt, H. M., Calhoun, K. S., & Arias, I. (1998). Prevalence of traumatic events and peritraumatic predictors of post-traumatic stress symptoms in a non-clinical sample of college students. *Journal of Traumatic Stress, 11*(4), 645–664.

Boudreaux, E., Kilpatrick, D. G., Resnick, H. S., Best, C. L., & Saunders, B. E. (1998). Criminal victimization, posttraumatic stress disorder, and comorbid psychopathology among a community sample of women. *Journal of Traumatic Stress, 11*(4), 665–678.

Bouffard, J. A. (2000). Predicting type of sexual assault case closure from victim, suspect, and case characteristics. *Journal of Criminal Justice, 28*, 527–542.

Breslau, N., Davis, G. C., Andreski, P., & Peterson, E. (1991). Traumatic events and posttraumatic stress disorder in an urban population of young adults. *Archives of General Psychiatry, 48*, 216–222.

Breslau, N., Kessler, R. C., Chilcoat, H. D., Schultz, L. R., Davis, G. C., & Andreski, P. (1998). Trauma and posttraumatic stress disorder in the community: The 1996 Detroit area survey of trauma. *Archives of General Psychiatry, 55*(7), 626–632.

Brewin, C. R. Andrews, B., Rose, S., & Kirk, M. (1999). Acute stress disorder and posttraumatic stress disorder in victims of violent crime. *American Journal of Psychiatry, 156*(3), 360–366.

Brewin, C. R., Andrews, B., & Valentine, J. D. (2000). Meta-analysis of risk factors for posttraumatic stress disorder in trauma-exposed adults. *Journal of Consulting and Clinical Psychology, 68*(5), 748–766.

Brunello, N., Davidson, J. R. T., Deahl, M., Kessler, R. C., Mendlewicz, J., Racagni, G., Shalev, A. Y., & Zohar, J. (2001). Posttraumatic stress disorder: Diagnosis and epidemiology, comorbidity and social consequences, biology and treatment. *Neuropsychobiology, 43*, 150–162.

Byrne, C. A., Kilpatrick, D. G., Howley, S. S., & Beatty, D. (1999). Female victims of partner versus nonpartner violence: Experiences with the criminal justice system. *Criminal Justice and Behavior, 26*(3), 275–292.

Campbell, J. C., & Alford, P. (1989). The dark consequences of marital rape. *American Journal of Nursing, 89*, 946–949.

Campbell, J. C., & Martin, P. Y. (2001). Services for sexual assault survivors: The role of rape crisis centers. In C. M. Renzetti, J. L. Edleson, & R. K. Bergen (Eds.), *Sourcebook on violence against women* (pp. 227–241). Thousand Oaks, CA: Sage.

Campbell, J. C., & Soeken, K. L. (1999). Forced sex and intimate partner violence: Effects on women's risk and women's health. *Violence Against Women, 5*(9), 1017–1035.

Campbell, R., Ahrens, C. E., Sefl, T., Wasco, S. M., & Barnes, H. E. (2001). Social reactions to rape victims: Healing and hurtful effects on psychological and physical health outcomes. *Violence and Victims, 16*(3), 287–302.

Campbell, R. C., Wasco, S. M., Ahrens, C. E., Sefl, T., & Barnes, H. E. (2001). Preventing the "second rape": Rape survivors' experiences with community service providers. *Journal of Interpersonal Violence, 16*(12), 1239–1259.

Cloutier, S., Martin, S. L., & Poole, C. (2002). Sexual assault among North Carolina women: Prevalence and health risk factors. *Journal of Epidemiology and Community Health, 56*, 265–271.

Clum, G. A., Calhoun, K. S., & Kimerling, R. (2000). Associations among symptoms of depression and posttraumatic stress disorder and self-reported health in sexually assaulted women. *Journal of Nervous and Mental Disease, 188,* 671–678.

Culbertson, K. A., & Dehle, C. (2001). Impact of sexual assault as a function of perpetrator type. *Journal of Interpersonal Violence, 16*(10), 992–1007.

Dancu, C. V., Riggs, D. S., Hearst-Ikeda, D., & Shoyer, B. G. (1996). Dissociative experiences and posttraumatic stress disorder among female survivors of criminal assault and rape. *Journal of Traumatic Stress, 9*(2), 253–267.

Davidson, J. T., Hughes, D., Blazer, D. G., & George, L. K. (1991). Post-traumatic stress disorder in the community: An epidemiological study. *Psychological Medicine, 21,* 713–721.

Del Bove, G., & Stermac, L. (2002). Psychological evidence in sexual assault court cases: The use of expert testimony and third-party records by trail judges. In J. F. Hodgson & D. S. Kelley (Eds.), *Sexual violence: Policies, practices, and challenges in the United States and Canada* (pp. 119–134). Westport, CT: Praeger.

DuMont, J., & Myhr, T. L. (2000). So few convictions: The role of client-related characteristics in the legal processing of sexual assaults. *Violence Against Women, 6*(10), 1109–1136.

Ettner, S. L., Frank, R. G., & Kessler, R. C. (1997). The impact of psychiatric disorders on labor market outcomes. *Industrial and Labor Relations Review, 51*(1), 64–81.

Feehan, M., Nada-Raja, S., Martin, J. A., & Langley, J. D. (2001). The prevalence and correlates of psychological distress following physical and sexual assault in a young adult cohort. *Violence and Victims, 16*(1), 49–63.

Feeny, N. C., Zoellner, L. A., & Foa, E. B. (2000). Anger, dissociation, and posttraumatic stress disorder among female assault victims. *Journal of Traumatic Stress, 13*(1), 89–100.

Fisher, B. S., & Cullen, F. T. (2000). Measuring the sexual victimization of women: Evolution, current controversies, and future research. In D. Duffee (Ed.), *Measurement and analysis of crime and justice* (pp. 317–390). Rockville, MD: National Institute of Justice/NCJRS.

Foa, E. B., Ehlers, A., Clark, D. M., Tolin, D. F., & Orsillo, S. M. (1999). The posttraumatic cognitions inventory (PTCI): Development and validation. *Psychological Assessment, 11*(3), 303–314.

Foa, E. B., Hearst-Ikeda, D., & Perry, K. J. (1995). Evaluation of a brief cognitive-behavioral program for the prevention of chronic PTSD in recent assault victims. *Journal of Consulting and Clinical Psychology, 63*(6), 948–955.

Foa, E. B., Zoellner, L. A., & Feeny, N. C. (2003). *An evaluation of three brief prevention programs for facilitating recovery.* Manuscript under review.

Frazier, P. A., & Haney, B. (1996). Sexual assault cases in the legal system: Police, prosecutor, and victim perspectives. *Law and Human Behavior, 20*(6), 607–628.

Friedman, M. J., & Schnurr, P. P. (1995). The relationship between trauma, PTSD, and physical health. In M. J. Friedman, D. S. Charney, & A. Y. Deutch (Eds.), *Neurobiological and clinical consequences to stress: From normal adaptation to PTSD* (pp. 507–524). New York: Lippincott-Raven.

Geist, R. F. (1988). Sexually related trauma. *Emergency Medicine Clinics of North America,* 6(3), 439–466.

Gilboa-Schechtman, E., & Foa, E. B. (2001). Patterns of recovery after trauma: The use of intraindividual analysis. *Journal of Abnormal Psychology, 110,* 392–400.

Golding, J. M. (1996a). Sexual assault history and limitations in physical functioning in two general population samples. *Research in Nursing and Health, 19,* 33–44.

Golding, J. M. (1996b). Sexual assault history and women's reproductive and sexual health. *Psychology of Women Quarterly, 20,* 101–121.

Golding, J. M (1999a). Sexual assault history and headache: Five general population studies. *Journal of Nervous and Mental Disease, 187*(10), 624–629.

Golding, J. M. (1999b). Sexual-assault history and long-term physical health problems: Evidence from clinical and population epidemiology. *Current Directions in Psychological Science, 8*(6), 191–194.

Golding, J. M., Cooper, M. L., & George, L. K. (1997). Sexual assault history and health perceptions: Seven general population studies. *Health Psychology, 16*(5), 417–425.

Gostin, L., Lazzarini, Z., Alexander, D., Brandt, A. M., Mayer, K. H., & Silverman, D. C. (1994). HIV testing, counseling, and prophylaxis after sexual assault. *Journal of the American Medical Association, 271*(18), 1436–1444.

Green, B. L., Goodman, L. A., Krupnick, J. L., Corcoran, C. B., Petty, R. M., Stockton, P., & Stern, N. M. (2000). Outcomes of single versus multiple trauma exposure in a screening sample. *Journal of Traumatic Stress, 13*(2), 271–286.

Gregory, J., & Lees, S. (1999). *Policing sexual assault.* New York: Routledge.

Harlow, C. W. (1989). *Injuries from crime.* Washington, DC: Department of Justice, Bureau of Justice Statistics.

Helzer, J. E., Robine, L. N., & McEvoy, L. (1987). Post-traumatic stress disorder in the general population: Findings of the Epidemiological Catchment Area survey. *New England Journal of Medicine, 317*(26), 1630–1634.

Hodgson, J. F., & Kelley, D. S. (2002). Sexual violence: Policies, practices, and challenges. In J. F. Hodgson & D. S. Kelley (Eds.), *Sexual violence: Policies, practices, and challenges in the United States and Canada* (pp. 1–13). Westport, CT: Praeger.

Holmes, M. M., Resnick, H. S., Kilpatrick, D. G., & Best, C. L. (1996). Rape-related pregnancy: Estimates and descriptive characteristics from a national sample of women. *American Journal of Obstetrics and Gynecology, 175*(2), 320–324.

Jordan, J. (2001). Worlds apart: Women, rape, and the police reporting process. *British Journal of Criminology, 41,* 679–706.

Kelley, D. S. (2002). The measurement of rape. In J. F. Hodgson & D. S. Kelley (Eds.), *Sexual violence: Policies, practices, and challenges in the United States and Canada* (pp. 15–33). Westport, CT: Praeger.

Kessler, R. C. (2000). Posttraumatic stress disorder: The burden to the individual and to society. *Journal of Clinical Psychiatry, 61*(Suppl. 5), 4–12.

Kessler, R. C., Berglund, P. A., Foster, C. L., Saunders, W. B., Stang, P. E., & Walters, E. E. (1997). Social consequences of psychiatric disorders, II: Teenage parenthood. *American Journal of Psychiatry, 154*(10), 1405–1411.

Kessler, R. C., Foster, C. L., Saunders, W. B., & Stang, P. E. (1995). Social consequences of psychiatric disorders, I: Educational attainment. *American Journal of Psychiatry, 152*(7), 1026–1032.

Kessler, R. C., & Frank, R. G. (1997). The impact of psychiatric disorders on work loss days. *Psychological Medicine, 27*, 861–873.

Kessler, R. C., Sonnega, A., Bromet, E., Hughes, M., & Nelson C. B. (1995). Posttraumatic stress disorder in the national comorbidity survey. *Archives of General Psychiatry, 52*, 1048–1060.

Kessler, R. C., Walters, E. E., & Forthofer, M. S. (1998). The social consequences of psychiatric disorders, III: Probability of marital stability. *American Journal of Psychiatry, 155*(8), 1092–1096.

Kilpatrick, D. G., Acierno, R., Resnick, H. S., Saunders, B. E., & Best, C. L. (1997). A 2-year longitudinal analysis of the relationships between violent assault and substance abuse in women. *Journal of Consulting and Clinical Psychology, 65*(5), 834–847.

Kilpatrick, D. G., Best, C. L., Saunders, B. E., & Veronen, L. J. (1988). Rape in marriage and in dating relationships: How bad is it for mental health? *Annals of the New York Academy of Sciences, 528*, 335–344.

Kilpatrick, D. G., Edmunds, C. N., & Seymour, A. K. (1992). *Rape in America: A report to the nation.* Charleston, SC: National Victim Center and the National Crime Victims Research Center at the Medical University of South Carolina.

Kilpatrick, D. G., Saunders, B. E., Amick-McMullan, A., Best, C. L., Veronen, L. J., & Resnick, H. S. (1989). Victim and crime factors associated with the development of crime-related post-traumatic stress disorder. *Behavior Therapy, 20*, 199–214.

Kilpatrick, D. G., Saunders, B. E., Veronen, L. J., Best, C. L., & Von, J. M. (1987). Criminal victimization: Lifetime prevalence, reporting to police, and psychological impact. *Crime and Delinquency, 33*(4), 479–489.

Kilpatrick, D. G., & Veronen, L. J. (1984). Treatment for rape-related problems: Crisis intervention is not enough. In L. Cohen, W. Claiborn, & G. Specter (Eds.), *Crisis intervention: Community clinical psychology series* (2nd ed., pp. 165–185). New York: Human Services Press.

Kimerling, R., & Calhoun, K. S. (1994). Somatic symptoms, social support, and treatment seeking among sexual assault victims. *Journal of Consulting and Clinical Psychology, 62*(2), 333–340.

Kimerling, R., Clum, G. A., & Wolfe, J. (2000). Relationships among trauma exposure, chronic posttraumatic stress disorder symptoms, and self-reported health in women: Replication and extension. *Journal of Traumatic Stress, 13*(1), 115–128.

Kingsworth, R. F., MacIntosh, R. C., & Wenworth, J. (2002). Sexual assault: The role of prior relationship and victim characteristics in case processing. *Justice Quarterly, 16*(2), 275–301.

Konradi, A. (2001). Pulling strings doesn't work in court: Moving beyond puppetry in the relationship between prosecutors and rape survivors. *Journal of Social Distress and Homeless, 10*(10), 5–28.

Koss, M. P., Figueredo, A. J., & Prince, R. J. (2002). Cognitive mediation of rape's mental, physical, and social health impact: Tests of four models in cross-sectional data. *Journal of Consulting and Clinical Psychology, 70*(4), 926–941.

Koss, M. P., & Heslet, L. (1992). Somatic consequences of violence against women. *Archives of Family Medicine, 1,* 53–59.

Krakow, B., Artar, A., Warner, T. D., Melendez, D., Johnston, L., Hollifield, M., Germain, A., & Koss, M. (2000). Sleep disorder, depression, suicidality in female sexual assault survivors. *Crisis, 21*(4), 163–170.

Ledray, L. E. (2001). Sexual assault nurse examiner (SANE) program. In C. M. Renzetti, J. L. Edleson, & R. K. Bergen (Eds.), *Sourcebook on violence against women* (pp. 243–246). Thousand Oaks, CA: Sage.

Leserman, J., Drosman, D. A., Li, Z., Toomey, T. C., Nachman, G., & Glogau, L. (1996). Sexual and physical abuse history in gastroenterology practice: How types of abuse impact health status. *Psychosomatic Medicine, 58,* 4–15.

Leserman, J., Li, Z., Drossman, D. A., & Hu, Y. J. B. (1998). Selected symptoms associated with sexual and physical abuse history among female patients with gastrointestinal disorders: The impact on subsequent health care visits. *Psychological Medicine, 28,* 417–425.

Letourneau, E. J., Resnick, H. S., Kilpatrick, D. G., Saunders, B. E., & Best, C. L. (1996). Comorbidity of sexual problems and posttraumatic stress disorder in female crime victims. *Behavior Therapy, 27,* 321–336.

Litz, B. T., Gray, M. J., Bryant, R. A., & Adler, A. B. (2002). Early intervention for trauma: Current status and future directions. *Clinical Psychology: Science and Practice, 9*(2), 112–134.

Lord, V. B., & Rassel, G. (2002). Law enforcement's response to sexual assault: A comparative study of nine counties in North Carolina. In J. F. Hodgson & D. S. Kelley (Eds.), *Sexual violence: Policies, practices, and challenges in the United States and Canada* (pp. 155–172). Westport, CT: Praeger.

Mahoney, P. (1999). High rape chronicity and low rates of help-seeking among wife rape survivors in a nonclinical sample. *Violence Against Women, 5*(9), 993–1016.

Martin, L., Rosen, L. N., Durand, D. B., Knudson, K. H., & Stretch, R. H. (2000). Psychological and physical health effects of sexual assaults and nonsexual traumas among male and female United States Army soldiers. *Behavioral Medicine, 26,* 23–33.

Maruschak, L. M. (2002). *HIV in prisons, 2000.* Washington, DC: Bureau of Justice Statistics, U.S. Department of Justice.

Meredtih, T., Speir, J. C., & Johnson, M. (2000). Using research to improve services for victims of sexual assault. *Justice Research and Policy, 2*(2), 1–17.

Miller, T. R., Cohen, M. A., & Wiersema, B. (1996). *Victim cost and consequences: A new look.* Washington, DC: National Institute of Justice Research Report.

Murphy, W. J. (2001). The Victim Advocacy and Research Group: Serving a growing need to provide rape victims with personal legal representation to protect privacy rights and to fight gender bias in the criminal justice system. *Journal of Social Distress and the Homeless, 11*(1), 123–138.

Nacci, P., & Kane, T. (1982). *Sex and sexual aggression in federal prisons.* Washington, DC: Federal Bureau of Prisons.

Nisith, P., Mechanic, M. B., & Resick, P. A. (2000). Prior interpersonal trauma: The contribution to current PTSD symptoms in female rape victims. *Journal of Abnormal Psychology, 109*(1), 20–25.

Norris, F. H. (1992). Epidemiology of trauma: Frequency and impact of different potentially traumatic events on different demographic groups. *Journal of Consulting and Clinical Psychology, 60*(3), 409–418.

Rauch, S. A. M., Hembree, E. A., & Foa, E. B. (2001). Acute psychosocial preventative interventions for posttraumatic stress disorder. *Advances in Mind–Body Medicine, 17,* 187–191.

Rennison, C. (2002). *Criminal victimization, 2001.* Washington, DC: U.S. Department of Justice, Bureau of Justice Statistics.

Resnick, H., Acierno, R., Holmes, M., Dammeyer, M., & Kilpatrick, D. (2000). Emergency evaluation and intervention with female victims of rape and other violence. *Journal of Clinical Psychology, 56*(10), 1317–1333.

Resnick, H., Acierno, R., Holmes, M., Kilpatrick, D. G., & Jager, N. (1999). Prevention of post-rape psychopathology: Preliminary findings of a controlled acute rape treatment study. *Journal of Anxiety Disorders, 13*(4), 359–370.

Resnick, H. S., Acierno, R., & Kilpatrick, D. G. (1997). Health impact of interpersonal violence. 2: Medical and mental health outcomes. *Behavioral Medicine, 23,* 65–78.

Resnick, H. S., Kilpatrick, D. G., Dansky, B. S., Saunders, B. E., & Best, C. L. (1993). Prevalence of civilian trauma and posttraumatic stress disorder in a representative national sample of women. *Journal of Consulting and Clinical Psychology, 61,* 984–991.

Rothbaum, B. O., Foa, E. B., Riggs, D. S., Murdock, T., & Walsh, W. (1992). A prospective examination of post-traumatic stress disorder in rape victims. *Journal of Traumatic Stress, 5*(3), 455–475.

Russell, D. E., & Bolen, R. M. (2000). *The epidemic of rape and child sexual abuse in the United States.* Thousand Oaks, CA: Sage.

Sadler, A. G., Booth, B. M., Nielson, D., & Doebbeling, B. N. (2000). Health-related consequences of physical and sexual violence: Women in the military. *Obstetrics and Gynecology, 96*(3), 473–480.

Schuller, R. A., & Stewart, A. (2000). Police responses to sexual assault complaints: The role of perpetrator/complainant intoxication. *Law and Behavior, 24*(5), 535–551.

Solomon, S. D., & Davidson, J. R. T. (1997). Trauma: Prevalence, impairment, service use, and cost. *Journal of Clinical Psychiatry, 58*(Suppl. 9), 5–11.

Spitzberg, B. H. (1999). An analysis of empirical estimates of sexual aggression victimization and perpetration. *Violence and Victims, 14*(3), 241–260.

Statistics Canada. (1993). *The violence against women survey: Survey highlights.* Ottawa: Author.

Stein, M. B., & Barrett-Connor, E. (2000). Sexual assault and physical health: Findings from a population-based study of older adults. *Psychosomatic Medicine, 62,* 838–843.

Tjaden, P., & Thoennes, N. (2000). *Full report of the prevalence, incidence, and consequences of violence against women: Findings from the National Violence Against Women Survey.* Washington, DC: National Institute of Justice and Centers for Disease Control and Prevention.

Ullman, S. E. (1996a). Correlates and consequences of adult sexual assault disclosure. *Journal of Interpersonal Violence, 11*(4), 554–571.

Ullman, S. E. (1996b). Social reactions, coping strategies, and self-blame attributions in adjustment to sexual assault. *Psychology of Women Quarterly, 20,* 505–526.

Ullman, S. E. (1996c). Do social reactions to sexual assault victims vary by support provider? *Violence and Victims, 11,* 143–156.

Ullman, S. E. (1999). Social support and recovery from sexual assault: A review. *Aggression and Violent Behavior, 4*(3), 343–358.

Ullman, S. E., & Filipas, H. A. (2001). Correlates of formal and informal support seeking in sexual assault victims. *Journal of Interpersonal Violence, 16*(10), 1028–1047.

Ullman, S. E., & Seigel, J. M. (1995). Sexual assault, social reactions, and physical health. *Women's Health: Research on Gender, Behavior, and Policy, 1,* 289–308.

Valentiner, D. P., Foa, E. B., Riggs, D. S., & Gershuny, B. S. (1996). Coping strategies and posttraumatic stress disorder in female victims of sexual and nonsexual assault. *Journal of Abnormal Psychology, 105*(3), 455–458.

Weldon, S. L. (2002). *Protest, policy, and the problem of violence against women: A cross-national comparison.* Pittsburgh, PA: University of Pittsburgh Press.

Winfield, I., George, L. K., Swartz, M., & Blazer, D. G. (1990). Sexual assault and psychiatric disorders among a community sample of women. *American Journal of Psychiatry, 147*(3), 335–341.

Zoellner, L. A., Goodwin, M. L., & Foa, E. B. (2000). PTSD severity and health perceptions in female victims of sexual assault. *Journal of Traumatic Stress, 13*(4), 635–649.

12

When the Helpers Need Help

*Early Intervention for Emergency
and Relief Services Personnel*

CYNTHIA B. ERIKSSON
DAVID W. FOY
LINNEA C. LARSON

The events of 9-11-01 introduced a new perspective of terror to the United States and to the world. However, the response of thousands of emergency service personnel and relief workers in the immediate and prolonged aftermath of the terrorist attacks also rekindled a sense of awe in the acts of selfless heroism of emergency services and relief personnel that saved many lives. The terrorist attacks on 9-11-01 provide a tragic and stark example of the sacrifices, dangers, and demands of emergency and relief work, which happen everyday around the world.

Most emergency or relief workers respond to needs in their "hometowns." They are a few miles away from their own homes, families, and day-to-day responsibilities of caring for loved ones. The emergency may have touched their own social circle or damaged their own property. Other emergency or relief workers make the decision to travel to an environment that may be unfamiliar or quite culturally different, to support a community recovering from a natural or human-made disaster. They contribute countless hours in a short time span, hoping that their efforts can help make a difference. These traveling workers may or may not have the benefit of a close team to make up for the lack of nearby family and social support.

The rescue and recovery work in the aftermath of the 9-11 terrorist attacks also demonstrates the organizational challenges of disaster and relief efforts. Emergency mental health services were provided for many New York City firefighters, and critical incident stress management (CISM) teams came from locations across the United States to participate in this staff support process (Gulliver et al., 2002). However, the physical and emotional toll of the work continues to affect workers. Epidemiological reports indicate that 11 months after the attacks, 250 New York City Fire Department rescue workers remained on leave from duty due to stress-related illnesses, including post-traumatic stress disorder (PTSD), depression, anxiety, and bereavement (Centers for Disease Control and Prevention, 2002).

The agencies that employ emergency service or relief workers, or provide structure for volunteer workers, have begun to identify the need for an organizational policy and response to the possible consequences of emergency work. Several agencies and individuals have proposed programs oriented to select, train, and/or support staff through critical work-related events (Danieli, 2002; Mitchell, 1983). It is a complex task to respond effectively to this distinctive community, and continued work is required to clarify the optimal intervention strategies appropriate across different work and cultural contexts.

In this chapter, we first outline the empirical evidence for acute and long-term distress in both professional and volunteer service workers. Then, we discuss the unique risk and resilience factors associated with disaster or emergency service. In light of the evidence of distress, risk, and resilience, we review intervention strategies and highlight outcome research on early interventions for traumatic exposure. In conclusion, we propose recommendations for research, clinical intervention, and organizational response to help the helpers recover from the consequences of their traumatic exposure during emergency service.

EVIDENCE OF DISTRESS IN EMERGENCY AND RELIEF WORKERS

The majority of studies of distress in emergency and relief services personnel have focused on firefighters, police, paramedics, and military or civilian rescue workers. Only a few studies have examined distress in humanitarian aid workers in international contexts, although this is an area of growing research. Event-related distress in these populations has been measured weeks, months, or years postdisaster using a variety of measures and methods ranging from self-report questionnaires to face-to-face clinical interviews.

Military rescue workers are one group of emergency personnel in which distress has been identified. Johnsen, Eid, Lovstad, and Michelson (1997) studied 133 members of a Norwegian military company after an avalanche and found that spontaneous rescuers scored as high as victims for posttraumatic symptoms on the Impact of Event Scale (IES) both 2 weeks and 4 months postdisaster, and at 4 months both rescuers and victims still reported IES symptoms at the level of medium clinical concern (mean total scores of 19.0 and 19.7, respectively). In addition, both rescuers and victims scored significantly higher on posttraumatic symptoms than did nonexposed company members who were at the site of the disaster but were not involved in rescue efforts. Among rescuers surveyed 2 weeks postincident, 10% had a posttraumatic stress reaction (significant posttraumatic symptomatology, defined as a score of 5 or higher on at least four items of the Post Traumatic Stress Scale–10), whereas none met criteria for significant symptomatology on the PTSS at 4 months. Grieger et al. (2000) examined distress among 45 Air National Guard workers 6 months after an air disaster in which they were involved in the recovery and identification of human remains. In this sample, two of the workers (4.9%) met criteria for PTSD diagnosis defined as endorsement of all DSM-IV criteria and a "high" symptom level on the IES.

Ursano, Fullerton, Kao, and Bhartiya (1995) found that military mortuary volunteers (body handlers) reported significantly higher IES intrusion and avoidance scores 1 month after a gun turret explosion than a comparison group of volunteers who did not handle bodies. Forty-three percent of the body handlers endorsed total IES scores in the range of high clinical concern, and 6 (11%) met criteria for probable PTSD (defined by scores on an augmented Symptom Checklist 90—Revised [SCL-90-R] plus total score on the IES). There were significant reductions in IES scores at 4 and 13 months postexplosion, but, at 13 months, 15.8% of the body handlers still reported posttraumatic symptomatology in the range of high clinical concern, although probable PTSD had dropped to 2% (one worker). In another study of 355 military medical personnel responding to a crash at an air show (Epstein, Fullerton, & Ursano, 1998), 13.5 % had probable PTSD (defined by scores on an augmented SCL-90-R plus total score on the IES) at 6, 12, or 18 months, and the frequency of probable PTSD cases peaked at 12 months (12.1%). By 18 months, probable PTSD frequency had decreased to 7.3%, but posttraumatic stress symptoms had not decreased as quickly as PTSD cases.

Firefighters and police officers are two other groups in which distress has been documented. North et al. (2002) identified a PTSD rate of 13% in a sample of firefighters who were volunteer rescue workers after the Oklahoma City bombing compared to primary victims, who had a PTSD rate of 23%. PTSD was diagnosed by a structured interview 34 months postbombing. The rate of alcohol use disorder in the firefighters was 24% postdisaster and 47% lifetime, with only 2% of new cases occurring postbombing. The PTSD rate of 13% among these firefighters is high compared to that documented in military rescue workers, and the high rate of alcohol use disorder is also of concern.

A longitudinal study of Australian firefighters exposed to a bushfire disaster examined patterns of expression of morbidity over time (McFarlane, 1988). In this sample, the prevalence of significant posttraumatic morbidity as defined by the General Health Questionnaire was 32% at 4 months, 27% at 11 months, and 30% at 29 months, and the course of morbidity varied over time in three patterns. Morbidity only at 4 months postdisaster was seen in 9.2% of the firefighters (defined as the "acute group"); 21% of the firefighters had significant posttraumatic symptoms at 4 months as well as at 11 and/or 29 months (defined as the "chronic group"); and 19.7% of the firefighters did not have significant morbidity at 4 months but did have it at 11 and/or 29 months (defined as the "delayed-onset group"). This study points to the need for later intervention for those service workers who do not display posttraumatic symptoms in the early months after a disaster. However, the fact that 49.8% of the firefighters did not have significant posttraumatic morbidity at any of the three times highlights the practicality of targeting interventions for those displaying symptomatology.

Carlier, Lamberts, and Gersons (1997) studied Dutch police officers who had experienced a variety of duty-related critical incidents and found an overall PTSD rate of 7%, with 6% diagnosed via a structured interview at 3 months postevent, and an additional 1% diagnosed at 12 months. Subclinical PTSD symptoms were reported by 34% of the officers at some point during the study. In contrast, Hodgins, Creamer, and Bell (2001) conducted a prospective study of 223 junior police officers with a mean length of service of 15 months and found that levels of distress were relatively low, with none of the officers scoring above cutoff for PTSD (measured by the PTSD Checklist—Civilian Version).

Among firefighters, police, and other emergency services personnel, distress levels may be high regardless of whether or not they have recently been exposed to a critical incident. For example, Marmar, Weiss, Metzler, Ronfeldt, and Foreman (1996) documented no significant differences in posttraumatic stress symptoms (IES scores) 1½ years postevent between emergency services personnel (firefighters, police, EMT personnel, transportation rescue workers) involved in rescue efforts for a freeway collapse after an earthquake, a local control group not involved in rescue efforts, and another control group of emergency personnel geographically distant from the earthquake. When the three groups were combined, 5% were above threshold for intrusive and avoidant symptoms and for general psychological distress. At follow-up with this sample 2 years later, IES scores significantly decreased but general psychiatric symptoms (SCL-90-R Global Severity and Somatization indices) increased significantly among all three groups (Marmar et al., 1999). This evidence suggests the potential long-term adverse psychological effects of exposure to traumatic events in this population.

Indeed, Boxer and Wild (1993), in a study of 145 urban firefighters in the United States, found that 39% scored in the range suggesting high emotional distress on the General Health Questionnaire–12 (GHQ-12). Bryant and Harvey (1996) documented similar levels of distress on the GHQ-12 (27%) among 751 volunteer firefighters in Australia. In this same study, Bryant and Harvey also examined IES scores related to any firefighting-related event for which the firefighters reported associated symptoms, and found that 17% had IES scores greater than 19 (significant posttraumatic distress) and 9% reported IES scores greater than 29 (severe posttraumatic distress).

Studies of humanitarian aid workers have documented levels of distress similar to those of emergency services personnel and rescue workers. Eriksson, Vande Kemp, Gorsuch, Hoke, and Foy (2001) surveyed 113 humanitarian aid staff recently returned to the United States and found that 10% met full diagnostic criteria for PTSD in their first 6 months of reentry, defined as endorsement of moderate symptomatology across the three DSM-IV symptom categories on the Los Angeles Symptom Checklist. In addition, 19% of this sample met criteria for "partial PTSD"—endorsement of significant symptoms in two of the three symptom categories. Another study was completed in an active relief field. Expatriate and national staff from several international aid agencies completed a survey during their work in the complex humanitarian emergency in Kosovo (Cardozo & Salama, 2002). The participants in this study reported lower levels of PTSD as measured by the Harvard Trauma Questionnaire, with only 2% of expatriate and 7% of national staff meeting diagnostic levels. However, aid staff did report high levels of depression, anxiety, and alcohol use. In a study of a subsample of 70 human rights workers in Kosovo (mostly national staff), Holtz, Salama, Cardozo, and Gotway (2002) found a PTSD rate of 7.1% measured by the Harvard Trauma Questionnaire. Elevated symptoms of anxiety and depression, as measured by the Hopkins Symptom Checklist, were found in 17.1% and 8.6% of the workers, respectively. More research is needed among humanitarian aid workers to fully examine patterns of distress in this specialized group of service workers.

UNIQUE RISK AND RESILIENCE FACTORS

The Reality of Direct and Indirect Exposure to Trauma

One of the most distinctive characteristics of emergency service or relief work is the reality that one's work requires exposure to trauma. By the nature of the job, emergency personnel respond to large- and small-scale tragedy and disaster. They see the devastation, smell the odor of lost life, and hear the cries of families and victims alike. Confronting this horror can create a tremendous burden of indirect exposure to the traumatic aftermath. What might not be clear in initial recruitment is the fact that emergency workers might themselves become direct victims of the tragedy or violence. The deaths and injuries of many emergency rescue workers responding to the terrorist attacks on 9-11-01 underscore that risk. In addition, an increase in acts of violence against international humanitarian aid workers has created a situation in which it is more dangerous to be a civilian U.N. aid worker than a soldier deployed to peacekeeping duty in a conflict zone (Turner, 1998). Both emergency service workers and humanitarian aid personnel are at significant risk for extensive indirect and direct exposure to heinous traumatic events.

Recent research with domestic emergency service workers such as firefighters, police, military rescue workers, and emergency room nurses has identified the prevalence of direct and indirect exposure, as well as common types of critical events. In a study of volunteer firefighters, Bryant and Harvey (1996) reported that 56% of the sample had felt their personal safety was threatened during their work, and 15% believed that they had "come close to dying" while on duty (p. 55). In a survey of emergency room nurses, over half of the participants in this study had confronted the death of a child patient in the past year (Burns & Harm, 1993). It was also noted that several participants wrote in events on the survey that suggested personal threat (e.g., gang activity, patients with weapons in the emergency room, or violent patients who were acutely psychotic). Corneil, Beaton, Murphy, Johnson, and Pike (1999) found that groups of firefighters in different areas of service confronted different types and numbers of traumatic events. Their sample of 205 U.S. firefighters in an urban environment reported significantly more exposure to crime victims, as well as a higher mean level of exposure to traumatic incidents, than a comparison group of 625 Canadian urban firefighters. Finally, Alexander and Klein (2001) found road traffic accidents and medical emergencies were rated as the most disturbing events for a sample of Scottish ambulance workers.

Other research has sought to identify characteristics of work-related stressors that may be considered traumatogenic. Carlier et al. (1997) operationalized direct and indirect exposure to trauma in law enforcement by hypothesizing that police officers are commonly confronted with two types of stressors: "very violent" experiences, where the officer is an active participant in the event or "very depressing" experiences, where the officer must respond to the aftermath or consequences of such violence (p. 499). Later, related research utilized a dimensional analysis to identify three cognitive dimensions police officers used to interpret meaning in critical events: "emotional reactivity," "vulnerability and physical integrity," and "moral responsibility" (Carlier,

Lamberts, & Gersons, 2000, p. 34). Brown, Fielding, and Grover (1999) used factor analysis to consider the constructs underlying work-related stressors in British police officers. They discovered a similar set of factors which they labeled "exposure to death and disaster," "violence and injury," and "sexual crime" (p. 319). Beaton, Murphy, Johnson, Pike, and Corneil (1998) asked 173 urban firefighters and paramedics to rank-order a list of 33 possible duty-related critical events. The five events rated as most stressful were: "Witness duty related death of co-worker," "Co-worker firefighter fire fatality (not witnessed)," "Experience career ending injury (self)," "Render aid to seriously injured friend/relative," and "Sudden infant death incident" (p. 824). Principal components analysis applied to the ranked list of 33 events revealed five relevant components of duty-related stressors: serious injury to oneself or one's coworker, exposure to horrific consequences of events, providing care to seriously injured victims, limited injury to oneself, and exposure to death or dying.

Only a small number of empirical studies have been published identifying the level of exposure to trauma common in humanitarian aid workers. Eriksson et al. (2001) surveyed North American aid workers from five aid agencies who had recently returned from field locations. The most common traumatic events participants confronted directly included: "being threatened with serious physical harm by someone"; "life-threatening illness or chronic condition"; "being within the range of gunfire, being shot at"; and "road accidents" (Eriksson et al., 2001, p. 208). One-quarter to almost one-third of staff in this study had had personal experience of these events. Cardozo & Salama (2002) surveyed expatriate and national staff from several international aid agencies during the complex humanitarian emergency in Kosovo. The most common direct traumatic stressors included "a situation that was very frightening," "verbal or physical threats to life," "hostility of the local population," "armed attack or robbery," and "handling dead bodies" (p. 245). In the related study by Holtz et al. (2002), national and expatriate human rights workers in Kosovo reported the following most common personal traumatic events: "bombing of workplace or residence," "being close to death," "verbal or physical threats to your life," and a "situation that was very frightening" (p. 391). Ninety-three percent of these human rights workers were Kosovar Albanian, which highlights the reality of national workers experiencing traumas in the war or disaster itself, as well as later in the humanitarian work.

Each professional or volunteer service person has made a choice to face the human loss and physical devastation that accompany disasters. The outcome of this choice implies the distinctive risk of facing certain types of tasks that have been identified as particularly traumatogenic. A group of studies examining the effects of disaster and relief service on emergency workers has identified key trauma characteristics that are either commonly reported as the "most disturbing" event or statistically related to higher levels of emotional distress. Burns and Harm (1993) surveyed 682 emergency room nurses; their results indicated that the death of a child and the death of a coworker were considered the most critical events on the job. Navy divers recovering bodies after a plane crash reported that exposure to remains, especially the remains of a child, was more stressful than any of the safety hazards present in the recovery effort (Leffler & Dembert, 1998). Body recovery has been noted as a particularly traumatogenic disaster task; a key issue is the traumatic impact of a sense of personal identification with the deceased (Jones, 1985; Ursano et al., 1995). In a sample of 355 military health care workers responding to the aftermath of an air disaster, exposure to burn victims (grotesque injury) was associated with higher levels of posttraumatic distress (Epstein et al., 1998). In addition, human rights workers who had experienced an armed attack or hostile responses from the local community were at higher risk for elevated anxiety symptoms (Holtz et al., 2002).

In other studies of emergency workers, distress was not related to certain types of trauma but to the severity of threat of the trauma. For example, Carlier et al. (1997) identified that posttraumatic symptoms were not significantly related to the type of police trauma, but that the severity of the traumatic event was the only variable associated with PTSD symptoms at both the 3-month and 12-month assessment periods. Hodgins et al. (2001) also found severity of the incident to be significantly related to PTSD in police. Bryant and Harvey (1995) reported that a significant amount of variance in PTSD symptomatology in volunteer firefighters was associated with event specific factors: the severity of the personal threat, the closeness to death, and the level of fear involved.

Due to the nature of emergency service, a worker is often exposed to a number of traumatic incidents within a short period of time. Research with emergency service workers responding to the Loma Prieta earthquake in 1989 demonstrated that higher levels of exposure to critical incidents and higher levels of perceived personal threat were significantly related to posttraumatic distress (Marmar et al., 1996; Weiss, Marmar, Metzler, & Ronfeldt, 1995). In addition, the cumulative number of traumatic incidents reported by a sample of urban police officers was found to be significantly related to increased nightmares (Neylan et al., 2002). Furthermore, Dougall, Herberman, Delahanty, Inslicht, and Baum (2000) identified that prior exposure to traumatic events dissimilar to the stressors related to airline disasters put workers at risk for greater posttraumatic distress after participating in a large-scale air disaster response. Moreover, in a sample of North American aid workers returned from service, the amount of both direct and indirect exposure to life-threatening traumatic events was significantly related to the report of PTSD symptoms

(Eriksson, et al., 2001). Direct exposure for aid workers in Kosovo was also related to psychological distress; participants who identified exposure to more than six traumatic events were significantly more likely to report higher levels of anxiety symptoms (Cardozo & Salama, 2002).

Personal Risk Characteristics

In addition to event-related variables, empirical research has also suggested risk factors that the individual brings to his or her work and response. These factors include both background and personality characteristics. Pre-event and subsequent stressful life events (unemployment or loss of a loved one) increase risk for posttraumatic adjustment problems (Bryant & Harvey, 1995; Carlier et al., 1997; Epstein et al., 1998). Demographic variables such as lower education level (e.g., in military responders to air disaster; Epstein et al., 1998) and Hispanic-American ethnicity (e.g., urban police officers; Pole et al., 2001) have been identified as risk factors in certain discrete samples. There are conflicting reports of the influence of earlier psychiatric history as a risk factor. In two samples of firefighters, previous counseling or psychiatric treatment was associated with posttraumatic distress (Corneil et al., 1999; McFarlane, 1988), whereas in another sample of firefighters previous psychiatric history was not significantly related to higher levels of PTSD symptoms (Bryant & Harvey, 1995).

A few personality and emotional functioning variables have also been identified as risk factors that may be important in applicant screening and/or training. In an early longitudinal study of firefighters responding to a catastrophic bushfire, McFarlane (1988) identified that the group of workers exhibiting persistent, chronic PTSD symptoms scored higher on a scale of neuroticism. Traumatized police officers who acknowledged having difficulty expressing their emotions were also at higher risk for reporting PTSD symptoms at 3 months postcritical incident (Carlier et al., 1997). Several studies have indicated an increased risk for posttraumatic symptoms in those reporting peritraumatic dissociation symptoms (Epstein et al., 1998; Hodgins et al., 2001; Marmar et al., 1996; Marmar et al., 1999) and in those emergency workers reporting higher levels of posttraumatic distress at earlier time periods (Carlier et al., 1997; Marmar et al., 1996).

Organizational Risk Factors

The organizational context is a key aspect of unique risk for emergency service and relief workers. Two areas have been identified in particular: work strain and insufficient time to recover from critical incidents. Sloan, Rozensky, Kaplan, and Saunders (1994) reported that emergency responders endorsement of a "qualitatively heavy work load" was related to higher levels of intrusion and avoidance symptoms (p. 565). Emergency workers in this study expected that they would experience critical events and a challenging environment. However, the stressful part of the workload was the time pressure and number of events to respond to. Higher distress related to work strain and number of response events were also demonstrated in firefighters (Corneil et al., 1999), volunteer emergency medical personnel (Moran & Britton, 1994), and ambulance workers (Alexander & Klein, 2001). The pressure to respond to many events may also help explain the risk inherent in insufficient time to resolve exposure to critical events. Several studies specifically highlighted the deleterious effects of exhaustion when confronting a traumatic event and inadequate time between deployments to particularly critical events (Alexander & Klein, 2001; Bryant & Harvey, 1996; Carlier et al., 1997).

Research with humanitarian aid workers has not specifically examined these organizational factors. However, there is a clear risk for overwork and time pressure in the urgent response in international aid. Ager, Flapper, van Pietersom, and Simon (2002) write: "the culture of humanitarian work is no payment for extra work; being present and available 24 hours, 7 days a week, especially in emergencies" (p. 197). In the context of a complex humanitarian emergency, the level of need is overwhelming, and the response must be urgent. Choices that can have life-and-death consequences are commonplace (e.g., food aid distribution, rescue attempts with large numbers of injured, or limited medical services in areas such as refugee camps). Smith, Agger, Danieli, and Weisaeth (1996) describe the overwhelming needs during relief efforts in Goma, Zaire in 1994. The people of Goma were dying by the thousands due to dehydration. The sheer size of the need made it impossible for any relief effort to make a visible impact on the suffering. "When relief workers opted to define a small goal to devote all their energy to, their choice necessitated ignoring and literally driving by or walking over thousands of dying people every day" (Smith et al., 1996, p. 401). As a result of these conditions, emergency workers can struggle with a keen sense of helplessness or powerlessness. An inappropriate sense of guilt about not meeting overwhelming demands over time may contribute to overwork and exhaustion that jeopardizes individual and group well-being. In fact, Holtz et al. (2002) found that national and expatriate human rights workers were more at risk for elevated anxiety symptoms when they had worked for their organization longer than 6 months.

Social Support

One of the primary factors related to decreased distress and increased resilience in emergency service and relief personnel is social support. First, the area of support from colleagues has been identified as an often used and effective coping strategy (Alexander & Klein, 2001; Alexander & Wells, 1991). Urban firefighters report high levels of support at work and with family (Corneil et al., 1999), and U.S. Navy divers recovering remains after an air disaster rated telephone contact with family as one of the most successful coping strategies (Leffler & Dembert, 1998). In addition, higher levels of social support have been statistically related to lower levels of PTSD symptoms in air disaster workers (Dougall, Hyman, Hayward, McFeeley, & Baum, 2001) and emergency medical service workers (Weiss et al., 1995). Conversely, limited social interaction in a police officer's private life was associated with increased PTSD symptoms 12 months postcritical event (Carlier et al., 1997). International humanitarian aid workers' report of social support was found to buffer the experience of posttraumatic distress; staff with high levels of exposure to traumatic events and high perceived social support reported fewer PTSD symptoms than those endorsing high exposure and low social support (Eriksson et al., 2001).

In some cases, social networks may create a unique conflict for the emergency worker. Gibbs, Drummond, and Lackenmeyer (1993) emphasize the potential role conflict for local disaster workers. Emergency response, even in one's hometown, can isolate workers from their social support network or put unusual stress on those supportive relationships. Marmar et al. (1996) identified the complex needs regarding support and family as they described the context of the Loma Prieta earthquake response. First, staff were often preoccupied by thoughts for the welfare of their own friends and family who were affected by the earthquake. Then, being part of the response team meant being separated from loved ones. Emergency workers may feel a conflicting sense of duty to their community and duty to family.

International humanitarian aid workers often do not have the benefit of unit cohesion or team development that other emergency service personnel have created. It is common for international workers to be sent out to relief sites as individuals (McCall & Salama, 1999), and the aid worker's community is quite transient. It is rare for an aid worker to stay in one location for several years (Smith, 2002). In their research in Kosovo, Cardozo and Salama (2002) identified separation from family, lack of access to communication outside the field, and team conflicts as key, chronic, interpersonal stressors.

Training and Preparation

Another area of possible resilience is in training and preparation. Just as each recruit for emergency service makes a choice to face a challenging work environment, there is a choice to become as prepared as possible for the tasks at hand. Unfortunately, the results of empirical work are not as convincing as one might expect. In their research with emergency service personnel responding to the Loma Prieta earthquake, Marmar et al. (1996) found that increased posttraumatic distress was related to less preparation for a critical incident. In particular, paramedics/emergency medical technicians and California highway workers reported higher levels of symptoms than the police and firefighters. Alexander and Wells (1991) found that all but one of their sample of police officers doing body recovery reported that previous experience with dead bodies was helpful. However, in a statistical analysis, there was no difference in distress levels between the less experienced workers and the more experienced workers. In a survey of humanitarian aid agency administrators, McCall and Salama (1999) reported that the key areas for training aid workers, stress management, conflict resolution, team cohesion skills, cultural competency, and responding to the media, were often not included in current agency training programs or manuals.

EVIDENCE FOR EARLY INTERVENTIONS

Early interventions can be conceptually classified as following debriefing or cognitive-behavioral models (Litz, Gray, Bryant, & Adler, 2002). At present, controlled trials supporting the efficacy of early interventions of either type for psychological distress experienced by emergency service and international relief personnel are lacking. Many agencies, nevertheless, have policies and procedures in place for providing these services to their staff members (Danieli, 2002). Whether empirical support for the effectiveness of early intervention in preventing or reducing trauma-related distress ever emerges, the need to provide humanitarian workers with essential support and information is widely recognized. This vital information includes education about their traumatic stress reactions, as well as efforts to normalize these reactions and to promote positive coping (e.g. Ruzek, 2002).

Although debriefing is widely used, and is often described as helpful by recipients, its effectiveness is hotly debated. Recent comprehensive reviews of the efficacy research on debriefing illuminate the current status of our empirical knowledge (e.g., Bisson, McFarland, & Rose, 2000; Litz et al., 2002; Neria & Solomon, 2000). While proponents argue for its effectiveness in reducing traumatic distress, opponents argue that debriefing is ineffective, and perhaps even harmful. When examined critically, it is clear that most of the studies are plagued by methodological problems, including inconsistencies in intervention methods, timing, duration, trauma type, recipients, and facilitator training. In addition, few of the studies include appropriate control groups. The lack of randomization of participants to treatment and control conditions, absence of baseline data on symptom type and duration, and limited statistical power, as well as apparent self-selection of participants, are also problematic (Foy, Eriksson, & Trice, 2001).

At present there are fewer than 10 randomized controlled trials of debriefing, and only one of these (Deahl et al., 2000) deals with a population (military peacekeepers) similar to emergency or relief personnel. Most current studies have been clinical in nature, conducted with direct victims of recent traumatic experiences such as car accidents and sexual assaults (Litz et al., 2002). Findings from these studies are consistent in providing no support for the hypothesis that debriefing prevents or reduces PTSD symptoms. In contrast, findings from two randomized controlled trials of early intervention using a multisession cognitive-behavioral model have been more positive (Bryant, Harvey, Dang, Sackville, & Basten, 1998; Bryant, Sackville, Dang, Moulds, & Guthrie, 1999). Both studies showed significant reductions in PTSD severity in those treated with cognitive-behavioral therapy, compared to those randomized to supportive therapy alone. The extent to which findings from these studies can be generalized to emergency and humanitarian relief applications is not yet established.

Because the empirical literature on early intervention effectiveness in humanitarian aid workers is virtually nonexistent, relief agencies must make decisions about the nature of early intervention programs to be offered on the basis of "best judgment." Recent reports of various early interventions provided to emergency mental health service personnel working with families of Pentagon 9-11 victims illustrate a mixture of debriefing and cognitive-behavioral models in the descriptions of services provided by different military and other governmental agencies. For example, Ruzek (2002) presents a description of a brief cognitive-behavioral early intervention approach, provided by Veterans Administration mental health professionals, to staff of the Pentagon Family Assistance Center. Conversely, military mental health providers appeared more likely to employ methods taken from a debriefing perspective (e.g., Rowan, 2002; Schwerin, Kennedy, & Wardlaw, 2002).

Several international relief agencies have been in the forefront of developing and providing early intervention services for their staff (Danieli, 2002). Recent descriptions of the types of programs and organizational policies found among these agencies reflect the growing awareness of psychological risk associated with field relief work, along with increased emphasis on organizational responsibility for implementing policies that protect and restore the mental health of their workers. For example, the Antares Foundation, located in Amsterdam, is organized to provide a range of prevention and early intervention services to nongovernmental agencies, individual field workers, as well as staff training, organization development, and interlinking among relief agencies in Europe and Africa (Ager et al., 2002).

Médecins Sans Frontières Holland is another international agency that has a lengthy history of providing psychosocial support, including early intervention services, for its field workers. Using an eclectic approach to selecting early intervention services is described as a key element in the agency's procedures (van Gelder & van den Berkhof, 2002). Similarly, a large, faith-based relief agency, World Vision International, has developed a multifaceted early intervention approach for national staff that features elements of debriefing, presence of senior World Vision managers to provide immediate organizational support, and replenishment of basic necessities (e.g., money, child care, shelter, and other employment options). Feedback from World Vision staff after receiving early intervention services suggests that the level of organizational response was perceived as more important than personal debriefing services (Fawcett, 2002).

Taken together, these descriptions of early intervention programs from Antares, MSF-Holland, and World Vision International provide some encouragement that international relief agencies are taking active steps toward protecting the mental health of their most valuable human resources—their field workers. Providing a basic level of early intervention services to workers is an important beginning that needs to be followed by systematic efforts to empirically evaluate the actual services rendered. In the next section we provide conclusions and recommendations for "best practices" and "needed research" in early intervention for relief workers.

CONCLUSIONS AND RECOMMENDATIONS FOR PRACTICE AND RESEARCH

The empirical evidence offers strong support for the presence of posttraumatic distress in the diverse groups of workers providing rescue and relief support. PTSD has been identified in firefighters, police, body recovery workers, and humanitarian aid workers. The research methodology has not yet allowed for a consistent analysis of early acute stress disorder symptoms; most studies begin assessment after 30 days and/or use retrospective report to assess peritraumatic response. Several important risk and resilience factors have been identified in these studies. First, the levels of both direct and indirect exposure to trauma have been shown to be consistent stressors across several emergency and relief populations. In addition, critical trauma characteristics have also been identified: personal threat, exposure to child victims, body handling, and exposure to grotesque injury. Finally, other nonevent factors have also been linked to increased posttraumatic distress: higher work strain, less recovery time between deployment to critical events, increased levels of earlier or subsequent stressful events, and lower social support. Randomized controlled trials of early interventions for emergency and relief workers are lacking. Research with clinical populations appears to support a model of multisession early intervention to reduce PTSD symptoms, rather than a strict, single-session debriefing model. In the absence of specific research examining early intervention in emergency and relief workers, organizations have a responsibility to create structures and policy for staff support and intervention that consider the empirical evidence for distress, risk, and resilience.

Practice Recommendations

The literature on risk and resilience suggests that, even before a critical event occurs, organizations have a responsibility to create the best possible scenario for response. One of the most critical issues in "best practice" appears to be the benefit of working in a team. Social support and talking with colleagues are seen as key resilience factors for emergency workers. Preparing the team centers on (1) selecting and training the best team and (2) using that team in a sensitive and efficient manner. Selection procedures should be clear and consistent across units or branches of the service organization. The selection assessment may include personality variables, aspects of psychiatric history, and levels of current life stressors. To reduce levels of general psychiatric distress, Hodgins et al. (2001) recommend that applicants for emergency service positions (specifically police officers) be screened for the tendency to dissociation. In addition, they identify personality variables such as low agreeableness and low conscientiousness that may contribute to difficulties adjusting and coping effectively with the demands and structure of the work.

Training teams for emergency and relief work can address issues related to the reality of direct and indirect exposure. Managers and team members should be made aware of critical events that have been identified as particularly traumatogenic for their area of service. Training in large-scale disaster response may also be helpful for staff who may be used as "volunteers" when communitywide tragedies overwhelm smaller emergency teams. Security training for urban rescue workers or international humanitarian aid workers provides skills in recognizing the possibility of personal threat and managing potentially unstable social circumstances. Once a team is prepared, these men and women must be deployed in an effective manner. Organizations should establish protocols that require appropriate rest or recovery between response to critical events, as well as policies to reduce the level of work-related stresses that exist outside trauma exposure (e.g., job security, low income, excessive shift requirements, or poor management). In addition, policy that recognizes the practical needs of the worker must be established before the emergency (Ager et al., 2002). Plans for emergency financial resources, child care, health care, and alternative employment are critical to meet basic human needs in the midst of a crisis (Fawcett, 2002).

A unique area of need for organizational response to supporting traumatized emergency and relief workers is the recognition of the volunteer or "civilian" status of the majority of service workers. Research that examines risk and distress in active-duty emergency service personnel, particularly after a large-scale, highly publicized event, may misrepresent the experience of the larger population of local, volunteer service personnel (Moran & Britton, 1994). Many domestic disaster response programs depend on community volunteers (Red Cross volunteers, volunteer firefighters, community crime prevention programs, etc.). In addition, the vast majority of relief and development workers serving in areas of complex humanitarian emergencies are actually citizens of that country of service. Emergency workers responding to a disaster in their own community come to "work" each day with the knowledge that their own family or loved ones may be at risk. In a context of limited resources, working for an aid agency may actually limit access to certain goods and services (so that the organization avoids the risk of conflict of interest). The local emergency or relief staff person also has to deal with his or her own personal exposure to the critical event. In addition, if a new danger arises, local staff are not "sent home"; they are already home. Organizations face a complex set of financial and ethical dilemmas when establishing policy for this critical resource in emergency or relief response.

Early Clinical Intervention

Research examining early interventions suggests that early clinical interventions may be best suited for a select subset of individuals exposed to critical events (Litz, et al., 2002). Levels of posttraumatic distress in emergency service or relief workers are strongly associated with the traumatic incident or post-incident variables. Managers and clinicians involved in posttrauma intervention should screen workers for severity of the incident and initial, peri-traumatic psychological adjustment which contribute significantly to levels of PTSD distress (Hodgins et al., 2001).

The limited literature examining early intervention methodology has not demonstrated the efficacy of any particular model for this population of service workers. In fact, it would be difficult to suggest a circumscribed intervention strategy to respond to the needs of emergency service and relief personnel. These workers represent diverse organizational cultures, as well as cultures of origin. Instead, Raphael and Ursano (2002) recommend a set of core elements to be incorporated into early intervention methods: (1) "sharing and making meaning of experiences," (2) "trauma and loss," and (3) "learning" (pp. 346–347). The first element of sharing emphasizes the importance of talking about the experience. An early intervention should offer the individual or group an opportunity to express thoughts, memories, and experiences related to the event. Perhaps the benefit of talking is reflected in the strong evidence of social support as a resilience factor and preferred coping strategy in response to emergency and relief work related traumatic exposure. The second element for early intervention hinges on the issue of screening for severity and type of exposure to trauma and allowing appropriate timing for intervention. Those reporting bereavement and significant traumatic threat can be considered at higher risk for distress and therefore may be part of a group offered appropriately timed mental health intervention.

The final, basic element Raphael and Ursano (2002) suggest for early intervention, "learning," underscores the benefits of education in the aftermath of the event. An operational type of debriefing can identify areas of emergency response that were executed well, as well as areas for continued growth. The information provided in early intervention can also educate staff about common traumatic responses, helpful coping methods, and avoidance of harmful coping mechanisms (e.g., recognizing the risk of excessive alcohol use in humanitarian aid and rescue workers; Cardozo & Salama, 2002; North et al., 2002).

The early intervention procedures for emergency and relief personnel that have been described in published literature vary across service type and organization. Models for emergency service can follow a strict debriefing framework, or a brief cognitive-behavioral treatment approach (Rowan, 2002; Ruzek, 2002; Schwerin et al., 2002) Two models described by humanitarian aid organizations emphasize flexibility; there are established elements of response that are tailored to the specific context of the emergency. The interventions can include both debriefing and cognitive-behavioral treatment models, but debriefing is not conceived as a single-session, one-size-fits-all model (Fawcett, 2002; van Gelder & van den Berkhof, 2002). In fact, a humanitarian aid team is often made up of persons from a number of different cultures, which requires flexibility and sensitivity in creating culturally relevant interventions.

Recommendations for Further Research

Researchers face several areas of challenge in order to implement the randomized, controlled trials necessary to identify effective early intervention strategies for emergency and relief personnel. First, the urgency of the critical event itself must not circumvent the necessity of systematic, preintervention assessment. This will require a significant commitment on the part of the researchers, the organization, and the service personnel to invest in the work of outcome research in the midst of high organizational demands. When intervention is offered, the selection criteria for participation should be clearly outlined. Key risk and resilience factors may be part of the strategy for offering different types service to subgroups of personnel. Each aspect of intervention should also include pre- and postassessment. McFarlane (1988) and Marmar et al. (1999) have identified the potential chronic nature of emotional distress in emergency service personnel. Follow-up assessments for service workers who participate in early interventions would provide valuable information regarding the expression of distress over time and, ideally, the mitigating effects of successful early intervention.

The current research on epidemiology, risk, and resilience provides a rich foundation for the next step of randomized controlled trials. However, providing effective early intervention to emergency service and relief personnel creates an intriguing conundrum: Successful treatment allows for more exposure to trauma. Empirical research needs to inform the multiple levels of opportunity for intervention: at selection, during training, in the midst of exposure to critical incidents, and through organizational management. Helping the helpers is a long-term commitment.

REFERENCES

Ager, A., Flapper, E., van Pietersom, T., & Simon, W. (2002). Supporting and equipping national and international humanitarian non-governmental organizations and their workers. In Y. Danieli (Ed.), *Sharing the front line and the back hills: Peacekeepers, humanitarian aid workers and the media in the midst of crisis* (pp. 194–200). Amityville, NY: Baywood.

Alexander, D. A., & Klein, S. (2001). Ambulance personnel and critical incidents: Impact of accident and emergency work on mental health and emotional well-being. *British Journal of Psychiatry, 178,* 76–81.

Alexander, D. A., & Wells, A. (1991). Reactions of police officers to body-handling after a major disaster: A before-and-after comparison. *British Journal of Psychiatry, 159,* 547–555.

Beaton, R., Murphy, S., Johnson, C., Pike, K., & Corneil, W. (1998). Exposure to duty-related incident stressors in urban firefighters and paramedics. *Journal of Traumatic Stress, 11*(4), 821–828.

Bisson, J. I., McFarland, A. C., & Rose, S. (2000). Psychological debriefing. In E. B. Foa, T. M. Keane, & M. J. Friedman (Eds.), *Effective treatments for PTSD* (pp. 39–59). New York: Guilford Press.

Boxer, P. A., & Wild, D. (1993). Psychological distress and alcohol use among firefighters. *Scandinavian Journal of Environmental Health, 19,* 121–125.

Brown, J., Fielding, J., & Grover, J. (1999). Distinguishing traumatic, vicarious, and routine operational stressor exposure and attendant adverse consequences in a sample of police officers. *Work and Stress, 13*(4), 312–325.

Bryant, R. A., & Harvey, A. G. (1995). Posttraumatic stress in volunteer firefighters: Predictors of distress. *Journal of Nervous and Mental Disease, 183*(4), 267–271.

Bryant, R. A., & Harvey, A. G. (1996). Posttraumatic stress reactions in volunteer firefighters. *Journal of Traumatic Stress, 9*(1), 51–62.

Bryant, R. A., Harvey, A. G., Dang, S., Sackville, T., & Basten, C. (1998). Treatment of acute stress disorder: A comparison of cognitive-behavioral therapy and supportive counseling. *Journal of Consulting and Clinical Psychology, 66,* 862–866.

Bryant, R. A., Sackville, T., Dang, S. T., Moulds, M., & Guthrie, R. (1999). Treating acute stress disorder: An evaluation of cognitive-behavioral therapy and counseling techniques. *American Journal of Psychiatry, 156,* 1780–1786.

Burns, C., & Harm, N. J. (1993). Emergency nurses' perceptions of critical incidents and stress debriefing. *Journal of Emergency Nursing, 19*(5), 431–436.

Cardozo, B. L., & Salama, P. (2002). Mental health of humanitarian aid workers in complex emergencies. In Y. Danieli (Ed.), *Sharing the front line and the back hills: Peacekeepers, humanitarian aid workers and the media in the midst of crisis* (pp. 242–255). Amityville, NY: Baywood.

Carlier, I. V. E., Lamberts, R. D., & Gersons, B. P. R. (1997). Risk factors for posttraumatic stress symptomatology in police officers: A prospective analysis. *Journal of Nervous and Mental Disease, 185*(8), 498–506.

Carlier, I. V. E., Lamberts, R. D., & Gersons, B. P. R. (2000). The dimensionality of trauma: A multidimensional scaling comparison of police officers with and without posttraumatic stress disorder. *Psychiatry Research, 97,* 29–39.

Centers for Disease Control and Prevention. (2002). Injuries and illnesses among New York City fire department rescue workers after responding to the World Trade Center attacks. *Morbidity and Mortality Weekly Report: Special Issue, 51,* 1–5.

Corneil, W., Beaton, R., Murphy, S., Johnson, C., & Pike, K. (1999). Exposure to traumatic incidents and prevalence of posttraumatic stress symptomatology in urban firefighters in two countries. *Journal of Occupational Health Psychology, 4*(2), 131–141.

Danieli, Y. (Ed.). (2002). *Sharing the front line and the back hills: Peacekeepers, humanitarian aid workers and the media in the midst of crisis.* Amityville, NY: Baywood.

Deahl, M., Srinivasan, M., Jones, N., Thomas, J., Neblett, C., & Jolly, A. (2000). Preventing psychological trauma in soldiers: The role of operational stress training and psychological debriefing. *British Journal of Medical Psychology, 73,* 77–85.

Dougall, A. L., Herberman, H. B., Delahanty, D. L., Inslicht, S. S., & Baum, A. (2000). Similarity of prior trauma exposure as a determinant of chronic stress responding to an airline disaster. *Journal of Consulting and Clinical Psychology, 68*(2), 290–295.

Dougall, A. L., Hyman, K. B, Hayward, M. C., McFeeley, S., & Baum, A. (2001). Optimism and traumatic stress: The importance of social support and coping. *Journal of Applied Social Psychology, 31*(2), 223–245.

Epstein, R. S., Fullerton, C. S., & Ursano, R. J. (1998). Posttraumatic stress disorder following an air disaster: A prospective study. *American Journal of Psychiatry, 155*(7), 934–938.

Eriksson, C. B., Vande Kemp, H., Gorsuch, R., Hoke, S., & Foy, D. W. (2001). Trauma exposure and PTSD symptoms in international relief and development personnel. *Journal of Traumatic Stress, 14*(1), 205–212.

Fawcett, J. (2002). Preventing broken hearts, healing broken minds. In Y. Danieli (Ed.), *Sharing the front line and the back hills: Peacekeepers, humanitarian aid workers and the media in the midst of crisis* (pp. 223–232). Amityville, NY: Baywood.

Foy, D. W., Eriksson, C. B., & Trice, G. A. (2001). Introduction to group interventions for trauma survivors. *Group Dynamics: Theory, Research and Practice, 5*, 246–251.

Gibbs, M. S., Drummond, J., & Lackenmeyer, J. R. (1993). Effects of disasters on emergency workers: A review, with implications for training and postdisaster interventions. *Journal of Social Behavior and Personality, 8*(5), 189–212.

Grieger, T. A., Staab, J. P., Cardena, E., McCarroll, J. E., Brandt, G. T., Fullerton, C. S., & Ursano, R. J. (2000). Acute stress disorder and subsequent posttraumatic stress disorder in a group of exposed disaster workers. *Depression and Anxiety, 11*, 183–184.

Gulliver, S., Knight, J., Munroe, J., Wolfsdorf, B., Baker-Morrissette, S., & Mattuchio, T. (2002, November). *Secondary trauma in disaster relief clinicians at ground zero.* Paper presented at the 18th annual meeting of the International Society for Traumatic Stress Studies, Baltimore, MD.

Hodgins, G. A., Creamer, M., & Bell, R. (2001). Risk factors for posttrauma reactions in police officers: A longitudinal study. *Journal of Nervous and Mental Disease, 189*(8), 541–547.

Holtz, T. H., Salama, P., Cardozo, B. L., & Gotway, C. A. (2002). Mental health status of human rights workers, Kosovo, June 2000. *Journal of Traumatic Stress, 15*(5), 389–395.

Johnsen, B. H., Eid, J., Lovstad, T., & Michelson, L. T. (1997). Posttraumatic stress symptoms in nonexposed, victims, and spontaneous rescuers after an avalanche. *Journal of Traumatic Stress, 10*(1), 133–140.

Jones, D. R. (1985). Secondary disaster victims: The emotional effects of recovering and identifying human remains. *American Journal of Psychiatry, 142*(3), 303–307.

Leffler, C. T., & Dembert, M.L. (1998). Posttraumatic stress symptoms among U.S. Navy divers recovering TWA flight 800. *Journal of Nervous and Mental Disease, 186*(9), 574–577.

Litz, B. T., Gray, M. J., Bryant, R. A., & Adler, A. B. (2002). Early interventions for trauma: Current status and future directions. *Clinical Psychology: Science and Practice, 9*, 112–134.

Marmar, C. R., Weiss, D. S., Metzler, T. J., DeLucchi, K. L., Best, S. R., & Wentworth, K. A. (1999). Longitudinal course and predictors of continuing distress following critical incident exposure in emergency services personnel. *Journal of Nervous and Mental Disease, 187*(1), 15–22.

Marmar, C. R., Weiss, D. S., Metzler, T. J., Ronfeldt, H. M., & Foreman, C. (1996). Stress responses of emergency services personnel to the Loma Prieta earthquake interstate 880 freeway collapse and control traumatic incidents. *Journal of Traumatic Stress, 9*(1), 63–85.

McCall, M., & Salama, P. (1999). Selection, training, and support of relief workers: An occupational health issue. *British Medical Journal, 318*, 113–116.

McFarlane, A. C. (1988). The longitudinal course of posttraumatic morbidity: The range of outcomes and their predictors. *Journal of Nervous and Mental Disease, 176*(1), 30–40.

Mitchell, J. T. (1983). When disaster strikes. . . The critical incident stress debriefing process. *Journal of Emergency Medical Services, 8*(1), 36–39.

Moran, C., & Britton, N. R. (1994). Emergency work experience and reactions to traumatic incidents. *Journal of Traumatic Stress, 7*(4), 575–585.

Neria, Y., & Solomon, Z. (2000). Prevention of posttraumatic reactions: Debriefing and frontline treatment. In P.A. Saigh & J.D. Bremner (Eds.), *Posttraumatic stress disorder: A comprehensive text* (pp. 309–326). Boston: Allyn & Bacon.

Neylan, T. C., Metzler, T. J., Best, S. R., Weiss, D. S., Fagan, J. A., Liberman, A., Rogers, C., Vedantham, K., Brunet, A., Lipsey, T. L., & Marmar, C. R. (2002). Critical incident exposure and sleep quality in police officers. *Psychosomatic Medicine, 64,* 345–352.

North, C. S., Tivis, L., McMillen, J. C., Pfefferbaum, B., Spitznagel, E. L, Cox, J., Nixon, S., Bunch, K., & Smith, E. (2002). Psychiatric disorders in rescue workers after the Oklahoma City bombing. *American Journal of Psychiatry 159*(5), 857–859.

Pole, N., Best, S. R., Weiss, D. S., Metzler, T., Liberman, A. M., Fagan, J., & Marmar, C. R. (2001). Effects of gender and ethnicity on duty-related posttraumatic stress symptoms among urban police officers. *Journal of Nervous and Mental Disease, 189*(7), 442–448.

Raphael, B., & Ursano, R. (2002) Psychological debriefing. In Y. Danieli (Ed.), *Sharing the front line and the back hills: Peacekeepers, humanitarian aid workers and the media in the midst of crisis* (pp. 343–352). Amityville, NY: Baywood.

Rowan, A. B. (2002). Air Force critical incident stress management outreach with Pentagon staff after the terrorist attack. *Military Medicine, 167,* 33–35.

Ruzek, J. I. (2002). "Brief Education and Support" for emergency response workers: An alternative to debriefing. *Military Medicine, 167,* 73–75.

Schwerin, M. J., Kennedy, K., & Wardlaw, M. (2002). Counseling support within the Navy Mass Casualty Assistance Team post-September 11. *Military Medicine, 167,* 76–78.

Sloan, I. H., Rozensky, R. H., Kaplan, L., & Saunders, S. M. (1994). A shooting incident in an elementary school: Effects of worker stress on public safety, mental health, and medical personnel. *Journal of Traumatic Stress, 7*(4), 565–574.

Smith, B. (2002). The dangers of aid work. In Y. Danieli (Ed.), *Sharing the front line and the back hills: Peacekeepers, humanitarian aid workers and the media in the midst of crisis* (pp. 171–176). Amityville, NY: Baywood.

Smith, B., Agger, I., Danieli, Y., & Weisaeth, L. (1996). Emotional responses of international humanitarian aid workers: The contribution of non-governmental organizations. In Y. Danieli, N. Rodley, & L. Weisaeth (Eds.), *International responses to traumatic stress: Humanitarian, human rights, justice, peace and development contributions, collaborative actions, and future initiatives* (pp. 397–423). Amityville, NY: Baywood.

Turner, C. (1998, August 2). Humanitarian U.N. work is risky business. *The Los Angeles Times,* pp. A1, A8, A9.

Ursano, R. J., Fullerton, C. S., Kao, T., & Bhartiya, V. R. (1995). Longitudinal assessment of posttraumatic stress disorder and depression after exposure to traumatic death. *Journal of Nervous and Mental Disease, 183*(1), 36–42.

van Gelder, P., & van den Berkhof, R. (2002). Psychological care for humanitarian aid workers: The Médecins Sans Frontières Holland Experience. In Y. Danieli (Ed.), *Sharing the front line and the back hills: Peacekeepers, humanitarian aid workers and the media in the midst of crisis* (pp. 179–185). Amityville, NY: Baywood.

Weiss, D. S., Marmar, C. R., Metzler, T. J., & Ronfeldt, H. M. (1995). Predicting symptomatic distress in emergency services personnel. *Journal of Consulting and Clinical Psychology, 63*(3), 361–368.

13

Evaluating and Treating Injured Trauma Survivors in Trauma Care Systems

DOUGLAS ZATZICK
AMY WAGNER

$\mathbf{N}$atural or man-made disasters, motor vehicle crashes, and violent trauma all entail the threat of physical injury. In the United States, approximately 37 million individuals visit emergency departments each year after sustaining traumatic injuries (Bonnie, Fulco, & Liverman, 1999). Approximately 2.5 million Americans sustain injuries so severe that they require inpatient hospitalization (Bonnie et al., 1999; McCaig, 1994; Rice, MacKenzie, & Associates, 1989). In 1987, injuries accounted for 12% of medical expenditures in the United States (Miller, Galbraith, Lestina, & Viano, 1994). From a global perspective, approximately 16% of the world's burden of disease is attributable to traumatic injuries (Krug, Sharma, & Lozano, 2000).

Most patients injured in the United States receive their initial treatment via the trauma care system—a system is an organized and coordinated effort in a defined geographic area designated to deliver care to injured trauma victims (Bonnie et al., 1999). Care begins immediately after the injury and includes paramedic and ambulance service, emergency department triage, and inpatient hospitalization. Trauma centers are acute care hospitals designed to treat emergent medical complications related to physical injury. Level I trauma centers are designated and equipped to care for the most severely injured patients, while level II–IV centers are designed to treat less severely injured patients. After the acute care episode, injured patients continue on to receive surgical and primary care outpatient services and are ultimately rehabilitated in the community; these outpatient and community services constitute the rehabilitative component of the trauma care system.

The events of 9-11 reinforce the importance of systematically addressing the treatment needs of injured trauma survivors who receive their treatment within trauma care systems. The Centers for Disease Control report that within 48 hours of the attack, 1,103 physically injured survivors were seen at five Manhattan trauma centers/hospitals (Centers for Disease Control and Prevention, 2002). Over 15% of these trauma survivors were so severely injured that they required inpatient hospital admission. From a mental health perspective, injured trauma patients triaged in acute care medical settings after a mass attack are high risk for posttraumatic psychiatric complications. Recent consensus guidelines recommend that injured trauma survivors who receive medical/surgical attention after a mass attack undergo early mental health screening and evaluation procedures (National Institute of Mental Health, 2002). Although physical injuries incurred from mass violence highlight the need for special public health approaches to secondary prevention, physical injuries of any kind incurred during a traumatic event should trigger an in-hospital mental health strategy to evaluate risk and provide early intervention, when appropriate. Indeed, we argue that mental health screening and evaluation procedures established, tested, and honed in acute care settings are useful models for the care required after larger-scale mass violence events.

The reason that the mental health needs of any injured patient require special attention is that trauma exposure, when coupled with physical injury, carries a markedly elevated risk for the development of posttraumatic stress disorder (PTSD; e.g., Abenhaim, Dab, & Salmi, 1992; Green, 1993; Helzer, Robins, & McEvoy, 1987; Koren et al., 2002). Between 10 and 40% of U.S. civilians admitted to the hospital after sustaining intentional injuries (e.g., injuries associated with human malice such as physical assaults) and unintentional injuries (e.g., motor vehicle crashes and job-related injuries) may go on to develop symptoms consistent with a diagnosis of PTSD (Blanchard et al., 1996; Holbrook, Anderson, Sieber, Browner, & Hoyt, 1999; Michaels et al., 1998; Ursano et al., 1999; Zatzick et al., 2001). Variations in rates of PTSD have been reported across injured populations ranging from less than 5% in European survivors of unintentional injuries (Malt, 1988; Schnyder, Moergeli, Klaghofer, & Buddeberg, 2001) to 10–30% among trauma survivors in Australia, England, and Israel (Harvey & Bryant, 1998; Mayou, Bryant, & Duthie, 1993; Shalev, Peri, Canetti, & Schreiber, 1996).

PTSD is frequently characterized by multiple, comorbid conditions (Kessler, Sonnega, Bromet, Hughes, & Nelson, 1995). For example, PTSD is often comorbid with depressive symptoms (Blanchard, Hickling, Taylor, & Loos, 1995; Holbrook et al., 1999; Shalev et al., 1998; Zatzick et al., 2002). As with other populations exposed to trauma, injured patients with PTSD and depression report more frequent and intense somatic symptoms (Zatzick, Russo, & Katon, in press). In addition, it has been reported that between 20 and 55% of trauma survivors hospitalized on surgical wards may meet diagnostic criteria for current or lifetime substance abuse or dependence (e.g., Li, 2000; Soderstrom et al., 1997).

In veterans (e.g., Zatzick, Marmar, et al., 1997; Zatzick, Weiss, et al., 1997), refugees (Mollica et al., 1999), and physically injured civilians (Greenspan & Kellermann, 2002; Holbrook et al., 1999; Michaels et al., 1999; Zatzick, Jurkovich, Gentilello, Wisner, & Rivara, 2002), PTSD makes a unique contribution to posttraumatic functional limitations and diminished quality of life above and beyond the impact of injury severity and comorbid medical conditions. For example, in a representative sample of physically injured trauma survivors, PTSD 1 year after the injury was the strongest independent predictor of impairments in role, social, and emotional functions at 1 year (Zatzick, Jurkovich, et al., 2002).

Thus, early interventions that address the secondary prevention of PTSD after traumatic injury may be an essential component of public health efforts targeting injury control (Bonnie et al., 1999). Although there is a growing body of evidence to support cognitive-behavioral therapy (CBT) as a secondary prevention intervention (Bryant, Harvey, Dang, Sackville, & Basten, 1998; Foa, Hearst-Ikeda, & Perry, 1995), there are no randomized controlled trials of any psychological or psychopharmacological intervention specifically tailored to meet the early intervention needs of physically injured trauma survivors. We now share a conceptual framework that can guide future controlled early intervention research in the acute care medical context. This framework is derived from a quality of care paradigm frequently employed in mental health services research.

EARLY INTERVENTIONS THAT INCORPORATE THE INSTITUTE OF MEDICINE'S QUALITY-OF-CARE CRITERIA

Although effective psychotherapeutic and psychopharmacological treatments for PTSD have been developed, these intervention strategies, and the guidelines that describe them, have yet to be translated to injured trauma survivors treated within trauma care systems (Zatzick, Roy-Byrne, et al., 2001). The Institute of Medicine (IOM) has published quality-of-care criteria that are explicitly designed to influence the development of health care interventions in the United States (Committee on Quality of Health Care in America, 2001).

According to the IOM, high-quality care must be evidence-based—that is, founded on the best scientific knowledge available (Committee on Quality of Health Care in America, 2001). This is consistent with the general consensus that clinicians should only employ early interventions for trauma that have sufficiently rigorous evidence to support their efficacy (e.g., Litz, Gray, Bryant, & Adler, 2002). A body of mental health efficacy research that aims to maximize the internal validity of investigations is derived from the evidence-based paradigm. The requisite elements of rigorous controlled efficacy research include random allocation of participants, state-of-the-art diagnostic assessment methods, the delivery of standardized treatments with treatment integrity/quality checks, and independent blind outcome assessment (e.g., Foa & Meadows, 1997).

Patients treated within trauma care systems are remarkably heterogeneous with regard to injury, demographic, and clinical characteristics (Figure 13.1). This heterogeneity begins with patient background characteristics and injury type, cause, and severity and extends to postinjury clinical characteristics and trajectory. The end result is a service delivery sector with multiple, complex contextual variables that may prove daunting for trials that aim to exclusively maximize internal validity (Figure 13.1). Thus, a challenge for future early intervention trials conducted within trauma care systems is to simultaneously maximize standards for internal and external validity (Hoagwood, Burns, Kiser, Ringeisen, & Schoenwald, 2001; Schoenwald & Hoagwood, 2001).

In addition to being evidence-based, the IOM criteria also mandate that health care delivered in the United States be equitable and patient-centered (Committee on Quality of Health Care in America, 2001). Equitable care suggests a population-based approach that does not discriminate in the delivery of medical resources because of socioeconomic, ethnocultural, or gender-related criteria.

Patient-centered care is customized to meet patients' needs, incorporate patients' values, and allow patients to share knowledge and information and participate in decision making (Charles, Gafni, & Whelan, 1999; Emanuel & Emanuel, 1992; Zatzick, Kang, et al., 2001). The IOM criteria explicitly state that high-quality, patient-centered care builds on the foundation of a continuous healing relationship. Providing continuous care from inpatient settings through outpatient clinics and community rehabilitation has been a concentrated focus in the movement toward patient-centered care delivery (Ellers &

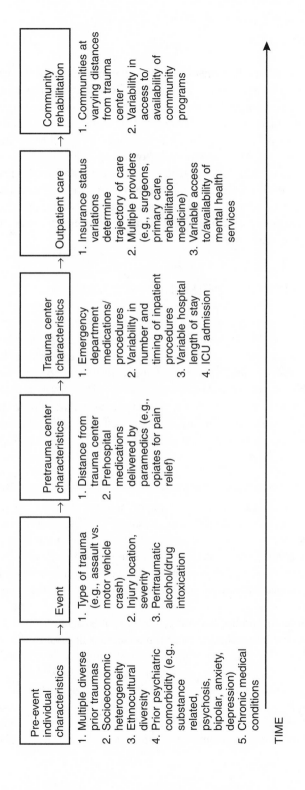

FIGURE 13.1. Injury, demographic, and clinical characteristics that contribute to the heterogeneity of patients treated in trauma care systems.

Walker, 1993). Finally, high-quality care, according to the IOM, is also characterized as being collaborative; the IOM criteria explicitly state that clinicians and institutions should actively collaborate and communicate in order to ensure an appropriate exchange of information and coordination of care (Committee on Quality of Health Care in America, 2001). To date, few early intervention trials have developed methods for incorporating the IOM's multifaceted, patient-centeredness criteria. Next, we present a new method of customizing the care of physically injured trauma survivors. The elicitation, tracking, and targeting for amelioration of each patient's unique and evolving posttraumatic concerns constitute an initial step in meeting the IOM's patient-centered quality of care criteria.

ELICITING AND TRACKING POSTTRAUMATIC CONCERNS

A prerequisite to the delivery of patient-centered care is the development of an assessment approach that captures the unique needs and concerns of individual trauma survivors. Although epidemiological studies have shown physical injury to be a risk factor for PTSD, clinical needs assessment research is necessary to appreciate the varied and unique concerns of physically injured trauma survivors. Unfortunately, standardized psychiatric interviews and quality-of-life assessments are not up to the task because fixed-choice formats constrain participant response options (Gill & Feinstein, 1994; Villasenor & Waitzkin, 1999).

We developed a method of assessing patient's posttraumatic concerns that was based on procedures recommended by Kleinman, Eisenberg, and Good (1978) and advocates of clinimetric approaches to outcome and quality-of-life assessments (Feinstein, 1987; Gill & Feinstein, 1994). A series of brief, open-ended questions were developed that allowed patients an unconstrained opportunity to describe their posttraumatic illness experiences. Prior investigations with cancer and end-stage renal disease patients has found that asking broadly about concerns allowed patients to address both medical and non-medical aspects of their quality of life and illness experience (Bass et al., 1999; Spencer, Frank, & Mcguire, 1996; Wang, Cosby, Harris, & Liu, 1999). In addition, our focus on posttraumatic concerns resonated with prior qualitative investigations that have identified themes of disruption and preoccupation in the narratives of trauma survivors (Jenkins & Cofresi, 1998; Lifton, 1993; Uehara, Farris, Morelli, & Ishisaka, 2001; Waitzkin & Magana, 1997; Zatzick & Johnson, 1997).

Our goal was to generate questions that could be immediately interpretable, or "sensible" to the spectrum of surgical, primary care, and mental health providers who deliver posttraumatic care in a medical setting (Feinstein, 1987). With this in mind, three brief, open-ended questions regarding patients' posttraumatic concerns were conceived during multidisciplinary discussions that included a psychiatrist, psychologist, internist, and a consulting trauma surgery clinical nurse specialist, all of whom had clinical experience with trauma survivors. The items were comprehensible, face valid, and easy to use (Feinstein, 1987).

The three concern questions were: "Of all the things that have happened to you since you were injured, what concerns you the most?" "What about this worries you?" and "How concerning is this to you?" The first two questions were designed to elicit and explore the patient's concerns, whereas the third question was designed to allow the patient to rate the importance of each concern (Gill & Feinstein, 1994). For research purposes, the answers to these questions were transcribed verbatim, and themes were extracted from the narratives.

At 1, 4, and 12 months postinjury, 99% of a randomly selected cohort of injured trauma survivors expressed one or more concerns. Six categories of posttraumatic concerns were identified, with 73% of patients expressing physical health concerns, 58% psychological concerns, 53% work and finance concerns, 40% social concerns, 10% legal concerns, and 10% medical concerns over the course of a year (Zatzick, Kang, et al., 2001). The psychological concerns endorsed by the injured trauma survivors were diverse, including anxiety and depressive symptoms, substance abuse, concerns about personnel safety, and existential considerations in the wake of the trauma. The number of concerns expressed gradually decreased over time, which suggests that the trajectory of general complaints remit with the passage of time, similar to acute symptoms of PTSD (Zatzick, Kang, et al., 2001).

Most injured patients report clinically significant PTSD symptoms while they are in the hospital but at 1-year follow-up they frequently report that the distress derived solely from their PTSD symptoms was not serious enough to seek treatment (Kessler, 2000; Zatzick, 2003b). It has been established that patients have other pressing needs to attend to or with which they might need assistance (e.g., pain management, financial loss, legal problems, or disruptions in social networks; Zatzick, Kang, et al., 2001). This highlights the importance of eliciting and tracking needs and concerns. Early interventions that target only PTSD symptoms may fail to adequately engage injured trauma survivors who endorse multiple concerns. If injured trauma survivors are to be treated successfully using early intervention, then patient-centered treatments that address the full spectrum of posttraumatic suffering in physically injured trauma survivors must be developed and tested in randomized controlled trials.

INTRODUCING COLLABORATIVE CARE INTERVENTIONS
INTO TRAUMA CARE SYSTEMS

A fundamental tension can exist between patients' evolving posttraumatic needs and the concerns, values, and goals of medical providers, the trauma care system, and society. The resolution of these tensions in a clinical model of the patient–provider relationship is an overarching conceptual issue that can inform the development of early interventions for injured trauma survivors treated acutely within trauma care systems (Zatzick, 2003a).

For mental health professionals, acute stress disorder represents a debilitating disturbance that should be addressed with evidence-based secondary prevention interventions. From both a societal and provider perspective there is a strong impetus for effective treatment because PTSD is associated with a broad spectrum of functional disabilities, as noted earlier.

In contrast, for the individual patient, other non–mental health-related concerns may outweigh the initial posttraumatic focus of mental health professionals and society (Zatzick, Kang, et al., 2001). Mental health professionals may impose their value system by stressing early intervention to prevent chronic PTSD. This potentially paternalistic view of the patient–provider relationship threatens to undermine patient autonomy and ignores other potential posttraumatic concerns that may take priority over specific mental health treatments (Emanuel & Emanuel, 1992; Kessler, 2000; Zatzick, Kang, et al., 2001). At the other end of the spectrum is the idea that patients should be allowed to choose their own course of PTSD treatment, completely independent of guidance from mental health professionals. The drawback to this approach is that lack of knowledge of the condition and treatment may increase the probability of the patient developing chronic PTSD, which is extremely difficult to treat.

The collaborative care model addresses these tensions by framing posttraumatic care delivery as an ongoing deliberation between patient and provider in the context of an engaging helping relationship. A deliberation is defined as a discussion between patient and provider that serves to help the patient determine and choose the best health-related treatments/values that can be attained at a particular time point postevent (Emanuel & Emanuel, 1992).

Collaborative care is a disease-management strategy that seeks to find the optimal roles for primary care providers, specialists, and allied health professionals in the delivery of care for patients with psychiatric disorders and chronic medical conditions. Essential elements of collaborative care include shared patient–provider treatment planning, the provision of medical support services, such as case management, and the delivery of evidence-based PTSD treatments such as cognitive-behavioral therapies and pharmacological treatments.

A key feature of the collaborative approach is the mental health team's maintenance of a continuous helping relationship. The team performs an initial evaluation and then treats the patient longitudinally, facilitating care provision across service delivery sectors (e.g., acute care, primary care, and mental health specialty care). The collaborative team's central objective is to help patients understand why certain health-related decisions, and the values that underlie them, are advantageous to the patient. The collaborative team may therefore deliberate with the patient around multiple areas of concern such as the long-term risk of functional impairment related to chronic PTSD, or the prevention of high-risk behaviors such as alcohol intoxication that may lead to injury recurrence.

Previous investigation suggests that collaborative interventions can improve clinical outcomes for patients with complex, comorbid presentations, while flexibly integrating patients' perspectives into the delivery of care (Katon et al., 1999; Von Korff, Schaefer, Curry, & Wagner, 1997). Recent randomized trials have documented the effectiveness of collaborative care models for patients with depressive and anxiety disorders in primary care (Katon et al., 1996; Katon et al., 1999; Roy-Byrne, Katon, Cowley, & Russo, 2001; Unutzer et al., 2002). It makes sense that early intervention for trauma provided in a similar vein could be successful; however, this is an issue that needs to be resolved through future research.

ADDRESSING THE DELIVERY OF EQUITABLE CARE THROUGH STEPPED COLLABORATIVE CARE

Population-based care implies delivering optimal care to injured trauma survivors treated within trauma care systems. In a system with unlimited resources, this would be a relatively straightforward process. However, medical resources are limited within trauma care systems, with demand for care far exceeding ability to provide service.

Prior longitudinal investigations demonstrate that a substantial percentage of patients initially symptomatic with PTSD spontaneously remit over the course of the year postinjury (Mayou, Tyndel, & Bryant, 1997; Rothbaum & Foa, 1994; Shalev et al., 1996; Zatzick, Kang, et al., 2002). This suggests that a stepped-care approach to posttraumatic interventions is indicated. Stepped care involves the allocation of increasingly greater resources to patients who do not remit spontaneously or respond to initial, low-intensity interventions (Katon et al., 1999). In addition, a stepped-care approach may simultaneously address the unique needs of the individual trauma survivor while also taking into consideration the mandate to equitably distribute limited mental health resources to all patients treated within a trauma care system.

AN EXAMPLE OF A COLLABORATIVE INTERVENTION FOR INJURED TRAUMA SURVIVORS TREATED WITHIN TRAUMA CARE SYSTEMS

Our group has conducted two pilot intervention trials designed to assess specific components of a collaborative intervention (Zatzick, Roy-Byrne, et al., 2001; Zatzick, Russo, et al., 2002). The first investigation was conducted at the UC Davis Medical Center (UCD) level 1 academic trauma center. The investigation was a pilot randomized controlled trial of a 4-month-long collaborative intervention (Zatzick, Roy-Byrne, et al., 2001). The rationale for the design of the investigation was strongly influenced by the results of a 1999 study by Gentillelo et al. (1999). This work demonstrated that a PhD-level, trauma center-based clinician could successfully deliver a brief motivational interviewing intervention that was found to reduce posttraumatic alcohol use and injury recurrence. The UCD pilot sought to establish the feasibility of having seasoned trauma center workers deliver a brief intervention that targeted PTSD symptoms and alcohol use.

Three highly experienced, multidisciplinary providers were the interventionists for the study. On a surgical ward, each patient was assigned to an interventionist who met each patient at his or her bedside. To establish a basis for collaborative problem definition and shared patient–provider treatment planning, the trauma support specialists were instructed to elicit and track patients' posttraumatic concerns. The interventionists also received a 4-hour training in the delivery of psychoeducational interventions for PTSD and cognitive-behavioral interventions for alcohol treatment.

To better understand factors that served to modify the delivery of the collaborative intervention, a clinical ethnographic component used in past studies was attached to the initial pilot intervention (Zatzick & Johnson, 1997). The principal investigator supervised the collection of extensive logs by each of the study's interventionists and also took extensive notes when conducting clinical activities and reviewing intervention cases. These logs were then used to augment quantitative data derived from standardized assessments.

A total of 105 patients were screened for study participation. Of the 57 patients randomly approached for the protocol, 8 refused participation. Eleven subjects completed the interview but were discharged before they could be enrolled in the clinical trial, leaving 34 patients in the trial. Sixteen subjects were assigned to the collaborative care intervention and 18 subjects were assigned to the usual care control group. The investigation was able to follow up over

75% of the participants at 4-month follow-up and 88% of patients had data from at least two time points.

Levels of PTSD symptoms were assessed using the civilian version of the Post-Traumatic Stress Disorder Checklist (PCL-C; Weathers, Huska, & Keane, 1991). The Center for Epidemiological Studies Depression Scale was used to assess depressive symptoms (Radloff, 1977). Alcohol and drug use at the time of the traumatic event was assessed with blood alcohol and urine toxicology screens. Because alcohol intoxication is a risk factor for recurrent traumatic injury (Hingson, Heeren, Jamanka, & Howland, 2000; Rivara, Koepsell, Jurkovich, Gurney, & Soderberg, 1993), patient self-reports of drinking to the point of intoxication were assessed with a single item from the Addiction Severity Index (ASI; McLellan, Luborsky, Woody, & Obrien, 1980).

Trauma support specialists spent an average of 90 minutes per patient delivering the intervention over the course of the 4-month study. Examination of trauma support specialists' logs and field notes revealed that 75% of the patient contact occurred between hospital admission and 1-month follow-up, while 25% of patient contact occurred between 1 and 4 months. Virtually all the surgical ward contact occurred as face-to-face counseling, while after hospital discharge the vast majority of contacts with the patient, family members, and surgical and primary care providers were over the telephone. Review of study logs revealed that patients' posttraumatic concerns were frequently discussed during multidisciplinary team meetings and targeted for amelioration by the trauma support specialists.

Comparisons of PTSD symptom levels between the intervention and control groups reflected the variations in the intensity of the intervention. From the time of the surgical ward admission through the 1-month follow-up, intervention subjects had significantly decreased PTSD symptoms when compared to controls. From the 1-month through the 4-month follow-up assessments, intervention patients' symptoms significantly increased relative to controls. Comparisons of depressive symptom levels between the intervention and control groups revealed similar results. There was no significant difference between the two groups with regard to drinking to the point of intoxication.

PILOTING OF THE COLLABORATIVE INTERVENTION WITH AN EMBEDDED COGNITIVE-BEHAVIORAL COMPONENT FOR POSTTRAUMATIC STRESS DISORDER

Our research group is currently conducting a second, larger-scale pilot study of the collaborative intervention that incorporates an evidence-based cognitive-behavioral intervention module (Zatzick, Russo, et al., 2002). The Trauma Survivors Outcomes and Support Study (TSOS) is a 12-month, stepped, collaborative care intervention conducted at the University of Washington's Harborview Level 1 Trauma Center (Harborview). This study is ongoing and aims to reduce PTSD symptoms in randomly selected, injured trauma survivors. The collaborative intervention begins with population-based screening for posttraumatic disturbances in the surgical inpatient ward (Step I). Next, a master's-level trauma support specialist meets symptomatic injured patients in the trauma ward and continues care during the days and weeks postinjury (Step II). Step II also includes a more in-depth assessment that elicits both posttraumatic concerns and PTSD symptoms, with the aim of developing a comprehensive treatment plan. Evidence-based psychotherapeutic and psychopharmacological treatments are delivered in Step III (1–3 months postinjury). Step IV (3–12 months postinjury) extends treatment to individuals with recalcitrant symptoms while also attempting to link injured patients to community resources that will facilitate ongoing physical and mental rehabilitation. Table 13.1 outlines the stepped-care approach.

To more directly treat PTSD symptoms, the collaborative intervention incorporates a cognitive-behavioral therapy module, in addition to an algorithm-driven pharmacological module and supportive case management. The outcome literature indicates that CBT interventions that incorporate the principles of exposure (imaginal and *in vivo*), response prevention, cognitive restructuring, and relaxation training are the most efficacious in the reduction of PTSD symptoms (Foa & Meadows, 1997). Further, some data suggest that these approaches significantly reduce comorbid conditions such as depression (Foa et al., 1995). Given the stepped approach to care, and recent data supporting the efficacy of short-term adaptations of exposure-based interventions (Bryant et al., 1998; Foa et al., 1995), our primary CBT intervention adheres closely to the formula used by Bryant et al. (1998) in their short-term treatment of acute stress disorder in recent survivors of motor vehicle and industrial accidents. The CBT treatment is designed to be delivered in four sessions by a trained nurse practitioner. If patients meet criteria for PTSD, CBT is also considered as an option for treatment 1–3 months postinjury (other options include medication, CBT that excludes imaginal exposure, or no treatment). Intervention does not begin until at least 1 month postinjury, as PTSD symptoms often naturally remit over time. Final determination of choice of treatment is based on deliberations between both the patient and the treatment provider, as well as the treatment provider and the broader treatment team.

To date, little research has examined the effectiveness of CBT for PTSD in real-world settings, despite the obvious and pressing need to do so (Litz et al., 2002). In our experience working in trauma centers and piloting this treatment approach, we have had to take into account many factors that can impede the delivery and effectiveness of CBT in recent injury survivors. Some of these

TABLE 13.1. Linking Stepped Collaborative Care to Quality Indicators within Trauma Care Systems

Step	Intervention components	Outcome/quality indicator
Step I (0–1 months)	Population-based screening	IOM equitable care criteria (Committee on Quality of Health Care in America, 2001)
Step II (0–1 months)	In-depth evaluation of symptomatic injured patients	In-depth evaluation for PTSD after injury as recommended by consensus conference guidelines (National Institute of Mental Health, 2002)
Step II (0–3 months)	Patient-centered trauma support • Continuous helping relationship • Posttraumatic concerns addressed • Care coordination across sectors	IOM patient-centered care criteria (Committee on Quality of Health Care in America, 2001)
Step III (1-3 months)	Delivery of evidence-based, guideline-level manualized treatments • CBT • Medications	• PTSD guidelines (Foa, Keane, & Friedman, 2000; Journal of Clinical Psychiatry Guidelines, 1999) • Trauma center treatment alcohol guidelines (P. Rostenberg, 1995) • IOM effectiveness criteria (Committee on Quality of Health Care in America, 2001)
Step III/IV (3–12 months)	Stepped-up care for patients who remain symptomatic Relapse prevention Community linkage	IOM effectiveness, patient-centeredness and efficiency criteria (Committee on Quality of Health Care in America, 2001)

factors were discussed earlier in the chapter with reference to the importance of assessing the full range of patients' concerns. We argued that treating the PTSD directly without considering other patient concerns may interfere with the development of an effective collaborative relationship (therapeutic alliance).

Additional factors may not be specifically identified by patients as concerns but nonetheless interfere with the delivery and effectiveness of the therapy. For example, the lives of many injury survivors are significantly disrupted following injury. They may experience significant changes in roles (e.g., temporary or permanent unemployment and assuming the "patient" role in families), they may be unable perform many of the tasks that they previously could (e.g., activities of daily living and pleasurable/meaningful activities), they may have significant financial stress, or they may be faced with ongoing and sometimes unpredictable medical procedures which can result in an uneven course of functional ability. Many patients manage ongoing physical pain with pain medication that can interfere with emotional and cognitive functioning. Further, substance abuse is common, afflicting up to half of injured trauma survivors in the United States (Soderstrom et al., 1997). In addition to PTSD, emotional reactions, including grief, anger, and depression, are also common among injury survivors. Likewise, physical injury can cause disfigurement, which can result in additional emotional reactions (e.g., loss, embarrassment, and frustration) and subsequent avoidance of people and activities.

These factors can impact the delivery and effectiveness of treatment (e.g., patients' ability to attend sessions and complete homework). Research suggests that effective exposure requires contact with traumatic cues and habituation to the cues (Jaycox, Foa, & Morral, 1998), and many of these factors would interfere with both (e.g., physical limitations or embarrassment over disfigurement may lead to avoidance; secondary emotions such as anger or guilt or substance use may interfere with habituation). Treatment is complicated even further by the fact that, as mentioned previously, many of the self-reported concerns of trauma survivors do not pertain to PTSD symptoms, even when they are objectively symptomatic. The discrepancy between subjective and objective problems can affect treatment compliance. Finally, it is important to note that the population of trauma survivors is heterogeneous. Traumatic injury affects all ethnic and cultural groups, age ranges, and socioeconomic classes. Thus, effective treatment must necessarily take into account the variety of factors that may maintain problems or interfere with change. As discussed, two aspects of our intervention directly address many of these issues: elicitation and attention to patient concerns occurs throughout the year postinjury; further, the deliberative process promotes patient understanding and compliance with any intervention, including CBT.

In addition, we have included the regular use of functional analyses to our CBT module to specifically assess the range of factors that can be related to the maintenance of PTSD symptoms in our population (in addition to standardized diagnostic instruments). This refers to a thorough assessment of the contextual, antecedent, and consequent circumstances that are directly related to the development and maintenance of the presenting problems. In any cognitive-behavioral therapy, functional analyses are the cornerstone of effective treatment planning (Goldfried & Davison, 1994), yet they are frequently dropped from standardized treatment protocols. This is because standardized treatments assume a standard, uncomplicated course, which, if it occurred in every instance would obviate the need for functional analyses.

However, individuals who have suffered traumatic injury in the real-world setting experience a number of unique factors related to the maintenance of their PTSD. We propose the reintroduction of functional analyses into protocol CBT treatment as a solution to the problems inherent in attempting to translate protocol treatments to the real-world setting. Functional analyses are used to develop individualized behavioral case formulations. These, in turn, guide minor modifications to our CBT protocol (Bryant et al., 1998). This approach is supported by Davison and others in the treatment of more complex patients and in the application of empirically supported treatments outside the laboratory (Davison, 2000; Newman, 2000).

The CBT module is consistent with the IOM, evidence-based, patient-centered, and equitable quality-of-care criteria in several key respects. First and foremost, the efficacy of CBT for PTSD is well established (Foa & Meadows, 1997). Second, the use of functional analyses in patient assessment and treatment planning is both patient-centered and equitable. As mentioned, functional analyses allow for the careful consideration of ideographic factors in case formulation and intervention, including ethnicity, culture, socioeconomic status, age, and specific life circumstances; this approach allows for the inclusion of all subgroups and can further individualize treatment within groups. The patient-centered nature of CBT is evident in additional aspects of the treatment. There is an emphasis in CBT on psychoeducation and orienting patients to the nature and purpose of interventions. This teaches patients strategies that they can then generalize to novel problems and situations, independent of the interventionist, thus promoting their overall well-being and inherent capabilities. Further, exposure-based interventions, particularly *in vivo* exposure, are tailored to the individual's unique goals for overcoming avoidance. The embedding of the CBT module within the larger collaborative approach with delivery by the same interventionist allows for the development of a continuous healing relationship with the patient. Finally, at every level in the intervention, collaboration and communication are emphasized. The CBT interventionists and supervisor routinely meet with the larger treatment team and treatment decisions are based on ongoing deliberations between team members. The CBT module described earlier is currently being tested in the randomized effectiveness design of the TSOS study.

FUTURE DIRECTIONS

In summary, no organized system of care exists for physically injured trauma survivors suffering from posttraumatic behavioral and emotional disturbances who are treated in the acute care medical sector. The results of pilot trials of the collaborative intervention suggest that these multifaceted interventions can be feasibly delivered within trauma care systems. Future investigations should develop and test high-quality, cost-effective, stepped collaborative care interventions that target trauma symptoms and a variety of functional impairments implicated by physical injury. Future research within trauma care systems should also link stepped care protocols to the rigorous development and assessment of quality indicators (Table 13.1). In this way evidence-based, patient-centered, population-based interventions for the secondary prevention of PTSD for injured victims of individual and mass events can be developed and tested within the context of the trauma care systems.

ACKNOWLEDGMENTS

Preparation of this chapter was supported in part by National Institute of Mental Health Grant No. 1K08 MH01610 and Centers for Disease Control Grant No. CCR303568.

REFERENCES

Abenhaim, L., Dab, W., & Salmi, L. R. (1992). Study of civilian victims of terrorist attacks (France 1982–1987). *Journal of Clinical Epidemiology, 45*, 103–109.

Bass, E. B., Jenckes, M. W., Fink, N. E., Cagney, K. A., Wu, A. W., Sadler, J. H., Meyer, K. B., Levey, A. S., & Powe, N. R. (1999). Use of focus groups to identify concerns about dialysis. *Medical Decision Making, 19*, 287–295.

Blanchard, E. B., Hickling, E. J., Taylor, A. E., & Loos, W. (1995). Psychiatric morbidity associated with motor vehicle accidents. *Journal of Nervous and Mental Disease, 183*, 495–504.

Blanchard, E. B., Hickling, E. J., Taylor, A. E., Loos, W., Forneris, C. A., & Jaccard, J. (1996). Who develops PTSD from motor vehicle accidents? *Behaviour Research and Therapy, 34*, 1–10.

Bonnie, R. J., Fulco, C. E., & Liverman, C. T. (1999). *Reducing the burden of injury: Advancing prevention and treatment.* Washington, DC: National Academy Press.

Bryant, R. A., Harvey, A. G., Dang, S. T., Sackville, T., & Basten, C. (1998). Treatment of acute stress disorder: A comparison of cognitive-behavioral therapy and supportive counseling. *Journal of Consulting Clinical Psychology, 66*, 862–866.

Centers for Disease Control and Prevention. (2002, January 11). Rapid assessment of injuries among survivors of the terrorist attack on the World Trade Center—New York City, September 2001. *Morbidity and Mortality Weekly Report, 51*, 1–4.

Charles, C., Gafni, A., & Whelan, T. (1999). Decision-making in the physician–patient encounter: Revisiting the shared treatment decision-making model. *Social Science and Medicine, 49*, 651–661.

Committee on Quality of Health Care in America. (2001). *Crossing the quality chasm:*

A new health system for the 21st century. Washington, DC: National Academy Press.

Davison, G. C. (2000). Stepped care: Doing more with less? *Journal of Consulting and Clinical Psychology, 68,* 580–585.

Ellers, B., & Walker, J. (1993). Facilitating the transition out of the hospital. In M. Gerteis, S. Edgman-Levitan, J. Daley, & T. Delbanco (Eds.), *Through the patient's eyes: Understanding and promoting patient-centered care* (pp. 204–226). San Francisco: Jossey-Bass.

Emanuel, E. J., & Emanuel, L. L. (1992). Four models of the patient-physician relationship. *The Journal of the American Medical Association, 267,* 2221–2226.

Feinstein, A. R. (1987). *Clinimetrics.* New Haven: Yale University Press.

Foa, E. B., Hearst-Ikeda, D., & Perry, K. J. (1995). Evaluation of a brief cognitive-behavioral program for the prevention of chronic PTSD in recent assault victims. *Journal of Consulting and Clinical Psychology, 63,* 948–955.

Foa, E. B., Keane, T. M., & Friedman, M. J. (2000). Guidelines for treatment of PTSD. *Journal of Traumatic Stress, 13,* 539–588.

Foa, E. B., & Meadows, E. A. (1997). Psychosocial treatments for posttraumatic stress disorder: A critical review. *Annual Review of Psychology, 48,* 449–480.

Gentilello, L. M., Rivara, F. P., Donovan, D. M., Jurkovich, G. J., Daranciang, E., Dunn, C. W., Villaveces, A., Copass, M., & Ries, R. R. (1999). Alcohol interventions in a trauma center as a means of reducing the risk of injury recurrence. *Annals of Surgery, 230,* 473–480.

Gill, T. M., & Feinstein, A. R. (1994). A critical appraisal of the quality of quality-of-life measurements. *Journal of the American Medical Association, 272,* 619–626.

Goldfried, M. R., & Davison, G. C. (1994). *Clinical behavior therapy.* New York: Wiley.

Green, B. L. (1993). Identifying survivors at risk. In J. P. Wilson & B. Raphael (Eds.), *International handbook of traumatic stress syndromes* (pp. 135–144). New York: Plenum Press.

Greenspan, A. I., & Kellermann, A. L. (2002). Physical and psychological outcomes 8 months after serious gunshot injury. *Journal of Trauma, 53,* 707–716.

Harvey, A. G., & Bryant, R. A. (1998). The relationship between acute stress disorder and posttraumatic stress disorder: A prospective evaluation of motor vehicle accident survivors. *Journal of Consulting and Clinical Psychology, 66,* 507–512.

Helzer, J. E., Robins, L. N., & McEvoy, L. (1987). Post-traumatic stress disorder in the general population: Findings of the epidemiological catchment area survey. *New England Journal of Medicine, 317,* 1630–1634.

Hingson, R., Heeren, T., Jamanka, A., & Howland, J. (2000). Age of drinking onset and unintentional injury involvement after drinking. *Journal of the American Medical Association, 284,* 1527–1533.

Hoagwood, K., Burns, B. J., Kiser, L., Ringeisen, H., & Schoenwald, S. K. (2001). Evidence-based practice in child and adolescent mental health services. *Psychiatric Services, 52,* 1179–1189.

Holbrook, T., Anderson, J., Sieber, W., Browner, D., & Hoyt, D. (1999). Outcome after major trauma: 12-month and 18 month follow-up results from the Trauma Recovery Project. *Journal of Trauma, 46,* 765–773.

Jaycox, L. H., Foa, E. B., & Morral, A. R. (1998). Influence of emotional engagement and habituation on exposure therapy for PTSD. *Journal of Consulting and Clinical Psychology, 66,* 185–192.

Jenkins, J., & Cofresi, N. (1998). The sociosomatic course of depression and trauma: A cultural analysis of resilience in the life of a Puerto Rican woman. *Psychosomatic Medicine, 60,* 439–447.

Journal of Clinical Psychiatry Guidelines. (1999). PTSD Expert consensus guidelines. *Journal of Clinical Psychiatry, 60*(Suppl. 16).

Katon, W., Robinson, P., Von Korff, M. V., Lin, E., Bush, T., Ludman, E., Simon, G., & Walker, E. (1996). A mulitfaceted intervention to improve treatment of depression in primary care. *Archives of General Psychiatry, 53,* 924–932.

Katon, W., Von Korff, M., Lin, E., Simon, G., Walker, E., Unutzer, J., Bush, T., Russo, J., & Ludman, E. (1999). Stepped collaborative care for primary care patients with persistent depression: A randomized trial. *Archives of General Psychiatry, 56,* 1109–1115.

Kessler, R. C. (2000). Posttraumatic stress disorder: The burden to the individual and society. *Journal of Clinical Psychiatry, 61*(Suppl. 5), 4–14.

Kessler, R. C., Sonnega, A., Bromet, E., Hughes, M., & Nelson, C. B. (1995). Posttraumatic stress disorder in the National Comorbidity Survey. *Archives of General Psychiatry, 52,* 1048–1060.

Kleinman, A., Eisenberg, L., & Good, B. (1978). Culture, illness, and care: Clinical lessons from anthropologic and cross-cultural research. *Annals of Internal Medicine, 88,* 251–258.

Koren, D., Tzarfati, A., Sheli-Vacnin, O., Mor, D., Goshen-Kita, Y., Ziv, L., & Klein, E. (2002, November 7–10). *Combat-related injury and PTSD: An event-based injured-control study.* Paper presented at the 18th annual meeting of Second Announcement, "Complex Psychological Trauma: Its Correlates and Effects," Baltimore, MD.

Krug, E., Sharma, G., & Lozano, R. (2000). The global burden of injuries. *American Journal of Public Health, 90,* 523–526.

Li, G. (2000). Epidemiology of substance abuse among trauma patients. *Trauma Quarterly, 14,* 353–364.

Lifton, R. J. (1993). From Hiroshima to the Nazi doctors: The evolution of psychoformative approaches to understanding traumatic stress syndromes. In J. Wilson & B. Raphael (Eds.), *International handbook of traumatic stress syndromes: The Plenum series on stress and coping* (pp. 11–23). New York: Plenum Press.

Litz, B. T., Gray, M. J., Bryant, R. A., & Adler, A. B. (2002). Early intervention for trauma: Current status and future directions. *Clinical Psychology: Science and Practice, 9,* 112–134.

Malt, U. F. (1988). The longterm psychiatric consequences of accidental injury a longitudinal study of 107 adults. *British Journal of Psychiatry, 153,* 810–818.

Mayou, R., Bryant, B., & Duthie, R. (1993). Psychiatric consequences of road traffic accidents. *British Medical Journal 307,* 647–651.

Mayou, R., Tyndel, S., & Bryant, B. (1997). Long-term outcome of motor vehicle accident injury. *Psychosomatic Medicine, 59,* 578–584.

McCaig, L. F. (1994). *National Hospital Ambulatory Medical Care Survey: 1992 emergency department summary* (Vol. 245). Hyattsville, MD: National Center for Health Statistics.

McLellan, A. T., Luborsky, L., Woody, G. E., & Obrien, C. P. (1980). An improved diagnostic evaluation instrument for substance abuse patients: The Addiction Severity Index. *Journal of Nervous and Mental Disease, 168,* 26–33.

Michaels, A. J., Michaels, C. E., Moon, C. H., Smith, J. S., Zimmerman, M. A., Taheri, P. A., & Peterson, C. (1999). Posttraumatic stress disorder after injury: Impact on general health outcome and early risk assessment. *Journal of Trauma, 47,* 460–467.

Michaels, A. J., Michaels, C. E., Moon, C. H., Zimmerman, M. A., Peterson, C., & Rodriguez, J. L. (1998). Psychosocial factors limit outcomes after trauma. *Journal of Trauma, 44,* 644–648.

Miller, T., Galbraith, M., Lestina, D., & Viano, D. (1994). Medical care spending, United States. *Morbidity and Mortality Weekly Report, 43,* 581–586.

Mollica, R. F., McInnes, K., Sarajlie, N., Lavelle, J., Sarajlie, I., & Massagli, M. P. (1999). Disability associated with psychiatric comorbidity and health status in Bosnian refugees living in Croatia. *Journal of the American Medical Association, 282,* 433–439.

National Institute of Mental Health. (2002). *Mental health and mass violence: Evidence-based early psychological intervention for victims/survivors of mass violence.* Washington, DC: Author.

Newman, M. G. (2000). Recommendations for a cost-offset model of psychotherapy allocation using generalized anxiety disorder as an example. *Journal of Consulting and Clinical Psychology, 68,* 549–555.

Radloff, L. S. (1977). The CES-D Scale: A self-report depression scale for research in the general population. *Applied Psychological Measurement 1,* 385–401.

Rice, D. R., MacKenzie, E. J., & Associates. (1989). *Cost of injury in the United States: A report to congress.* San Francisco: Institute for Health and Aging, University of California, and Injury Prevention Center, Johns Hopkins University.

Rivara, F. P., Koepsell, T. D., Jurkovich, G. J., Gurney, J. G., & Soderberg, R. (1993). The effects of alcohol abuse on readmission for trauma. *Journal of the American Medical Association, 270,* 1962–1964.

Rostenberg, P. O. (1995). *Treatment Improvement Protocol 16: Alcohol and other drug screening of hospitalized trauma patients.* Washington, DC: Substance Abuse and Mental Health Services Administration.

Rothbaum, B. O., & Foa, E. (1994). Subtypes of posttraumatic stress disorder and duration of symptoms. In J. Davidson & E. Foa (Eds.), *Posttraumatic stress disorder: DSM-IV and beyond* (pp. 23–36). Washington, DC: American Psychiatric Association Press.

Roy-Byrne, P., Katon, W., Cowley, D., & Russo, J. (2001). A randomized effectiveness trial of collaborative care for patients with panic disorder in primary care. *Archives of General Psychiatry, 58,* 869–876.

Schnyder, U., Moergeli, H., Klaghofer, R., & Buddeberg, C. (2001). Incidence and prediction of posttraumatic stress disorder symptoms in severely injured accident victims. *American Journal of Psychiatry, 158,* 594–599.

Schoenwald, S. K., & Hoagwood, K. (2001). Effectiveness, transportability, and dissemination of interventions: What matters when? *Psychiatric Services, 52,* 1190–1197.

Shalev, A. Y., Freedman, S., Peri, T., Brandes, D., Sahar, T., Orr, S. P., & Pitman, R. K. (1998). Prospective study of posttraumatic stress disorder and depression following trauma. *American Journal of Psychiatry, 155,* 630–637.

Shalev, A. Y., Peri, T., Canetti, L., & Schreiber, S. (1996). Predictors of PTSD in injured trauma survivors: A prospective study. *American Journal of Psychiatry, 153,* 219–225.

Soderstrom, C. A., Smith, G. S., Dischinger, P. C., McDuff, D. R., Hebel, J. R., Gorelick, D. A., Kerns, T. J., Ho, S. M., & Read, K. M. (1997). Psychoactive substance use disorders among seriously injured trauma center patients. *Journal of the American Medical Association, 277,* 1769–1774.

Spencer, C. S., Frank, R. G., & Mcguire, T. G. (1996). How should the profit motive be used in managed care? In A. Lazarus (Ed.), *Controversies in managed mental health care* (pp. 279–290). Washington, DC: American Psychiatric Association Press.

Uehara, E. D., Farris, M., Morelli, P. T., & Ishisaka, A. (2001). Eloquent chaos in the oral discourse of killing fields survivors: An exploration of atrocity and narrativization. *Culture, Medicine and Psychiatry, 25,* 29–61.

Unutzer, J., Katon, W., Callahan, C. M., Williams, J. W. Jr., Hunkeler, E., Harpole, L., Hoffing, M., Della Penna, R. D., Noel, P. H., Lin, E. H., Arena, P. A., Hegel, M. T., Tang, L., Berlin, T. R., Oishi, S., & Langston, C. (2002). IMPACT Investigators. Improving Mood-Promoting Access to Collaborative Treatment. Collaborative care management of late-life depression in the primary care setting: A randomized controlled trial. *Journal of the American Medical Association, 288,* 2836–2845.

Ursano, R. J., Fullerton, C. S., Epstein, R. S., Crowley, B., Kao, T., Vance, K., Craig, K. J., Dougall, A. L., & Baum, A. (1999). Acute and chronic posttraumatic stress disorder in motor vehicle accident victims. *American Journal of Psychiatry, 156,* 589–595.

Villasenor, Y., & Waitzkin, H. (1999). Limitations of a structured psychiatric diagnostic instrument in assessing somatization among Latino patients in primary care. *Medical Care, 37,* 637–646.

Von Korff, M. J. G., Schaefer, J., Curry, S. J., & Wagner, E. H. (1997). Collaborative management of chronic illness. *Annals of Internal Medicine, 127,* 1097–1102.

Waitzkin, H., & Magana, H. (1997). The black box in somatization: Unexplained physical symptoms, culture, and narratives of trauma. *Social Science and Medicine, 45,* 811–825.

Wang, X., Cosby, L. G., Harris, M. G., & Liu, T. (1999). Major concerns and needs of breast cancer patients. *Cancer Nursing, 22,* 157–163.

Weathers, F. W., Huska, J. A., & Keane, T. M. (1991). *The PTSD Checklist—Civilian Version.* Boston: National Center for PTSD, Boston VA Medical Center.

Zatzick, D. (2003a). Collaborative care for injured victims of individual and mass trauma: A health services research approach to developing early interventions. In R. J. Ursano, B. G. McCaughey, & C. S. Fullerton (Eds.), *Individual and community re-*

sponses to trauma and disaster: The structure of human chaos (pp. 189–205). New York: Cambridge University Press.

Zatzick, D. (2003b). Posttraumatic stress, functional impairment, and service utilization after injury: A public health approach. *Seminars in Clinical Neuropsychiatry, 8,* 149–157.

Zatzick, D. F., & Johnson, F. A. (1997). Alternative psychotherapeutic practice among middle class Americans: I. Case studies and follow-up. *Culture, Medicine and Psychiatry, 21,* 53–88.

Zatzick, D. F., Jurkovich, G. J., Gentilello, L. M., Wisner, D. H., & Rivara, F. P. (2002). Posttraumatic stress, problem drinking and functioning 1 year after injury. *Archives of Surgery, 137,* 200–205.

Zatzick, D. F., Kang, S. M., Hinton, W. L., Kelly, R. H., Hilty, D. M., Franz, C. E., Le, L., & Kravitz, R. L. (2001). Posttraumatic concerns: A patient-centered approach to outcome assessment after traumatic physical injury. *Medical Care, 39,* 327–339.

Zatzick, D. F., Kang, S. M., Muller, H. G., Russo, J. E., Rivara, F. P., Katon, W., Jurkovich, G. J., & Roy-Byrne, P. (2002). Predicting posttraumatic distress in hospitalized trauma survivors with acute injuries. *American Journal of Psychiatry, 159,* 941–946.

Zatzick, D. F., Marmar, C. R., Weiss, D. S., Browner, W., Metzler, T. J., Golding, J. M., Stewart, A., Schlenger, W. E., & Wells, K. B. (1997). Posttraumatic stress disorder, and functioning and quality of life outcomes in a nationally representative sample of male Vietnam veterans. *American Journal of Psychiatry, 154,* 1690–1695.

Zatzick, D. F., Roy-Byrne, P., Russo, J., Rivara, F. P., Koike, A., Jurkovich, G. J., & Katon, W. (2001). Collaborative interventions for physically injured trauma survivors: A pilot randomized effectiveness trial. *General Hospital Psychiatry, 23,* 114–123.

Zatzick, D., Russo, J., & Katon, W. (in press). The interrelationship of PTSD, depression and somatic complaints: Extending the study of symptoms to injured trauma survivors treated in trauma surgery. *Psychomatics.*

Zatzick, D. F., Russo, J., Roy-Byrne, P., Wagner, A. W., Fuchs, C. H., Rajotte, E., Mathison, S. M., Uehara, E., & Katon, W. (2002). *The association between posttraumatic stress disorder and functional impairment: Does the evidence support early intervention?* Paper presented at the National Institute of Mental Health Division of Services and Intervention Research, "Evidence in Mental Health Services Research Conference: What Types, How Much and Then What?" Washington, DC.

Zatzick, D. F., Weiss, D. S., Marmar, C. R., Metzler, T., Wells, K., Golding, J. M., Stewart, A., Schlenger, W. E., & Browner, W. S. (1997). Post-traumatic stess disorder and functioning and quality of life outcomes in female Vietnam veterans. *Military Medicine, 162,* 661–665.

14

Early Intervention for Psychological Consequences of Personal Injury Motor Vehicle Accidents

EDWARD B. BLANCHARD
EDWARD J. HICKLING
ERIC KUHN
JOHN BRODERICK

Arguably, the most common trauma experienced by people in the United States is involvement in a personal injury motor vehicle accident (MVA). More than 3 million Americans are injured in MVAs each year, a frequency that has recurred annually since 1990. In addition, over 41,000 individuals were killed each year in MVAs (U.S. Department of Transportation, 2000). Moreover, approximately 23% of survivors of personal injury MVAs will develop posttraumatic stress disorder (PTSD) in the first few months after their accident (e.g., Ehlers, Mayou, & Bryant, 1998), which extrapolates to about 750,000 new cases of MVA-related PTSD in the United States each year. About one-half of those with initial PTSD following a MVA will partially or fully remit in the first 6 months (e.g., Blanchard et al., 1996; Ehlers et al., 1998; Koren, Arnon, & Klein,

1999; Shalev, Freedman, et al., 1998; Ursano et al., 1999), and an additional one-fourth to one-third remit within 1 year (Blanchard & Hickling, 1997). Nevertheless, this translates conservatively to about 250,000 individuals each year who develop chronic PTSD related to their MVA.

These prevalence statistics illustrate the need for effective early secondary prevention interventions for MVA survivors. There are several reasons why early intervention for MVA survivors in particular is important to study:

1. MVA-related trauma tends to occur about equally in men and women alike, as opposed to the traumas of combat or sexual assault that tend to be confined primarily to one gender or the other.
2. MVAs are a widespread and prevalent problem, both in the United States and around the world (Evans, 2002).
3. A small literature on assessment and early treatment of the psychological difficulties accompanying MVAs exists that can be expanded on.
4. There is also a small but expanding literature on the development of acute stress disorder (ASD) in MVA survivors as well as the development of PTSD in those with MVA-related ASD.

In this chapter, we first review the literature on controlled early intervention trials with MVA survivors, MVA survivors with chronic PTSD, and early intervention for those injured as a result of a MVA. Then, we describe the rationale and procedures involved in our own early intervention work. Finally, we present preliminary data on the first group of MVA survivors who have received this new treatment and on a comparable group of untreated survivors.

Given the magnitude of the psychiatric morbidity problems that personal injury MVAs create, especially PTSD and major depression, it is not surprising that research efforts have begun to focus on treatments for this problem. Studies for the treatment of MVA-related psychological distress can be subdivided into early intervention studies, which begin treatment within the first month after the MVA, and studies that implement the intervention 3 months or more after the MVA. We focus here on the former type of study.

EARLY INTERVENTION TRIALS: PSYCHOLOGICAL THERAPY

Despite the tendency for PTSD symptomotology to remit over time, it is advantageous to provide early intervention for MVA survivors in order to reduce overall psychological distress and promote a faster return to pre-MVA psychological functioning than might occur naturally. Early intervention trials can be divided into those that provided a single treatment session, akin to psychological debriefing, and those with two or more treatment sessions spread out over time. Both types of early intervention are described later.

Early Intervention Trials: Single Session

The first psychological debriefing trial took place in the United Kingdom (Hobbs, Mayou, Harrison, & Worlock, 1996). A total of 106 MVA survivors were recruited from the hospital emergency department and were randomly assigned to either a one-hour debriefing session ($n = 54$) or to an assessment-only control condition ($n = 52$). Patients with head trauma who could not remember the accident or those who had no psychological symptoms were excluded. Overall, eight eligible MVA survivors (7%) declined participation. The sample was 62% male with a median age of 27. The median number of days in hospital was significantly lower for the controls (3.7) than for the experimental treatment group (6.3).

Treatment lasted for about 1 hour and usually took place on the second day after the MVA. It covered (1) a review of the traumatic experience, (2) encouraging participants to express emotions related to the MVA, (3) education on typical emotional reactions to trauma, (4) encouragement to think and talk about the trauma, and (5) encouragement to engage in an early, graded return to normal road travel. Participants were also given a written summary of the advice.

Treated participants (78%) and controls (94%) were reassessed at 4 months by telephone interview and self-report measures. There were no significant differences on the total score on the Impact of Event Scale (IES; Horowitz, Wilmer, & Alvarez, 1979) between the two conditions, although controls showed a trend toward improvement. There were no significant reductions on clinical ratings of mood disturbance, presence of diagnosable PTSD, travel anxiety, or intrusive thoughts indexed by the IES. In addition, the Global Severity Index (GSI) of the Brief Symptom Inventory (BSI; Derogatis & Melisaratos, 1983) was unchanged. However, the treated group reported an increase in general distress, while scores in the control group decreased slightly. On two scales of the BSI, the treated group was significantly worse than the controls. The brief treatment was clearly ineffective in comparison to an assessment-only (and routine medical care) control condition. Moreover, treated participants showed nonsignificant trends toward increased symptomotology when compared to the control group.

The team of researchers at Oxford followed up both groups 3 years after the accident, collecting data on 62 of 106 participants (58.5% of the total sample; Mayou, Ehlers, & Hobbs, 2000). Dropouts had significantly lower initial injury scores. Although there was a significant reduction in IES total scores at the 3-year follow-up, there was no significant difference in IES scores between the treated and control groups at this time point. The GSI scores showed no overall reduction at 3 years. However, when pretreatment distress was factored into the analysis, the treated group reported significantly greater distress when compared to the control group, during the 3-year follow-up.

Mayou et al. (2000) performed an additional analysis on IES scores by subdividing the groups, based on IES scores, and reanalyzed the results. The groups with low initial IES scores showed slight, nonsignificant increases. Control participants with high initial scores exhibited a significant reduction in IES scores at 4 months, which remained low at 3 years. Those in the treated group with high initial IES scores showed little initial reduction at 4 months, and a slight reduction at 3 years. This analysis suggests that the subgroup with high initial PTSD symptoms did not profit from the brief early intervention. In fact, treatment may have delayed natural recovery.

The second single-session early intervention study was also conducted in the United Kingdom (Conlon, Fahy, & Conroy, 1999). Forty MVA survivors with relatively minor injuries (none were admitted to hospital) were randomly assigned to a single-session intervention about 1 week after the MVA ($n = 18$) or to an assessment-only control condition ($n = 22$). All participants were assessed using the IES and the CAPS (Clinician-Administered PTSD Scale; Blake et al., 1995). The 30-minute intervention encouraged participants to express emotions and cognitions around the MVA, gave them information about PTSD, and offered coping strategies. Participants also received an advice leaflet. At reassessment 3 months later, there was differential loss of participants; 39% within the intervention group could not be contacted, versus 5% of the assessment-only controls.

The groups did not differ on initial IES or CAPS scores. Moreover, at the 3month reassessment, both IES and CAPS scores showed significant overall reductions; however there were no significant differences in scores between the two groups. The within group change on IES was from 35 to 26 for the treated group and 28.5 to 16 for the controls and thus favored the control condition. Categorical data favored the treatment group, with 0% of treated participants meeting criteria for PTSD at 3 months whereas 14% of those in the control group met criteria for PTSD. However, problems with retention in treatment group could have affected results. Nevertheless, in a less severely injured sample, there is further evidence for no advantage of early brief treatment, relative to no treatment, akin to Hobbs et al. (1996). We conclude that there appears to be no support for applying a brief (one session) early intervention to unselected MVA survivors.

Early Intervention Trials: Multiple Sessions

The first randomized controlled treatment study using MVA survivors was conducted in the Netherlands by Brom, Kleber, and Hofman (1993). Participants were recruited through the police who routinely compiled a list of MVA survivors along with ratings of the severity of the MVA. (This severity rating was only marginally reliable with interrater reliability.)

A total of 738 potentially eligible participants were randomly selected to receive one of two letters within the first month after the MVA. The first letter asked survivors to participate in a research project (assessment-only control group), while the second letter asked survivors to participate in a secondary prevention (early treatment) program. Thirty-six percent of those asked to participate in the control condition agreed ($n = 83$, mean age 39, 63.8% male) while only 13% of those asked to participate in the treatment trial consented to participate ($n = 68$, mean age 36, 52.9% male).

The treatment consisted of (1) practical help on financial and medical matters and education about reactions to trauma and what constituted normal coping; (2) support (reassurance that the trauma is over, assisting the participant in labeling their emotions, and assisting them in mobilizing their own social support network); and (3) attempts to facilitate coping through confrontation and reality testing. Treatment was delivered individually over several sessions (three to six) by one of two experienced therapists. At the follow-up assessment 6 months later, 24% ($n = 20$) of the monitoring control group had dropped out versus 16% ($n = 11$) of those in treatment.

At the initial assessment, using a Dutch version of the IES, about half of the total sample reported moderate to severe symptoms of intrusion and avoidance. On the reassessment, only 8% showed severe symptoms while another 10–17% showed moderate symptoms. However, there was no significant difference in degree of improvement on the IES between the treatment group and the monitoring control group. However, on a separate questionnaire, over 90% of the treatment completers indicated they were satisfied or very satisfied with treatment. Thus, this more intensive early intervention failed, as did the preceding brief trials, to show an advantage for treatment over the mere passage of time in survivors of severe MVAs, half of whom endorsed severe symptoms of avoidance and intrusion on the IES.

Gidron, Gal, Freedman, et al., (2001), working in Israel, expanded on this research by changing the focus of the early intervention to MVA survivors who had visited an emergency department (ED) and were thought to be at high risk for developing PTSD because of (1) high ED heart rate, greater than 95 beats per minute (bpm), (2) acknowledgment of peritraumatic dissociative symptoms, and (3) a history of psychological treatment prior to the MVA.

Seventeen MVA survivors deemed to be high risk (10 men, 7 women, average age 38) were randomly assigned to the treatment ($n = 8$) or control condition ($n = 9$). Treatment consisted of two structured telephone sessions, with homework assignments in between the calls. During the first session, the patient described the MVA fully; then, with the therapist's assistance, the patient described the MVA again in an organized, logical manner, with added detail. As homework, the patient was to practice telling family and friends the new structured version of the MVA to enhance the reorganized memory and reduce the avoidance of the memories. At the second phone call, the patient practiced the narrative again with the therapist and was told to seek out social support. For those in the control group, the therapist provided supportive listening (but no correction) as the patient described the MVA.

There was no pretreatment assessment; however, at a posttreatment follow-up approximately 3–4 months post-MVA, the participants were given the Posttraumatic Diagnostic Scale (Foa, Cashman, Jaycox, & Perry, 1997) as a structured interview by someone blind to condition. Based on one-tailed (liberal) statistical tests, the treated group reported significantly less frequent total PTSD symptoms. Moreover, of the cases with full PTSD (29%), four of nine (44%) were in the control condition versus one of eight (12.5%) in the treated condition. Thus, it appears that within the limitations of a small-scale study with no pretreatment measures, this telephone-based "memory restructuring" therapy was effective with a high-risk population.

By far the strongest results from intensive, early intervention trials are those from two studies conducted in Australia by Richard Bryant and colleagues (Bryant, Harvey, Dang, Sackville, & Basten, 1998; Bryant, Sackville, Dang, Moulds, & Guthrie, 1999). In the first study, 12 individuals (7 female, 5 male, average age 32.3 years) who had been hospitalized for MVAs or industrial accidents, and who met criteria for ASD, were randomized to receive five individually administered 90-minute sessions of cognitive-behavioral therapy (CBT) while 12 others (7 women, 5 men, average age 33) were randomized to receive supportive counseling for a comparable amount of time. Bryant and Harvey's (2000) book, *Acute Stress Disorder*, describes the CBT, which consists of education about trauma reactions, progressive muscle relaxation, imaginal exposure to traumatic memories, cognitive restructuring, and graded *in vivo* exposure to avoided situations. The supportive counseling consisted of education about trauma reactions and general problem solving. Participants were assessed at pretreatment, posttreatment, and 6-month followup with psychological tests and structured interviews. Mean IES scores were found to change differentially between the two groups (CBT: 53.5 to 15.5 to 15.6, support: 53.7 to 40 to 37.3). For categorical diagnoses, 1 of 12 (8.3%) participants in the CBT condition met criteria for PTSD at posttreatment versus 10/12 (83.3%) in support.

These results illustrate that the CBT condition was significantly superior to support at posttreatment and at the 6-month follow-up. In fact, the supportive counseling condition was ineffective and potentially detrimental. In their naturalistic follow-up of MVA-related cases of ASD (Harvey & Bryant, 1998), seven of nine (77.8%) cases with ASD at an initial assessment (about 1 week post-MVA) met criteria for PTSD at a follow-up assessment. Thus, the supportive psychotherapy was either equivalent to no treatment or possibly slightly worse. Nevertheless, it seems clear that the intensive CBT applied over the first 6 to 8 weeks post-MVA was effective in preventing high-risk patients from developing PTSD.

In the second study, Bryant et al. (1999) attempted to isolate the important components of the CBT package. A total of 66 individuals with either MVA- or non–sexual assault-related ASD, not all of whom had been hospitalized, were randomized to one of the three conditions described later. There were 11 (16.7%) dropouts evenly distributed across the three conditions.

The first condition was essentially a replication of the earlier CBT condition and emphasized prolonged exposure to trauma (both in imagination and *in vivo*) plus anxiety management procedures (such as relaxation training). The second condition included prolonged exposure and cognitive restructuring and correction but did not have the anxiety management components. The same supportive counseling condition described in the earlier study was the third condition. Participants received five 90-minute individual treatment sessions along with pretreatment, posttreatment, and 6-month follow-up assessment.

Bryant and colleagues found that there were comparable levels of improvement in both CBT conditions, and that both versions of CBT were significantly superior to supportive counseling. IES scores at the three assessments were as follows: (1) in the exposure-plus-anxiety-management condition (pre-: 54.9, post-: 23.5, follow-up: 18.8); (2) in the exposure-only condition (pre-: 54.1, post-: 16.5, follow-up: 19.5); and (3) the support-only condition (pre-: 49.2, post-: 44.1, follow-up: 35.8). A total of 23% of those in the exposure-plus-anxiety-management condition met criteria for PTSD at follow-up, while 15% of those in the exposure-only condition, and 67% of those in the supportive counseling condition met criteria at follow-up. Again, based on analysis of categorical diagnostic data, the experimental conditions did not differ and were significantly better than supportive counseling. In this study, the latter condition was not detrimental but was equivalent to no treatment.

Summary

Given the aforementioned studies discussed, the following conclusions seem warranted:

1. Early (first 2 weeks post-MVA) single-session interventions applied to all MVA survivors attending the emergency department are ineffective at best and possibly detrimental to those with high initial IES scores. This is true, despite the inclusion of apparently relevant treatment elements in the early brief intervention.
2. Early (beginning in first 2 weeks post-MVA) multisession intensive CBT interventions, applied to high-risk (ASD) MVA survivors, are effective at preventing the development of PTSD at 2 to 3 months post-MVA and at longer-term follow-up. This conclusion may also apply to a brief telephone cognitive restructuring treatment.
3. Early multisession supportive counseling, applied to high-risk (ASD) MVA survivors is ineffective at best, leading to no difference from a naturalistic (no treatment) follow-up and may even be slightly detrimental.

EARLY INTERVENTION: MEDICATION TRIALS

There has been one report of an early intervention medication trial for MVA survivors. Pitman et al. (2002) reported a double-blind, placebo-controlled trial of propranolol as a possible secondary prevention treatment for survivors of MVAs ($n = 29$) or other traumas ($n = 12$). Propranolol, a beta-adrenergic blocking agent, is used as a cardiac drug as well as a drug for prophylaxis of migraine headaches. Given the findings of several recent studies of the psychophysiology of MVA survivors described next, it is valid to examine the effects of an arousal reducing agent such as propranolol in the early intervention for trauma.

Shalev, Sahar, et al. (1998), in a prospective follow-up of MVA survivors attending an emergency department in Israel, assessed 70 MVA survivors (81.4%) and 15 survivors of other traumas in the emergency department and at 1 week, 1 month, and 4 months posttrauma. The sample included 52 males and 34 females averaging age 27.3 (no participants were admitted to the hospital). In addition to structured interviews to assess PTSD and other comorbid conditions, heart rate (HR; measured in bpm) was measured at each assessment point. Four months post-MVA, when those who met criteria for PTSD and those who did not were examined separately, a significant difference in HR was found at the initial assessment (PTSD: 95.1 bpm, non-PTSD: 84.7 bpm). At 1-week reassessment, a trend toward a significant difference ($p = .09$) was found (PTSD: 77.3 bpm, non-PTSD: 72.6 bpm), with no significant differences between groups at 1 month and 4 months. An emergency department HR of 90 bpm or greater discriminated well between those who eventually met criteria for PTSD and those who did not (75% of PTSD vs. 24% of non-PTSD cases).

Bryant, Harvey, Guthrie, and Moulds (2000) reported the results of a similar study of hospitalized MVA survivors. They assessed 146 individuals in the hospital on the day they were discharged and were able to reassess 113 for PTSD 6 months later. They found that those who met criteria for PTSD at 6 months had significantly higher hospital discharge HRs (82.9 bpm) than those who were not diagnosed with PTSD at 6 months (76.3 bpm).

These findings led Pitman et al. (2002) to hypothesize that blocking cardiac arousal pharmacologically with propranolol, might, in turn, prevent the development of PTSD. Participants in their study were selected if their HR in the emergency department was 80 bpm or greater, they were acknowledging great psychological distress, and propranolol was not contraindicated. Patients were given 40 mg of propranolol within the first 6 hours and then asked to take 160 mg per day for 10 days before tapering off over the next 9 days. They were then assessed with the CAPS at 1 month and 3 months after the trauma.

One-month results were available on 11 of the 18 (61%) in the active drug condition versus 20 of 23 (87%) in the placebo condition. Total CAPS scores were not different at 1 month (propranolol: 27.6, placebo: 35.5). At 3 months, 50% of those in the active drug condition and 65% of those in the placebo group were reassessed and CAPS scores were again found not to differ between groups (propranolol: 21.1, placebo: 20.5). There was no significant difference between groups in the number of people meeting criteria for full PTSD at 1 month posttrauma (18% of those in the propranolol condition vs. 30% of in the placebo condition met criteria). At 3 months, the rates were 11% (1/9) for propranolol and 13% (2/15) in placebo. These results can be interpreted as not supporting early beta-blockade as early intervention for MVA survivors at risk for developing PTSD, based on the direct comparisons of completers, and on a significantly greater dropout in the propranolol condition.

MULTISESSION PSYCHOLOGICAL TREATMENT
OF CHRONIC MVA-RELATED POSTTRAUMATIC STRESS DISORDER

To round out the picture of the psychological treatment of MVA-related psychological distress, we describe two recent controlled trials. The first, which involved 24 MVA survivors with chronic PTSD, was conducted in Canada by

Fecteau and Nicki (1999). With four participants dropping out, the final sample included 6 males and 14 females (average age = 41.3) whose time since the MVA ranged from 3 to 95 months, with a mean of 19 months. Ten were randomized to four 2-hour sessions of CBT treatment consisting of education about trauma; relaxation training; and exposure in imagination, cognitive reappraisal, and self-directed, graduated *in vivo* exposure. The other 10 were place in a wait-list control condition.

Results showed a significantly greater reduction in CAPS scores for the CBT group (from 70.9 to 37.5) than for the wait-list group (from 77.3 to 74.6). Five of the 10 participants in the CBT condition no longer met criteria for PTSD at posttreatment compared to 0 of 10 in the wait-list. A 3month follow-up by questionnaire showed good maintenance of reduced symptoms.

In addition, we recently reported a controlled evaluation of CBT versus supportive psychotherapy (SP) versus wait-list control for injured MVA survivors administered 6 to 24 months postMVA (Blanchard et al., 2003). The sample included 26 males and 72 females who were, on average, 13-months post-MVA (average age = 40). The vast majority, about 92%, had lingering physical problems and about 58% were engaged in litigation. Twenty individuals of the original 98 dropped out over the course of treatment. Treatment was administered by three practitioners from the community. The CBT treatment consisted of education about trauma and PTSD, exposure to a written description of the accident, relaxation training, cognitive therapy, graduated *in vivo* exposure, and behavioral activation for the numbing symptoms. Both CBT and SP were administered for 8 to 12 sessions, with a mean of 10.1. Evaluations were done by individuals blind to treatment condition using the CAPS interview.

The CBT was superior to SP, which was in turn superior to the wait-list control condition in reducing CAPS scores (CBT: 68.2 to 23.7, SP: 65.0 to 40.1, wait list: 65.8 to 54.0). CAPS scores at 3 months were relatively unchanged on the 96% of the treated samples who were reassessed. For CBT, 16 of 21 (76%) with initial full PTSD no longer met criteria at posttreatment; for SP, 10 of 21 (47.6%) recovered, and for wait list, 5 of 21 (23.8%) no longer met criteria. Thus, CBT was superior to SP which was clearly an active treatment with significant within-group improvement and greater improvement than shown by an assessment-only wait list.

BRIEF EARLY PSYCHOLOGICAL INTERVENTION FOR MVA SURVIVORS

A brief intervention for ASD was developed using the available literature and our own experience providing cognitive-behavioral treatments for MVA survivors (Blanchard & Hickling, 1997). In this section, we discuss the specific components of our intervention and an explanation of why we chose to include them.

Overall, we decided that we would need to decrease the total amount of treatment received in previous successful interventions (in terms of total sessions and number of therapist hours) in order to create a brief treatment. The treatment would include those elements of intervention we deemed most important, delivered in a more intensive fashion. The delivery of treatment therefore was to be less than four sessions in length (less than 4 hours of therapist time). This approach to treatment delivery would therefore place more burden on the MVA survivor and new demands on the therapist for flexible treatment strategies and methods of interaction. We decided to include handouts containing information about completing treatment and examples and suggestions for application of treatment. We also provided telephone follow-ups to encourage patients and midtreatment adjustments in the therapy as needed.

Session 1

The majority of treatment information and training was provided in the initial meeting. The session began with a review of the psychological assessment information and the reason that patients were seeking treatment. This included a description of the MVA and responses on the ASD interview. Patients' ASD symptoms were reviewed and discussed as they fit within the diagnosis of ASD. "Normal reactions" to trauma, cognitively, behaviorally, and emotionally, were discussed. The two-factor theory of PTSD (classical conditioning of the MVA, followed by reinforced avoidance of reminders of the trauma, e.g., not driving) was described in an effort to illustrate how the next few weeks might greatly affect subsequent psychological responses to the trauma.

We then offered a rationale for the treatment, which included exposure, both imaginally and *in vivo*. The initial exposure entailed having the MVA survivor provide a brief, audiotaped description of his or her MVA. They were then instructed to listen to the audiotape three times each day. This approach was modeled after Foa, Rothbaum, Riggs, and Murdock's (1991) approach to treating rape victims with PTSD. We thought that listening to an audiotape would be more efficient than having the MVA survivor write out the description as we had done in our controlled treatment studies.

Following the making of the audiotape, the MVA survivor was introduced to a basic model of how thoughts affect subsequent reactions, both emotionally and behaviorally. In fact, any significant emotional reaction that occurred during the description of the MVA was used to exemplify how "just talking or thinking about something" can lead to a powerful emotional and physical reaction.

Participants were then instructed to complete an *in vivo*/imaginal hierarchy of situations that provoke a reaction. They were taught subjective units of distress scale (SUDS) ratings and shown how to build a hierarchy that they were to use over the next week or so. The therapist then offered examples of imaginal and *in vivo* exercises.

To help patients cope with the situations they were to confront, on and off their hierarchy, they were taught two "tools": (1) adaptive cognitive self-talk to address their emotional and physical reactions and (2) relaxation to help moderate any physical reactions that might occur in times of stress. Participants were instructed to use these tools for any stress response created by the situations they were to place themselves in. A list of common cognitive distortions found in MVA survivors was then provided and reviewed. Various ways to deal with any cognitive distortions, using the new techniques they had just been taught, were modeled and discussed as needed.

The second skill/tool, relaxation training, which uses four-muscle relaxation with additional attention to diaphragmatic breathing techniques, was then introduced (see Blanchard & Hickling, 1997). An audiotape of this exercise was made ahead of time to give to the participant after the live demonstration of the technique.

The first session concluded with instructions for exposure, relaxation, and development and application of the *in vivo* driving/MVA hierarchy. Handouts on coping self-statements, cognitive reappraisal information, the SUDS-rated hierarchy (complete with instructions), and a rating system for relaxation effects and homework tasks were provided in addition to the handout on cognitive distortions common to MVA survivors. Accurate phone numbers were confirmed, and a time to call the MVA survivor in the next week to 10 days was set up.

Session 2 (Telephone Follow-Up)

At the arranged time, a telephone session was conducted. Major points covered during this contact included how the MVA survivor was progressing with the exposure audiotape of their MVA, imaginal and *in vivo* exposure to feared/anxiety-provoking situations on their MVA hierarchy, cognitive coping and cognitive reappraisal skills, relaxation skill, and, if needed, how to deal with intrusive thoughts. Suggestions for interventions were offered, as was clarification of any questions related to the material covered during the initial meeting. A second face-to-face meeting was arranged at the conclusion of the telephone conversation and the time and date confirmed.

Session 3 (and Session 4, If Needed)

These sessions were largely a review and extension of the first meeting. The primary goals were to make sure the MVA survivor followed the treatment plan provided and to determine whether any additional treatment would be needed. The third meeting once again involved reviewing all homework assignments and discussing interventions and any treatment-related situation brought up by the MVA survivor. The relaxation and cognitive techniques were also reviewed, particularly as they were used in application to provocative situations, either imaginally or *in vivo*. This session included having the MVA survivor describe his or her MVA aloud and rate and respond to any reactions using the cognitive-behavioral techniques provided.

While still in a preliminary stage of development, this treatment approach applied several important elements. First, the intervention provided a rationale for the MVA survivor's reaction and placed his or her reaction in an understandable context (i.e., ASD and a major trauma). Although this has not been shown to be a sufficient intervention to help prevent the development of subsequent PTSD symptoms, it nevertheless provides a good starting point for a cognitive-behavioral intervention. The learning theory–based rationale, based on the two-factor theory of PTSD, provides the basis for an exposure-based intervention drawing from behavioral principles. Employing an idiosyncratic description of each survivor's unique MVA is consistent with empirically derived treatments in the PTSD literature. A brief introduction to cognitive and relaxation techniques allows the MVA survivor to approach provocative tasks (e.g., driving) with a rationale and plan for success and an understanding of where and why their reactions are occurring. Finally, continued contact with the treating therapist allows for immediate revision of the treatment plan so that unforeseen difficulties can be dealt with. The therapist contact, although complemented with numerous handouts, also allows the MVA survivor to have professional contact and encouragement with the tasks and demands of an exposure-based intervention as needed.

Pilot Data on Our Brief Intervention

We have completed treatment on three MVA survivors with ASD using the new brief protocol and have data from three other accident survivors who were assessed on the same timetable but not offered treatment. The initial results look promising. The brief yet intensive CBT treatment appears to work as an early intervention (the difference in developing PTSD at 4 to 5 weeks post-MVA favors the treated group; $p = .20$, Fisher's exact test). However, more cases are needed before firm conclusions can be drawn.

Early Clinical Observations

The brief treatment combines traditional therapist-led psychological treatment with a selfdirected, patient-led treatment. MVA survivors can experience a wide range of difficulties that interfere with psychological treatments, including medical problems, disruption of work, financial concerns, and interpersonal challenges. This treatment addresses only the psychological symptoms that can follow a MVA. Patient-contact time is an important factor when providing brief interventions. If treatment time is spent on related but tangential problems (e.g., relationship difficulties), there will not be time to attend to all the details necessary for this particular method of intervention. It becomes necessary for the therapist to be firm at times about the purpose of the meeting, and how much there is to cover in a short period of time. The other problems are relegated to any time that remains in the session after the material regarding ASD has been covered. By the end of the first session, most are quite ready to proceed as we have outlined.

Telephone contact appears to be critical. Even when the time spent on the telephone is brief, anecdotal information from MVA survivors suggests how important such contact was, and how important it was to cover the material a second and third time. The material presented in the treatment is new to most MVA survivors. The MVA survivor's ability to appreciate the material is complicated by his or her powerful emotional reaction to the trauma. The telephone contact allows for greater information to be covered without the time needed for travel to and from appointments. The MVA survivors we have seen are agreeable to using the phone and do not see it as a limiting factor. One study from Israel (Gidron et al., 2001) supports the idea of the provision of therapy for memory restructuring by phone with trauma survivors. Our audiotape exposure, as well as the discussion and organization of the key elements in each survivor's story, appears to contain some of the same elements as the memory restructuring of Gidron et al.'s intervention.

The assessment process has also appeared to be a therapeutic experience. MVA survivors have commented that the assessment process allows them to see how they are changing (improving), and how treatment is focused directly on the symptoms they are experiencing. In a brief treatment this seems to be an important element for compliance with a quick, largely self-directed (therapist-guided) treatment.

CONCLUSION

It seems clear from our pilot work and from other larger-scale controlled trials that early intensive CBT intervention can reduce the likelihood of the development of PTSD in high-risk MVA survivors. In addition, studies have shown that intensive CBT can be effective in alleviating chronic PTSD in MVA survivors. Brief, one-session education interventions given to all injured MVA survivors appear to be counterproductive, as does supportive counseling given early and intensively. Nevertheless, supportive counseling for those with chronic PTSD is significantly better than mere assessment. Brief, self-directed and self-paced CBT appears to be a very promising secondary prevention intervention for MVA survivors, which promotes change while lowering costs (e.g., therapist time and effort).

ACKNOWLEDGMENTS

Preparation of this chapter was supported in part by National Institute of Mental Health Grant No. MH-48476.

REFERENCES

Blake, D. D., Weathers, F. W., Nagy, L. M., Kaloupek, D. G., Gusman, F. D., Charney, D. S., & Keane, T. M. (1995). The development of a Clinician-Administered PTSD Scale. *Journal of Traumatic Stress, 8,* 75–90.

Blanchard, E. B. & Hickling, E. J. (1997). *After the crash: Assessment and treatment of motor vehicle accident survivors.* Washington, DC: American Psychological Association.

Blanchard, E. B., Hickling, E. J., Barton, K. A., Taylor, A. E., Loos, W. R., & Jones-Alexander, J. (1996). One-year prospective follow-up of motor vehicle accident victims. *Behaviour Research and Therapy, 34,* 775–786.

Blanchard, E. B., Hickling, E. J., Devineni, T., Veazey, C. H., Galovski, T. E., Mundy, E., Malta, L. S., & Buckley, T. C. (2003). A controlled evaluation of cognitive behavioral therapy for posttraumatic stress in motor vehicle accident survivors. *Behaviour Research and Therapy, 41,* 79–96.

Brom, D., Kleber, R. J., & Hofman, M. C. (1993). Victims of traffic accidents: Incidence and prevention of post-traumatic stress disorder. *Journal of Clinical Psychology, 49,* 131–140.

Bryant, R. A., & Harvey, A. G. (2000). *Acute stress disorder: A handbook of theory, assessment, and treatment.* Washington, DC: American Psychological Association.

Bryant, R. A., Harvey, A. G., Dang, S. T., Sackville, T., & Basten, C. (1998). Treatment of acute stress disorder: A comparison of cognitive-behavioral therapy and supportive counseling. *Journal of Consulting and Clinical Psychology, 66,* 862–866.

Bryant, R. A., Harvey, A. G., Guthrie, R. M., & Moulds, M. L. (2000). A prospective study of psychophysiological arousal, acute stress disorder and posttraumatic stress disorder. *Journal of Abnormal Psychology, 109*(2), 341–344.

Bryant, R. A., Sackville, T., Dang, S. T., Moulds, M., & Guthrie, R. (1999). Treating acute stress disorder: An evaluation of cognitive behavior therapy and supporting counseling techniques. *American Journal of Psychiatry, 156,* 1790–1786.

Conlon, L., Fahy, T. J., & Conroy, R. (1999). PTSD in ambulant RTA victims: A randomized controlled trial of debriefing. *Journal of Psychosomatic Research, 46,* 37–44.

Derogatis, L. R., & Melisaratos, N. (1983). The Brief Symptom Inventory: An introductory report. *Psychological Medicine, 13,* 595–605.

Ehlers, A., Mayou, R. A., & Bryant, B. (1998). Psychological predictors of chronic posttraumatic stress disorder after motor vehicle accidents. *Journal of Abnormal Psychology, 107,* 508–519.

Evans, L. (2002). Traffic crashes: Measures to make traffic safer are most effective when they weigh the relative importance of factors such as automotive engineering and driver behavior. *American Scientist, 90,* 244–253.

Fecteau, G., & Nicki, R. (1999). Cognitive behavioral treatment of posttraumatic stress disorder after motor vehicle accidents. *Behavioral and Cognitive Psychotherapy, 27,* 201–214.

Foa, E. B., Cashman, L., Jaycox, L., & Perry, K. (1997). The validation of a self-report measure of posttraumatic stress disorder: The Posttraumatic Diagnostic Scale. *Psychological Assessment, 9,* 445–451.

Foa, E. B., Rothbaum, B. O., Riggs, D. S., & Murdock, T. B. (1991). Treatment of posttraumatic stress disorder in rape victims: A comparison between cognitive behavioral procedures and counseling. *Journal of Consulting and Clinical Psychology, 59,* 715–723.

Gidron, Y., Gal, R., Freedman, S., Twiser, I., Lauden, A., Snir, Y., & Benjamin, J. (2001). Translating research findings to PTSD prevention: Results of a randomized-controlled pilot study. *Journal of Traumatic Stress, 14,* 773–780.

Harvey, A. G., & Bryant, R. A. (1998). The relationship between acute stress disorder and posttraumatic stress disorder: A prospective evaluation of motor vehicle accident survivors. *Journal of Consulting and Clinical Psychology, 66,* 507–512.

Hobbs, M., Mayou, R., Harrison, B., & Worlock, P. (1996). A randomized controlled trial of psychological debriefing for victims of road traffic accidents. *British Medical Journal, 313,* 1438–1439.

Horowitz, M. J., Wilmer, N., & Alvarez, N. (1979). Impact of Event Scale: A measure of subjective stress. *Psychosomatic Medicine, 41,* 209–218.

Koren, D., Arnon, I., & Klein, E. (1999). Acute stress response and posttraumatic stress disorder in traffic accident victims: A one-year prospective, follow-up study. *American Journal of Psychiatry, 156,* 367–373.

Mayou, R. A., Ehlers, A., & Hobbs, M. (2000). Psychological debriefing for road traffic accident victims: Three-year follow-up of a randomized controlled trial. *British Journal of Psychiatry, 17,* 589–593.

Pitman, R. K., Sanders, K. M., Zusman, R. M., Healy, A. R., Cheema, F., Lasko, N. B., Cahill, L., & Orr, S. P. (2002). Pilot study of secondary prevention of posttraumatic stress disorder with propranolol. *Society of Biological Psychiatry, 51,* 190–192.

Shalev, A. Y., Freedman, S., Peri, T., Brandes, D., Sahar, T., Orr, S. P., & Pitman, R. K. (1998). Prospective study of posttraumatic stress disorder and depression following trauma. *American Journal of Psychiatry, 155,* 630–637.

Shalev, A. Y., Sahar, T., Freedman, S., Peri, T., Glick, N., Brandes, D., Orr, S. P., & Pitman, R. K. (1998). A prospective study of heart rate response following trauma and the subsequent development of posttraumatic stress disorder. *Archives of General Psychiatry, 55,* 553–559.

Ursano, R. J., Fullerton, C. S., Epstein, R. S., Crowley, B., Kao, T., Vance, K., Craig, K. J., Dougall, A. L., & Baum, A. (1999). Acute and chronic posttraumatic stress disorder in motor vehicle accident victims. *American Journal of Psychiatry, 156*(4), 589–595.

U.S. Department of Transportation. (2000). *National Highway Traffic Safety Administration: "Crashes, Fatalities, Injuries and Costs," 2000, 1999, 1998* [On-line]. Available: *www.transportation.gov.*

15

The Challenge of Providing Mental Health Prevention and Early Intervention in the U.S. Military

CARL ANDREW CASTRO
CHARLES C. ENGEL, JR.
AMY B. ADLER

The military specializes in preparing individuals to encounter potentially traumatic events. These traumatic events may occur in the context of combat and peacekeeping missions (e.g., Adler, Litz, & Bartone, in press; Southwick, Morgan, Nicolaou, & Charney, 1997; Stretch et al., 1996; Thomas & Castro, in press) or even during humanitarian missions (e.g., Gifford, Jackson, & DeShazo, 1993; McRae-Bergeron et al., 1999), when exposure to traumatic events is initially unexpected. Such traumatic events may include the perpetration of violence, witnessing violence, being victimized by violence, or some combination thereof. Military personnel also risk training or other work-related accidents and are targets of terrorist violence. Exposing military personnel to such critical incidents has the potential to affect their physical health

The views expressed in this chapter are those of the authors and do not necessarily represent the official policy or position of the Department of Defense or the U.S. Army Medical Command.

and psychological well-being, and thereby their readiness for subsequent military operations. Thus, for the military, providing effective early intervention following exposure to potentially traumatizing events in order to minimize their impact on well-being is a top priority. Although selection and training are also key components to helping military personnel cope with these potentially traumatic events, early intervention programs are critical for optimizing the coping of service members in the wake of such events.

Providing these services in the military, however, presents some unique challenges. First, preventive and early intervention services need to be administered on a large scale. Finely tailored, highly individualized programs of intervention are not likely to be well suited given the complexity and size of the U.S. military. The successful delivery of mental health services needs to be geared toward the entire population, must work within the military chain of command, and must consider the role of stigma (Britt, 2000) and the subsequent consequences of using mental health services on military careers (Hoge, Lesikar, et al., 2002). Besides the risk of encountering traumatic events, the military is also distinguished by a particular, if not idealized, sense of community. In the U.S. military, such concepts are frequently referred to as "taking care of our own" to describe the military's sense of commitment to the service member (Plummer, 1997). One natural extension of this cultural concept is the role of the Veterans Administration in providing care across the military life cycle of service members; the saying from "cradle to grave" now takes on a literal meaning.

It is within this context that we discuss the challenges involved in providing mental health prevention and early intervention programs to U.S. military personnel, always keeping in mind that we must balance the requirement for efficacious interventions given the risk of encountering potentially traumatic events with the cultural expectations that care will be provided. We begin by first discussing the important issue of how to evaluate the effectiveness of prevention and early intervention in military populations. Next, we critically review the several programs that the U.S. military has used or currently uses that fall within the prevention and early intervention framework. Specifically, we discuss (1) the selection and psychological screening program, (2) the psychological debriefing initiative, (3) the concept of "PIES," which has shaped how the U.S. military provides mental health services on the battlefield for at least the past 60 years, and (4) the emerging importance of command consultations for affecting the establishment of commandwide prevention and early intervention programs. Although our discussion is limited to the U.S. military, it is our hope that mental health care providers from the both the civilian sector as well as from other militaries will find our experiences, both our successes and our failures, useful.

EVALUATING EARLY INTERVENTION IN THE MILITARY

There are a number of questions and issues to consider when evaluating the effectiveness of prevention and early intervention efforts aimed to reduce or eliminate the effects of combat stress. Most of them remain unresolved and serve to highlight that the uncertainty associated with the utility of early battlefield mental health intervention mirrors the chaos and uncertainty of the battlefield. The first issue involves identifying the outcome of interest that will be useful in determining the effectiveness of the intervention program. There is a wide range of potential outcomes of interest when considering early battlefield mental health intervention; historically, discussion has focused primarily on the outcome of greatest interest to the operational commanders, maintaining the fighting strength. Indeed, mental health care providers often state that early intervention is a "force multiplier" in that it allows a large proportion of affected troops that seek or are referred for mental health support to be rapidly returned to battle (see Ingraham & Manning, 1980, for a historical discussion of the rationale for this thinking). Meanwhile, other important effects of battle stress, such as its intermediate and long-term impact on the health, functioning, and quality of life of military personnel, is much less well documented or understood.

Two key questions should be kept in mind when evaluating the appropriateness of implementing a selection or early mental health intervention program. The first question is whether there are any potential adverse effects of the early mental health intervention. The possible harms of early intervention with subsequent return to military duty may include harm to military discipline and unit cohesion when someone is returned to the unit who is functioning but near to psychological decompensation, increased mental and physical harm to the individual returned to duty who faces future combat, stigmatization of the soldier if it is known by others that he has received a mental health intervention, and heightening the expectation of posttraumatic symptoms in someone who might otherwise have done well.

Unfortunately, the question regarding the possibility of harm has received inadequate attention. During the post-World War II, Korean and Vietnam eras, it was presumed that combat trauma was likely to break everyone at some point (see Harris, Mayer, & Becker, 1955; Swank & Marchand, 1946). Over the past two decades, however, it has been clearly shown that while mental health outcomes are a function of the intensity of combat trauma, even under the most intense fighting, the majority of soldiers do not develop posttraumatic stress disorder. One critical implication of the fact that most military personnel do not develop chronic posttraumatic distress after experiencing combat is the potential for ostensibly preventive actions to cause harm among those who might have done well without the intervention. Although it is an intriguing hypothesis that early mental health intervention on the battlefield may in fact cause harm, we should make it clear that there is currently no evidence to support this possibility. Our point in raising this prospect is that "good intentions" should not be deemed sufficient justification for implementing early intervention strategies.

The second question to consider when deciding on whether a prevention and early intervention program is warranted is one of validation. Simply stated, is there an obligation or duty to provide early intervention when scientific evidence to support efficacy is lacking? The group that stands to gain the most from early intervention is the group at greatest risk of poor outcome after combat trauma. It seems clear that one important obligation is to target early intervention to those who are likely to have poor outcomes. Therefore, effective prognostic indicators besides the combat experience itself are needed. Unfortunately, existing evidence suggests that in the immediate aftermath of a traumatic event, distress is ubiquitous and is consistently but only weakly related to long-term mental health outcomes, a feature that also holds true for other potential predictors of outcome such as premorbid personality, age, gender, occupation, and time in military service (e.g., Rothbaum, Foa, Riggs, Murdock, & Walsh, 1992; see King, Vogt, & King, Chapter 3, this volume). North et al. (1999) have found that lifetime history of PTSD or other major Axis I mental disorders are a strong predictor of postdisaster mental health outcome, perhaps suggesting one way of identifying those most in need of early intervention. Prospective longitudinal studies are badly needed to investigate the use of specific prognostic measures. Substantial uncertainty remains in this area, though it seems fairly certain that our societal need to respond to those traumatized in combat as well as the need of the mental health profession to prove themselves valuable to the military and society will ensure that even in uncertainty, activity will trump passivity.

SELECTION AND PSYCHOLOGICAL SCREENING

Two of the most fundamental methods of early or prevention intervention, selection and screening, are also two of the more controversial interventions. Although it is frequently stated that the extensive effort during World War II to "select out" individuals who were least likely to tolerate the experience of combat was successful, a more detailed look suggests that the mental health screening process was, in fact, a failure, resulting in the exclusion of a large number of men from serving in the war effort (see Perkins, 1955). Indeed, a conservative estimate is that approximately 372,000 men, or the equivalent of 25 divisions, were needlessly excluded from military service due to an excessively narrow psychiatric screening process (Ginzberg, 1959). This loss in manpower is well in excess of all battlefield deaths suffered by U.S. forces during World War II.

A secondary reason for the apparent lack of success in this area has been the absence of normative data from military samples. In World War II, many prediction efforts were highly idiosyncratic, and even today, none have been appropriately validated to see whether particular baseline variables adequately predict militarily important health outcomes in the military context. A crucial requirement for completing this type of study correctly is that baseline data cannot be used to determine the fate of the soldier. For example, if the baseline "screen" is used to decide whether a soldier needs care, and care in some cases leads to administrative proceedings to separate the soldier from the military, an analysis of the baseline measure might suggest it is a good indicator of who leaves military service early, rendering the predictive value of such variables impossible to interpret.

There are indeed significant ethical concerns involved when using the results from mental health screens to select people out of military service or to select out military personnel from military missions. Recently, some have proposed to collect "baseline health data," on childhood abuse, borne out of perceived deficiencies in individual-level predeployment health status data among U.S. troops deployed to the 1991 Gulf War. The suggestion has been that early life abuse experiences will be useful for predicting who succeeds in the military and perhaps who develops medically unexplained symptoms such as those experienced by many after Gulf War deployment, the so-called Gulf War syndrome. Some would argue that the practice of selecting people out from military service based on past life experiences is a discriminatory practice, an argument bolstered by the fact that the rate of reported child sexual abuse among women is considerably higher than among men (National Center on Child Abuse and Neglect, 1992). Still others might suggest that there is an ethical obligation to select such people out to protect them from poor health outcomes.

The U.S. military's screening program today does not aim to "select out" personnel from service or military deployments, although certainly it may be viewed as both a mental health prevention and early intervention program. Developed in 1996, the current screening program can be applied to large military populations easily and unobtrusively. Further, the screening can be implemented during routine duties in garrison and prior to, during, or after a deployment. Although it has changed considerably since its inception, the basics of the screening process have remained the same. A primary screening survey, which includes a range of mental health scales, is administered to each service member; the survey is scored on-site. If an individual scores above a prescribed cutoff, the person is briefly interviewed by a mental health specialist who determines need for follow-up. In a review of the program, Wright, Huffman, Adler, and Castro (2002) discuss key programmatic changes that have occurred, including an expansion of the symptoms for which military personnel are screened, a change in the cutoffs used to identify those in need of an on-site interview, and a refinement of the brief interview process.

While many countries have integrated screening in either predeployment or postdeployment processing, some screening is regarded as relatively perfunctory whereas other screening programs are regarded as more credible (Thompson & Pastó, 2003). The U.S. screening program provides individuals with the chance to refer themselves for mental health care, identifies those in need of follow-up mental health evaluation, and projects patient load both in garrison and on deployment. The results from the screening are also part of a larger database and can be used to identify trends or compare screening results across deployments (e.g., Adler, Wright, Huffman, Thomas, & Castro, 2002; Martinez, Huffman, Adler, & Castro, 2000).

In many respects, the current screening program is a significant advancement in the delivery of preventive mental health services in the military. It is designed to bring mental health services to military personnel rather than wait for military personnel to seek out services. Clearly, mental health screening is emerging as a standard tool to ensure readiness. It is even being used for soldiers who experienced combat while deployed to Afghanistan as part of Operation Enduring Freedom to determine the need for follow-up mental health care. Whether screening works as a means of early intervention or prevention, however, has not yet been systematically evaluated. Nevertheless, screening is one more example of how the military's requirement for a particular mental health service has prompted a reaction from the mental health community before the empirical evidence supporting the intervention is available.

PSYCHOLOGICAL DEBRIEFING

One of the most widely used and controversial methods of early intervention is psychological stress debriefing, a semistructured review of a critical incident, typically extremely traumatic in nature. In debriefing, the goal is to provide participants a confidential setting that facilitates the cognitive and emotional processing of the event. In the military setting, a critical distinction is made between *psychological debriefing* and an *after-action debriefing*, a guided review of an operational mission in which the goal is to identify key information for the development of lessons learned for future operations.

Often confused as an early variant of the psychological debriefing were the *after-action* debriefings conducted by S.L.A. Marshall (1947) as a method of collecting military information for historical records (see Shalev, 2000). The first systematic psychological debriefing paradigm rightly belongs to the French, who developed the concept of far-forward treatment for psychological casualties during World War I, which was subsequently adopted by the British (see Salmon, 1929). During World War II and Korea, the United States adopted a similar far-forward "treatment" paradigm, where treatment involved talking about the horror and terror of the most recent battle and emphasizing that the powerful emotions resulting from battle such as fear, grief, guilt, and remorse were common (Baker, 1975). Also emphasized in these early psychological debriefings was the expectation that the soldier would soon return to battle. Noticeably absent from this debriefing approach was a discussion of the distant past, relations with one's family, and distant future planning.

In contrast, Marshall's historical debriefings did not specifically address the psychological aspects of combat at all, including the soldiers' emotional reactions to it. It is for this reason that Marshall's historical debriefing paradigm is categorized within the after-action debriefing framework. What Marshall's historical debriefing approach did suggest, however, is that these early psychological debriefings could be conducted on nonpsychiatric casualties who just returned from combat. The addition of the historical or informational aspect of the debriefings led to the hypothesis that psychological debriefings would create an opportunity for the correction of misperceptions about the event. Further, obtaining social support from fellow soldiers was now possible as the debriefings were conducted within the existing social group, namely, the military unit.

Mitchell and Everly (1996) developed one of the best known methods of psychological debriefing, critical incident stress debriefing (CISD). CISD is one component of the critical incident stress management (CISM) system; it refers to a specific process by which a group of individuals is guided through a series of stages in discussing a particular traumatic or series of traumatic events that they witnessed or participated in, but were not direct victims of the event (Everly & Mitchell, 2000).

Now considered the standard of care for small units exposed to potentially traumatizing events in the military (e.g., Harvey, 2002; Martin & Belenky, 1993), and integrated into the training and doctrine of military stress response teams (e.g., Dinneen, 1994; Harvey, 2002), psychological debriefing is met with considerable skepticism in the scientific community (e.g., Rose, Bisson, & Wessely, 2001). There is a disturbing lack of sound empirical evidence supporting its effectiveness and its potential for harm. Although well-designed studies support the therapeutic benefits of self-disclosure (Pennebaker & Susman, 1989) and anecdotal evidence suggests that debriefing may be beneficial (e.g., Dyregrov & Mitchell, 1992; Robinson & Mitchell, 1993), there is a dearth of controlled studies examining the impact of debriefing.

In a review of the existing controlled studies, a Cochrane collaboration review of the randomized controlled trials of one-session debriefing (Rose et al., 2001) concludes that there is no evidence supporting debriefing; and there is, in fact, evidence suggesting it may be detrimental to psychological well-being. The studies cited in the review, however, did not apply the psychological debriefing procedures in the way in which it was originally intended—with groups of preexisting work teams (Weisaeth, 2000) and with individuals who were not physically harmed during the incident (see Everly & Mitchell, 2000; Mitchell & Everly, 1996). Furthermore, the studies cited do not report the specific psychological debriefing model used nor analyze the content of the debriefings as a manipulation check (see Litz, Gray, Bryant, & Adler, 2002, for a complete critique and additional review).

Despite the frequent use of psychological debriefing across a range of militaries from other nations (Adler & Bartone, 1999), surprisingly little research, randomized controlled studies, or otherwise, has examined the impact of debriefing on military personnel. Deahl et al. (2000) conducted the only randomized controlled study of soldiers that was identified in the literature. In a study of male soldiers returning from peacekeeping duty in Bosnia, 106 soldiers were randomly assigned to a debriefing or a nondebriefing control-group condition. At the 6-month follow-up, soldiers in the debriefed group had lower anxiety and a higher score on a measure of alcohol problems than those in the nondebriefed group, but the nondebriefed soldiers reported a greater drop in traumatic stress. This complex pattern of results is further complicated by the fact that both groups actually had very low rates of psychological symptoms and thus meaningful comparisons are difficult. Furthermore, the degree to which the peacekeeping events were experienced as potentially traumatizing is unclear. Deahl, Srinivasan, Jones, Neblett, and Jolly (2001) emphasized, however, the importance of outcomes other than traumatic stress in debriefing effectiveness research.

There are a handful of other studies that addresses the impact of psychological debriefing on military personnel. Although not randomized control trials, they represent the present state of research on this topic. Shalev (1994; also reported by Shalev, Peri, Rogel-Fuchs, Rusano, & Marlowe, 1998) examined the impact of psychological debriefing on the adjustment of 39 Israeli soldiers exposed to combat along the Lebanese border over a 2-year period. Soldiers were assessed before and after units were debriefed using the historical group-debriefing model. Results indicated that debriefing was followed by a significant decrease in anxiety among those soldiers who were the most anxious, and a significant increase in self-efficacy among those soldiers who had the lowest self-efficacy. Shalev concluded that debriefing was effective for those soldiers who avoided thinking about the incident and who were anxious. Without a control group, there remains the possibility that the soldiers would have improved over time on their own. The Shalev study is unique, however, in that the debriefing occurred in existing military units. Combat evaluation scores, an assessment of unit functioning, did not change immediately after the debriefing, but there were no follow-up assessments to measure any long-term effects (Shalev et al., 1998).

In a quasi-experimental study of the effects of debriefing on a small group of military personnel, Eid, Johnsen, and Weisaeth (2000) compared the health and attitudes of Norwegian personnel who responded to a serious car accident in a tunnel. Nine soldiers who inadvertently became involved in the rescue efforts were provided a group psychological debriefing following the event; nine firefighters who also responded to the scene were not. Two weeks later, the debriefed soldiers had lower traumatic stress scores and reported learning more about themselves from the accident than the professional rescue workers. Whereas this study suggests there may be positive results from debriefing, the fact that the two groups were not comparable prior to the intervention phase limits the internal validity of the study, as the authors acknowledge.

In another nonrandomized control study, Swedish peacekeepers deployed to Bosnia who had a ventilation session, or "defusing," with their group leader reported better postdeployment adjustment than soldiers who reported support only from peers or from a formal psychological debriefing (Larsson, Michel, & Lundin, 2000). The study did not assess the content of the actual intervention and the analysis included soldiers who reported no traumatic experiences at all (65% reported no traumatic event).

In a survey study of more than 1,000 U.S. peacekeepers assessed 1 to 2 months after their return from a 6-month deployment on a peacekeeping mission in Kosovo (Adler, Dolan, & Castro, 2000), respondents were asked whether they had received a debriefing during their deployment. Soldiers who reported having experienced at least one potentially traumatizing deployment-related event and reported that they received a debriefing had lower posttraumatic stress symptoms than those who did not report being debriefed. In contrast, soldiers who reported having experienced no high-impact event and who were debriefed reported higher posttraumatic stress symptom scores than those who had not received a debriefing. The study is limited by the fact that the data are retrospective and there was also no control over the kind of debriefing the soldiers reported receiving (see also Orsillo, Roemer, Litz, Ehlich, & Friedman, 1998).

The need for well-designed studies assessing the effectiveness and procedures of psychological debriefing is critical, especially given the frequency with which psychological debriefing is used in the U.S. military. Until that time, however, various other forms of early intervention, such as "therapy by walking around," are being proffered as effective early mental health intervention paradigms. Unfortunately, these "improved" mental health intervention procedures are equally untested and unvalidated.

BATTLEFIELD MENTAL HEALTH INTERVENTION: "PIES"

The prevailing wisdom informing battlefield mental health intervention in the U.S. military today is the notion of Proximity—Immediacy—Expectancy—Simplicity, simply known as "PIES" (see Table 15.1). Though the acronym was first coined after the Korean War (Artiss, 1963), as noted earlier, it was Salmon who developed the concept for the U.S. military, based on the French and the British experience in World War I. While the British evacuated their psychiatric casualties back to Britain to be rehabilitated in sanitariums, the French treated their casualties near the lines in a military environment. The French were able to return 70% of their psychiatric casualties to duty, the British less than 5% (Baker, 1975).

TABLE 15.1. PIES: Basic Principles of Early Mental Health Intervention in Combat

Acronym	Principle	Description
P	Proximity	Supportive intervention in combat should occur as close to the battle and the soldier's unit as possible.
I	Immediacy	Support should occur as soon as possible after a psychiatric casualty is recognized.
E	Expectancy	Support should avoid pathologizing symptoms or medicalizing existing disability. Instead, the soldier is informed that this is a normal part of the combat experience, that they are "fatigued," and that they will respond well enough within days to return to their unit.
S	Simplicity	Support is based on "simple" and largely nonmedical principles: rest (occasionally with sedation), nutrition, and physical reactivation (i.e., "three hots and a cot").

The objective of PIES is to ensure that mental health support is readily and immediately available for those troops facing the most intense combat. The preference is to avoid "pathologizing," diagnostic labels such as acute stress disorder, psychosis, or posttraumatic stress disorder in favor of "battle fatigue" or "combat exhaustion" in an effort to normalize the experience in the eyes of both the affected soldier and his unit members. "Treatment" is similarly nonmedical and usually consists of 24–72 hours of rest, nutrition, and modest physical activity. Reported rates of successful return to duty have varied widely from a high of 90% to less than 40% (Collins, 1972; Peterson & Chambers, 1952; Shephard, 2001). Although the capacity for soldiers to remain with the unit for their full combat tour is unknown, during the Korean War it was estimated that 90% of the neuropsychiatric casualties treated under the PIES paradigm returned to combat and only 10% experienced a second breakdown (Peterson & Chambers, 1952). The theoretical principles behind PIES are to preserve supportive relationships between affected soldiers and unit members, to prevent soldiers from seeing themselves as ill or disabled, and to bolster their self-esteem by facilitating their capacity to fulfill their obligation to their unit and country.

Although PIES has essentially become reified in military mental health circles, there are reasons to question its goals and its effectiveness. There are no controlled clinical trials to support or refute its efficacy (some might argue for obvious reasons). Clearly, the immediate goal of PIES, returning people to the battle, is consistent with military objectives. In the absence of scientific evidence of efficacy, however, many have criticized the manner in which military psychiatrists have seemingly justified PIES by offering anecdotes suggesting that the approach is in the interest of the soldier because it improves the long-term mental status of treated soldiers. Indeed, it has been argued that the entire notion of PIES is specious in an age when battlefields are highly mobile or when guerrilla tactics render the "front line" indefinable (see Ingraham & Manning, 1980).

COMMAND CONSULTATION

Command consultation is another method of early intervention in the military that has not been specifically examined in randomized controlled trials. Similar to the concept of executive coaching (McCauley & Hezlett, 2001), command consultation is an interactive process in which a professional, usually from outside the command, provides support to a military commander in addressing particular issues or problems (see Thompson & Pastó, 2003, for a review). The consultant's approach can be formal or informal but generally involves some type of assessment, planning, implementation, and evaluation (Lenz & Roberts, 1991). The nature of that process is guided by the inherent power of the commander to accept or reject a particular recommendation. In addition, proximity to and experience in the theater of operations enhance the consultant's credibility.

Although there is evidence that military commanders often employ command consultation, some commanders may be reluctant to accept it because of concerns regarding confidentiality, the general stigma associated with mental health interventions (Thompson & Pastó, 2003), and lack of clarity about the role and services of such consultants. In addition, because command consultation covers such a wide spectrum of possible topics and interventions, the term itself has become excessively broad and difficult to conceptualize within the framework of an empirical study.

One type of command consultation of note is consultation following potentially traumatic events. Indeed, as a component of the CISM framework, command consultation is considered an integral part of a response to a critical incident (Everly & Mitchell, 2000). Several forms of command consultation were conducted, for example, following the terrorist attack on the Pentagon in September 2001. These included consulting with the Army Surgeon General about the best way to structure both on-site and follow-up mental health interventions, and the utility of a brief survey in assessing the impact of the trauma over time. Consultants also worked with senior military leaders at the Pentagon on effective ways to confront the emotional aftermath of the terrorist attack and provided them individualized support in the wake of the tragedy (Hoge, Engel, et al., 2002).

In responding to a potentially traumatic event, the role of a consultant from the mental health field is tailored to the specific situation. Nevertheless, there appear to be several consistent themes. The consultant serves as an outside support for organic mental health assets, provides suggestions for intervention management to the senior medical and operational leadership, and provides the senior leaders directly affected by the event an opportunity to discuss concerns they may have about their own experiences. Despite the importance and potential need for such services, again, there is no empirical evidence supporting this approach.

Another way in which command consultation may serve as a prevention tool is the use of human dimensions research teams to provide confidential and tailored feedback to commanders about their specific units. This feedback, typically based on soldier survey responses and interviews, consists of a personalized brief with mean scores on scales that provide comparisons to other units. The leaders are provided a personal code which allows them to compare their unit's score to those of other units. By providing feedback in real time, that is, before the mission is completed, it is hoped that the leaders can take the appropriate and feasible corrective mid-course action as a first preventive step (see, e.g., Castro, Bienvenu, Huffman, & Adler, 2000; Thomas & Castro, in press).

Finally, an emerging area of command consultation that remains largely unexplored is that of health risk communication, which has been defined as "an interactive process of exchange of information and opinion among individuals, groups, and institutions. It involves multiple messages about the nature of risk and other messages, not strictly about risk, that express concern, opinions, or reactions to risk messages or to legal and institutions arrangements for risk managers" (National Research Council, 1989). In the arena of clinical care, the field of risk communication has focused largely on helping patients understand the risks and benefits associated with medical therapies and diagnostic tests in an effort to enhance their ability to make good health decisions. Population-based approaches to risk communication have been adopted by government agencies and industry in an effort to collaborate more effectively with communities impacted by potentially hazardous exposures. Anecdotes abound regarding positive outcomes associated with effective risk communication (e.g., efforts by the maker of Tylenol to address public concern after some packages were tainted with cyanide) and negative outcomes associated with poor risk communication (e.g., the Exxon-Valdez disaster). These strategies remain unproven in careful studies but are the source of great interest among military medical experts attempting to mitigate the medical and psychosocial impact of what some have termed an "inherently dirty battlefield" (see Freeman, 2002). There is a long history of important but largely medically unexplained somatic consequences of war and trauma, including entities such as "soldier's heart," "nostalgia," "shell shock," "DaCosta's syndrome," and "Gulf War syndrome." More recent civilian concerns after terrorism have also revealed the need to carefully target communications regarding health risk (e.g., "World Trade Center syndrome," and persistent ailments among U.S. postal workers concerned regarding possible exposures to items containing anthrax or even to mail that has undergone irradiation to eliminate any residual anthrax spores).

The impact of command consultation, its role in early intervention, and the degree to which it provides support in the event of a critical incident need to be examined empirically. Although anecdotal evidence suggests it may be useful, there are no case-control studies demonstrating the impact of command consultation on performance, health, or other militarily relevant outcomes.

THE FUTURE OF MENTAL HEALTH PREVENTION
AND EARLY INTERVENTION

Providing mental health prevention and early intervention is a challenge because although combat is indeed both terrifying and horrifying even for those who perform exceedingly well (Murphy, 1956), most combat veterans do not develop significant mental health problems requiring intervention. Paradoxically, Audie Murphy, America's most decorated World War II veteran, apparently suffered from PTSD, suggesting that successful performance in combat alone does not "protect" one from subsequent mental health problems. In this chapter, we briefly reviewed the key prevention and early intervention programs, initiatives, and strategies adopted by the U.S. military to meet this challenge, paying particular attention to the evidence that merits their implementation. Surprisingly, there is very little systematic (i.e., scientific) evidence to support their use (or disuse).

Clearly, there is a need to conduct systematic, randomized control studies to determine the effectiveness (and safety) of our current mental health prevention and early intervention programs. Furthermore, these studies need to be prospective and longitudinal. Such studies will tell us not only whether our programs work but, more important, how our programs can be improved to meet the needs of the military personnel who are confronted with the stressors of combat, as well as other potentially traumatic events. Undoubtedly, such studies will be extremely difficult to conduct. However, only by relying on the findings of scientifically based studies in developing mental health prevention and early intervention programs will we be able to move beyond our reliance on personal experiences, opinions, and retrospective assessments to determine the best course of action. Our combat veterans deserve no less.

REFERENCES

Adler, A. B., & Bartone, P. T. (1999). International survey of military mental health professionals. *Military Medicine, 164*(11), 788–792.

Adler, A. B., Dolan, C. A., & Castro, C. A. (2000). U.S. soldier peacekeeping experiences and wellbeing after returning from deployment to Kosovo. In *Proceedings of the 36th International Applied Military Psychology Symposium* (pp. 30–34). Split, Croatia: Ministry of Defense of the Republic of Croatia.

Adler, A. B., Litz, B. T., & Bartone, P. T. (in press). The nature of peacekeeping stressors. In T. W. Britt & A. B. Adler (Eds.), *Psychology of the peacekeeper: Lessons from the field.* Westport, CT: Praeger.

Adler, A. B., Wright, K. M., Huffman, A. H., Thomas, J. L., & Castro, C. A. (2002). Deployment cycle effects on the psychological screening of soldiers. *U.S. Army Medical Department Journal, 4/5/6,* 31–37.

Artiss, K. L. (1963). Human behavior under stress—from combat to social psychiatry. *Military Medicine, 128,* 1011–1015.

Baker, S. L. (1975). Traumatic war neurosis. In A. M. Freedman, H. I. Kaplan, & B. J. Sadock (Eds.), *Comprehensive textbook of psychiatry II* (2nd ed., pp. 1618–1624). Baltimore, MD: Williams & Wilkins.

Britt, T. W. (2000). The stigma of psychological problems in a work environment: Evidence from the screening of service members returning from Bosnia. *Journal of Applied Social Psychology, 30,* 1599–1618.

Castro, C. A., Bienvenu, R. V., Huffman, A. H., & Adler, A. B. (2000). Soldier dimensions and operational readiness in U.S. Army forces deployed to Kosovo. *International Review of the Armed Forces Medical Services, 73,* 191–200.

Collins, J. L. (1972). Military psychiatry. *Journal of the National Medical Association, 64,* 32–34.

Deahl, M. P., Srinivasan, M., Jones, N., Neblett, C., & Jolly, A. (2001). Commentary: Evaluating psychological debriefing: Are we measuring the right outcomes? *Journal of Traumatic Stress, 14*(3), 527–529.

Deahl, M., Srinivasan, M., Jones, N., Thomas, J., Neblett, C., & Jolly, A. (2000). Preventing psychological trauma in soldiers: The role of operational stress training and psychological debriefing. *British Journal of Medical Psychology, 73,* 77–85.

Dineen, M. (1994, April). *Helping individuals and communities cope with overwhelming psychological trauma.* Garmish-Partekirschen, Germany: Army Medical Department Training Symposium.

Dyregrov, A., & Mitchell, J. T. (1992). Work with traumatized children. *Journal of Traumatic Stress, 5,* 5–17.

Eid, J., Johnsen, B. H., & Weisaeth, L. (2000, September). *Group psychological debriefings: Does it make a difference?* Paper presented at the meeting of the International Conference on Human Dimensions During Military Deployments, Heidelberg, Germany.

Everly, G. S., & Mitchell, J. T. (2000). *Critical incident stress management: Advanced group crisis interventions—A workbook.* Ellicott City, MD: International Critical Incident Stress Foundation.

Freeman, C. D. (2002). Risk communication: The leadership tool for the 21st Century. *U.S. Army Medical Department Journal, 1/2/3,* 40–43.

Gifford, R. K., Jackson, J. N., & DeShazo, K. B. (1993). *Report of the human dimensions research team Operation Restore Hope.* Unpublished report, Walter Reed Army Institute of Research.

Ginzberg, E. (1959). *The lost divisions.* New York: Columbia University Press.

Harris, F. G., Mayer, J., & Becker, H. A. (1955). *Experiences in the study of combat in the Korean theater: I. Psychiatric and psychological data.* Washington, DC: Walter Reed Army Institute of Research.

Harvey, S. C. (2002). Debriefing/decompression: Psychological support for OEF casualties. *U.S. Army Medical Department Journal, 10/11/12,* 14–20.

Hoge, C. W., Engel, C. C., Orman, D. T., Crandell, E. O., Patterson, V. J., Cox, A. L., Tobler, S. K., & Ursano, R. J. (2002). Development of a brief questionnaire to measure mental health outcomes among Pentagon employees following the September 11, 2001 attack. *Military Medicine, 167*(Suppl. 4), 60–63.

Hoge, C. W., Lesikar, S. E., Guevara, R., Lange, J., Brundage, J. F., Engel, C. C., Messer, S. C., & Orman, D. T. (2002). Mental disorders among U.S. military personnel in the 1990s: Association with high levels of health care utilization and early military attrition. *American Journal of Psychiatry, 159,* 1576–1583.

Ingraham, L. H., & Manning, F. J. (1980, August). Psychiatric battle casualties: The missing column in a war without replacements. *Military Review,* pp. 19–29.

Larsson, G., Michel, P., & Lundin, T. (2000). Systematic assessment of mental health following various types of posttrauma support. *Military Psychology, 12,* 121–135.

Lenz, E. J., & Roberts, B. J. (1991). Consultation in a military setting. In R. Gal & D. Mangelsdorff (Eds.), *Handbook of military psychology* (pp. 671–687). Chichester, UK: Wiley.

Litz, B. T., Gray, M., Bryant, R. A., & Adler, A. B. (2002). Early intervention for trauma: Current status and future directions. *Clinical Psychology: Science and Practice, 9*(2), 112–134.

Marshall, S. L. A. (1947). *Men against fire.* Glouchester, MS: Peter Smith.

Martin, J. A., & Belenky, G. L. (1993, November). *Operation Desert Storm after action stress debriefings.* Proceedings of the 35th annual conference of the Military Testing Association, Williamsburg, VA.

Martinez, J. A., Huffman, A. H., Adler, A. B., & Castro, C. A. (2000). Assessing psychological readiness in U.S. soldiers following NATO operations. *International Review of the Armed Forces Medical Services, 73,* 139–142.

McCauley, C. D., & Hezlett, S. A. (2001). Individual development in the workplace. In N. Anderson, D. S. Ones, H. K. Sinangil, & C. Viswesvaran (Eds.), *Handbook of industrial, work and organizational psychology* (Vol. I, pp. 313–335). London: Sage.

McRae-Bergeron, C. E., May, L., Foulks, R. W., Sisk, K., Chamings, P., & Clark, P. A. (1999). A medical readiness model of health assessment or well-being in first-increment air combat command medical personnel. *Military Medicine, 164,* 379–388.

Mitchell, J. T., & Everly, G. S., Jr. (1996). *Critical incident stress debriefing: An operations manual for the prevention of traumatic stress among emergency services and disaster workers* (2nd ed.). Ellicott City, MD: Chevron.

Murphy, A. (1956). *To hell and back.* London: Bartles.

National Center on Child Abuse and Neglect. (1992). *National child abuse and neglect data system* (No. ACF 92-30361). Washington, DC: Department of Health and Human Services.

National Research Council. (1989). *Improving risk communication.* Washington, DC: National Academy Press.

North, C. S., Nixon, S. J., Shariat, S., Mallonee, S., McMillen, J. C., Spitznagel, E. L., & Smith, E. M. (1999). Psychiatric disorders among survivors of the Oklahoma City bombing. *Journal of the American Medical Association, 282,* 755–762.

Orsillo, S. M., Roemer, L., Litz, B. T., Ehlich, P., & Friedman, M. J. (1998). Psychiatric symptomatology associated with contemporary peacekeeping: An examination of post-mission functioning among peacekeepers in Somalia. *Journal of Traumatic Stress, 11,* 611–625.

Pennebaker, J. W., & Susman, J. R. (1989). Disclosure of traumas and psychosomatic processes. *Social Science Medicine, 26,* 327–332.

Perkins, M. E. (1955). Preventive psychiatry during World War II. In J. B. Coates & E. C. Hoff (Eds.), *Preventive medicine in World War II: Vol. III. Personal health measures and immunization* (pp. 171–232). Washington, DC: Office of the Surgeon General, Department of the Army.

Peterson, D. B., & Chambers, R. E. (1952). Restatement of combat psychiatry. *American Journal of Psychiatry, 109,* 249–254.

Plummer, M. T. (1997, November). Quality of life is the most visible way of showing commitment to soldiers. *Army,* pp. 14–15.

Robinson, R. C., & Mitchell, J. T. (1993). Evaluation of psychological debriefings. *Journal of Traumatic Stress, 6,* 367–382.

Rose, S., Bisson, J., & Wessely, S. (2001). Psychological debriefing for preventing post-traumatic stress disorder (PTSD) (Cochrane review). In *The Cochrane Library* (Vol. 3). Oxford, UK: Update Software.

Rothbaum, B., Foa, E., Riggs, D., Murdock, T., & Walsh, W. (1992). A prospective examination of post-traumatic stress disorder in rape victims. *Journal of Traumatic Stress, 5,* 455–475.

Salmon, T. W. (1929). The care and treatment of mental diseases and war neurosis (shell shock) in the British Army. In *The Medical Department of the United States Army in the World War* (Vol. X, pp. 497–523). Washington, DC: U.S. Government Printing Office.

Shalev, A. Y. (1994). Debriefing following traumatic exposure. In R. J. Ursano, B. G. McCoughey, & C. S. Fullerton (Eds.), *Individual and community response to trauma and disaster: The structure of human chaos* (pp. 201–219). Cambridge, UK: Cambridge University Press.

Shalev, A. Y. (2000). Stress management and debriefing: Historical concepts and present patterns. In B. Raphael & J. P Wilson (Eds.), *Psychological debriefing* (pp. 17–31). Cambridge, UK: Cambridge University Press.

Shalev, A. Y., Peri, T., Rogel-Fuchs, Y., Ursano, R. J., & Marlowe, D. (1998). Historical group debriefing after combat exposure. *Military Medicine, 163,* 494–498.

Shephard, B. (2001). *A war of nerves.* Cambridge, MA: Harvard University Press.

Southwick, S. M., Morgan, C. A., Nicolaou, A. L., & Charney, D. S. (1997). Consistency of combat-related traumatic events in veterans of Operation Desert Storm. *American Journal of Psychiatry, 154,* 173–177.

Stretch, R. H., Bliese, P. D., Marlowe, D. H., Wright, K. M., Knudson, K. H., & Hoover, C. H. (1996). Psychological health of Gulf War-era military personnel. *Military Medicine, 161,* 257–261.

Swank, R., & Marchand, W. (1946). Combat neuroses: The development of combat exhaustion. *Archives of Neurology and Psychology, 55,* 236–247.

Thomas, J. L., & Castro, C. A. (in press). Organizational behavior and the U.S. peace-keeper. In T. W. Britt & A. B. Adler (Eds.), *Psychology of the peacekeeper: Lessons from the field*. Westport, CT: Praeger.

Thompson, M. M., & Pastó, L. (2003). Psychological Interventions in Peace Support Operations: Current Practices and Future Challenges. In T. W. Britt & A. B. Adler (Eds.), *Psychology of the peacekeeper: Lessons from the field*. Westport, CT: Praeger.

Weisaeth, L. (2000). Briefing and debriefing: group psychological interventions in acute stressor situations. In B. Raphael & J. P. Wilson (Eds.), *Psychological debriefing: Theory, practice and evidence* (pp. 43–57). Cambridge, UK: Cambridge University Press.

Wright, K. M., Huffman, A. H., Adler, A. B., & Castro, C. A. (2002). Psychological screening program overview. *Military Medicine, 167*(10), 853–861.

16

Closing Remarks

BRETT T. LITZ

I started this book with a series of chapters that laid the groundwork for understanding the acute psychological impact of trauma and traumatic loss that nearly everyone experiences and the chronic debilitating clinical problems that only a relatively small percentage of survivors will experience. A wealth of information was also provided about the current state of research that has attempted to examine the personal, cultural, and social factors that affect risk for developing chronic posttraumatic mental health problems as well as a roadmap for future research endeavors. Expanding our scientific knowledge is one of the most important challenges for the field. The more conclusive evidence we have about personal liabilities and risk factors for chronic posttraumatic problems, the greater our chances of meaningfully screening people who will have difficulty recovering on their own, and the greater confidence we can have in decisions about how secondary prevention resources should be used. Also, if future research can provide valid and useful information about the interpersonal, community, and cultural factors that affect recovery from trauma and traumatic loss, then ideas can be generated and tested to shift resources and modify practices to foster resilience in the family, school, and other public arenas.

In the next part, a series of chapters provided detailed descriptions of the epidemiology, phenomenology, mental health outcomes, and clinical care needs of individuals exposed to trauma and traumatic loss across the lifespan. Each chapter also provided a critique of current practices and summarized the available evidence for various early intervention strategies. One of the consistent messages throughout these chapters was the lack of sufficient research, particularly randomized controlled trials. Another conclusion of these chapters was that although there is sufficient evidence that secondary prevention is imperative for those particularly at risk for posttraumatic difficulties, there is not enough evidence to support specific strategies for a variety of contexts, particularly traumatic loss. The one exception is the generally positive evidence that cognitive-behavioral therapy (CBT) is effective as a secondary prevention intervention, if timed and implemented properly. Each chapter also emphasized that, because there is not sufficient evidence for a prescriptive or paradigmatic approach, all professional contacts with individuals soon after exposure to trauma or traumatic loss should be supportive, informational, and caring, and not intrusive or demanding of disclosure or emotional sharing. After some time has passed, if a person is still distressed and consumed by his or her loss and/or trauma, and he or she has difficulty reestablishing reasonable routines of daily living, then this person should be encouraged to seek professional assistance. There is sufficient empirical evidence to recommend a broad CBT approach as a secondary prevention intervention for adults suffering acutely from a relatively circumscribed traumatic event.

Every chapter in this part emphasized that although trauma and traumatic loss can be devastating and damaging across the lifespan, the majority of individuals exposed to even the most horrific and grotesque events eventually recover. Thus, the major challenge for the field is to find ways of providing empirically supported secondary prevention services to those most at risk for developing chronic posttrauma mental health problems. However, it should be underscored that research has revealed that only a small percentage of individuals exposed to trauma develop chronic posttraumatic stress disorder (PTSD), defined categorically using the diagnostic criteria established in the diagnostic nosology.

A categorical (yes/no) diagnosis of PTSD is not the only way to index the mental health impact of trauma. The number of symptoms required for a PTSD diagnosis is rather arbitrary; individuals could suffer considerably while failing to meet the diagnostic criteria by one or more symptoms. Indeed, there is growing empirical support for a dimensional (continuous severity) conceptualization of posttraumatic outcomes (e.g., Ruscio, Ruscio, & Keane, 2002; see also Moreau & Zisook, 2002). Generally, the field has focused on the risk for *diagnosable PTSD* and has failed to sufficiently account for how trauma impacts the quality of life, well-being, quality of relationships, self-esteem, and milder forms of mental health problems, such as periodic but functionally impairing depression and anxiety. Ideally, the course of a broader spectrum of posttrauma and postloss problems should be affected by early intervention.

On the other hand, it is important to appreciate individual and group (e.g., military personnel and emergency medical technicians) resilience and to respect individual and culture-based methods of recovery from trauma and traumatic loss where the elements of early intervention occur naturally or automatically. The trick is to allow for natural recovery and resilience while working hard at preventing stigma and shame in those who might need assistance. In addition, it is important to appreciate that some events are so enormous and heinous that no one would argue that special care is necessary in every circumstance. For example, being a prisoner of war, as well as other forms of captivity, torture, and severe sexual assault, is an event that requires a different approach and framework. For instance, imagine a prisoner of war and torture survivor who goes home right after being liberated, or imagine a child who loses his or her parents to homicide/suicide.

The last part of the book began with a depiction of how resources were marshaled after the horrific and tragic mass violence on 9-11 in New York City, and how the mental health response took shape over time. There was an enormous and impressive outpouring of volunteer counselors, therapists, and professional acute "trauma specialists" that descended upon lower Manhattan immediately after 9-11. However, the services provided recapitulated the status quo—typically, some variant of critical incident stress debriefing (CISD). Even academic medical centers and trauma researchers and experts were caught off guard (and unable to recommend a prescriptive approach). Chapter 10, by Neria, Suh, & Marshall, is rich with examples of lessons learned from this experience. There is no doubt that we are better prepared to address the immediate and acute aftermath of mass violence should such an event occur again in the United States, at the very least with respect to what not to do, which is an important start. However, at present, other than the group trained by the American Red Cross (ARC), it is unclear how much mental health professionals know about how they might be helpful, should a mass violence episode occur in their respective communities. To address this problem, we need a probability survey of mental health professionals across the country—what do mental health professionals know, and what might they need to learn if they were to be used as a resource in their communities? At present, the ARC is the only agency that provides "certified" training in mental health interventions after disasters. Although the ARC provides excellent and necessary training in the practical and logistical realities of disaster response, it uses CISD as its framework for early intervention. Given this, it seems prudent to work toward modernizing the training provided by the ARC. In addition, because many mental health professionals who are not formally trained end up assisting survivors after a disaster, some form of nationally mandated continuing education for the mental health professions could prepare clinicians, at least in a rudimentary fashion, for a disaster or mass violence event in every community throughout the United States.

In Chapter 11, in the "Special Topics" part, Rauch and Foa described what victims face in the immediate aftermath of sexual assault; the mental and physical toll that sexual assault takes on its victims; various strategies shown to be useful to help victims manage the medical, emotional, legal, interpersonal, and cultural impact of sexual assault; and the state-of-the-art, evidence-based secondary prevention interventions. While it is clear that the available services for sexual assault victims have improved greatly, too many women (and men) still suffer in isolation (and do not go to emergency rooms or rape crisis counseling centers). There still are subtle and nonsubtle forces that stigmatize, patronize, blame, and punish victims, which is unacceptable. Clinicians in emergency departments and rape crisis centers do a tremendous job supporting women through the various painful postassault demands imposed upon them. Sexual assault is an extreme trauma (often accompanied by horrific physical brutality, abuse, and injury) that requires special consideration in the immediate and acute phases (e.g., Resnick, Acierno, Holmes, Dammeyer, & Kilpatrick, 2000). Given the legal, medical, emotional, and stigmatizing effects of sexual assault, in an ideal world, no one would suffer this kind of experience alone. The care provided by rape crisis teams should be reinforced with empirical research (e.g., psychological first aid, advocacy, education, and family preparation). As argued by Gray, Prigerson, and Litz in Chapter 4, this kind of research is fraught with ethical dilemmas and methodological pitfalls, and it is enormously difficult to implement, but it is possible, and sorely needed.

Indeed, the only way that important research questions for the field can be answered rigorously and meaningfully is if the research occurs in real-world settings at every level of care (primary care, rape crisis centers, ARC, emergency rooms, etc.). At present, there is an unfortunate schism between academic researchers, front-line clinicians, organizations, advocates, and survivors. What is needed is rapprochement and collaboration. All clinicians, administrators, planners, funding agencies, and survivors should be concerned about the lack of evidence for various early interventions and the need for careful, externally valid research. Clinicians do not want to feel used; they want to be equal intellectual partners in research. They also feel an understandable need to be confident that their patients will be respected and cared for at a time of great tragedy and helplessness. Academics are suspicious of any form of intransigence. They also need to feel confident that data will be collected rigorously. Organizations, such as fire and police departments, need to feel that clinicians and researchers understand and respect the complexities of their organization and culture. Planners grow tired of the equivocation of scholars about the lack of evidence—in this context, established organizations or models, such as CISD, win out. Ultimately, everyone has the same agenda: Find the optimal way to help people in distress soon after trauma and traumatic loss, and find the most efficacious and efficient ways of preventing chronic posttraumatic impairment/dysfunction. The field will not advance unless there is openness to research findings; on the other hand, meaningful research is impossible without collaboration between researchers and others invested in helping trauma victims.

In Chapter 12, Eriksson, Foy, and Larson discussed the psychological risks related to emergency services and relief work and methods of preventing impairment and posttraumatic mental health problems. CISD is still the modal early intervention applied internationally specifically for emergency services personnel, who most often share events as a group and sometimes as an organization. Indeed, for a variety of reasons, there is tremendous support for CISD in emergency services organizations and considerable recalcitrance in the face of evidence that suggests that the intervention is inert. First, the language used to describe the intervention and its goals are reminiscent of the military origins of "debriefing" and thus are attractive to emergency services organizations that have a command structure like the military (e.g., fire departments). Second, emergency services personnel appreciate the model, and it is inculcated in the culture. Third, although controversial, CISD is provided to groups of individuals who have shared the same experiences, which can be efficient and morale enhancing. However, these attractive processes and goals do not provide secondary prevention of PTSD and other mental health problems implicated by exposure to trauma (as touted in the CISD literature). To date, there have been no randomized controlled trials of CISD in groups of emergency services personnel, which is extraordinary, given the growing consensus that CISD is inappropriate because it lacks empirical support.

In Chapter 13, Zatzick and Wagner discussed the intricacies of providing early intervention services for individuals hospitalized with more immediate and pressing physical injury-related demands and needs. Given that hospitalized trauma patients are captive for some period of time, it provides an important opportunity for mental health professionals to make some initial contact that may positively affect the trajectory of adaptation to trauma, including post-hospitalization care seeking. As emphasized by Zatzick and Wagner, this kind of work requires an appreciation of hospital care, physical injury, and the culture of the medical environment. In Chapter 14, Blanchard, Hickling, Kuhn, and Broderick described the toll that motor vehicle accidents take on survivors and their novel early intervention treatment protocol. With the work by Blanchard and colleagues and Bryant and colleagues, there is enough valid evidence to offer CBT prescriptively as an early secondary intervention for motor vehicle accident-related trauma. The new brief model of care offered by Blanchard is particularly attractive because it may save therapist resources. Because resources are often scarce in the aftermath of trauma, it will be important for the field to generate novel approaches to care that are effective, feasible, rapidly available, and efficiently delivered to the largest proportion of affected individuals possible.

CBT is typically labor- and therapist-intensive, which can be an obstacle to the provision of therapy to some. Also, typically, the availability of professionals trained in comprehensive CBT procedures is limited. Brief evidence-based interventions should be generated that are cost-effective and reach a larger number of victims. Given that gains from CBT are dependent on the completion of self-directed homework, it makes sense to consider broadening the homework basis of CBT and lessening the therapist role. In addition, the web or the telephone could be used to provide support and to ensure successful adherence to self-management CBT approaches. This approach has support from the treatment of other disorders that have used structured self-management programs to provide effective procedures to reduce psychological distress and psychopathology (e.g., Gould & Clum, 1993). For example, bibliotherapy with minimal therapist contact for panic disorder, which included an informational video about panic attacks and instruction in diaphragmatic breathing, and the provision of a relaxation tape that taught progressive muscle relaxation, was as effective as multisession behavior therapy (Gould & Clum, 1996; Lidren, Watkins, Gould, & Clum, 1995). Carlbring, Westling, Ljungstrand, Ekselius, and Andersson (2001) used the Internet, with minimal therapist contact via e-mail, to provide CBT for panic disorder, which was effective at ameliorating symptoms, relative to a wait-list control group. In an uncontrolled trial, Lange et al. (2000) successfully used a web-based program to treat PTSD and pathological grief. In addition, in a recent review, Marks, Shaw, and Parkin (1998) advocated use of the web for promoting mental health.

In Chapter 15, Castro, Engel, and Adler described the services provided to soldiers during and after combat to address war-zone-related stress reactions and acute stress disorder. Though it lacks empirical justification, CISD is doctrine in the military. Yet, employing evidence-based procedures for preventing the chronic personal and social dysfunction that inevitably comes after war for a small but salient percentage of veterans should be a critical mandate. What is clear from the information provided by Castro and colleagues is that the Department of Defense has built-in procedures and a wealth of well-trained mental health professionals to meet the challenges of screening, triage, assessment, and treatment of combat stress during and after deployment. Because these structures are in place, the military presents a fertile ground to conduct empirical research (e.g., randomized controlled trials) that could inform not only secondary prevention efforts for men and women who become exposed to the horrors and trauma of war but the entire field of early intervention for traumatic stress (and traumatic loss).

REFERENCES

Calbring, P., Westling, B. E., Ljungstrand, P., Ekselius, L., & Andersson, G. (2001). Treatment of panic disorder via the internet: A randomized trial of a self-help program. *Behavior Therapy, 32,* 751–764.

Gould, R. A., & Clum, G. A. (1993). A meta-analysis of self-help treatment approaches. *Clinical Psychology Review, 13,* 169–186.

Gould, R. A., & Clum, G. A. (1996). Self-help plus minimal therapist contact in the treatment of panic disorder: A replication and extension. *Behavior Therapy, 26,* 533–546.

Lange, A., Schrieken, B., van de Ven, J. P., Bredeweg, B., Emmelkamp, P. M. G., van der Kolk, J., Lydsdottir, L., Massaro, M., & Reuvers, A. (2000). "Interapy": The effects of a short protocolled treatment of posttraumatic stress and pathological grief through the Internet. *Behavioural and Cognitive Psychotherapy, 28,* 175–192.

Lindren, D. M., Watkins, P. L., Gould, R. A., & Clum, G. A. (1995). A comparison of bibliotherapy and group therapy in the treatment of panic disorder. *Journal of Consulting and Clinical Psychology, 62,* 865–869.

Marks, I., Shaw, S., & Parkin, R. (1998). Computer-aided treatments of mental health problems. *Clinical Psychology: Science and Practice, 5,* 151–170.

Moreau, C., & Zisook, S. (2002). Rationale for a posttraumatic stress spectrum disorder. *Psychiatric Clinics of North America, 25,* 775–790.

Resnick, H., Acierno, R., Holmes, M., Dammeyer, M., & Kilpatrick, D. (2000). Emergency evaluation and intervention with female victims of rape and other violence. *Journal of Clinical Psychology, 56,* 1317–1333.

Ruscio, A. M., Ruscio J., & Keane T. M. (2002). The latent structure of posttraumatic stress disorder: A taxometric investigation of reactions to extreme stress. *Journal of Abnormal Psychology, 111,* 290–301.

Index